# Nursing Care of the Pediatric
# Neurosurgery Patient

Cathy C. Cartwright    Donna C. Wallace

*Editors*

# Nursing Care of the Pediatric Neurosurgery Patient

With 119 Figures and 61 Tables

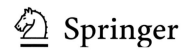 Springer

Cathy C. Cartwright, RN, MSN, PCNS
Pediatric Clinical Nurse Specialist
Neurosurgery
University of Missouri Health Care
Columbia, MO 65212
USA

Donna C. Wallace, RN, MS, CPNP
Pediatric Nurse Practitioner
Barrow Neurological Institute
St. Joseph's Hospital and Medical Center
500 West Thomas Road
Phoenix, AZ 85013
USA

ISBN    978-3-540-29703-1  Springer Berlin Heidelberg New York

Library of Congress Control Number: 2006936733

Springer is a part of Springer Science+Business Media
springer.com

© Springer-Verlag Berlin Heidelberg 2007
Printed in Germany

Editor: Gabriele M. Schröder, Heidelberg, Germany
Desk Editor: Stephanie Benko, Heidelberg, Germany
Production: LE-TeX, Jelonek, Schmidt & Vöckler GbR, Leipzig, Germany
Typesetting: Satz-Druck-Service (SDS), Leimen, Germany
Cover design: Frido Steinen-Broo, eStudio Calamar, Spain
Cover Illustration: Permission with compliments from PMT corporation, USA 2006 as well as patient's family.

Printed on acid-free paper    24/3100/YL      5 4 3 2 1 0

I wish to acknowledge my mentor, Dr. David Jimenez, for sharing his passion for pediatric neurosurgery and holding me to a higher standard. And to Zach, for his love, support and unfaltering belief that "I can do it."

**C.C.**


I wish to acknowledge Dr. Harold Rekate for his support and direction during the process of writing this book. He is unwavering in his mentorship of nurses who care for the patient with neurosurgical diagnoses. I certainly could not have completed this project without the love and understanding of my family and friends, which includes my son James.

**D.W.**

# Foreword

Nursing care of the pediatric neurosurgery patient and family can be extremely challenging and extraordinarily rewarding. Cathy Cartwright and Donna Wallace have edited a wonderful clinical resource to assist nurses in meeting the challenges. More than 32 contributors from 15 medical centers have shared their expertise in 12 chapters that delineate the etiology, pathophysiology, clinical presentation, and management of the most common neurosurgical problems. The text, tables, illustrations, photographs, radiographs, scans, "pediatric pearls," and "parent perspectives" combine to clearly present the essential information about each problem.

The more complex the illness or injury, the greater the potential contribution of the skilled and empathetic nurse to patient and family recovery. To paraphrase a parent quoted in this book, each child with a neurosurgical problem will have a unique life story. Although the child's life story will be affected by the neurosurgical problem, it will be shaped by the child's family and the valuable contributions of nurses such as those who have authored this book and those who will read it.

**Mary Fran Hazinski, MSN, RN, FAAN**
Clinical Nurse Specialist, Division of Trauma
Vanderbilt University Medical Center
Nashville, Tennessee, USA

# Preface

When we began working in pediatric neurosurgery as advanced practice nurses, we searched for a reference that would explain the different neurosurgical conditions affecting our patients and teach us how to care for them. There was nothing to be found. We asked our colleagues for a reference and they, too, had found none. "Someone should write a book about how to care for pediatric neurosurgery patients," we all said each time we met at the AANS pediatric neurosurgery section meeting.

Finally, it dawned on us. *We* were the *someone*. We were the ones that have cared for these children over the years. We were the ones that should share our experiences and write the book.

And, so, a number of pediatric neurosurgery nurses pooled our expertise to write this book to teach nurses how to care for children with neurosurgical conditions. Although not comprehensive in scope, it provides basic knowledge of the pathophysiology, medical-surgical intervention, nursing considerations and outcomes for the more common neurosurgical conditions. Each chapter reflects the authors' experience with a particular topic in addition to pediatric practice pearls that focus on important issues.

This book would not be possible without the tremendous effort of all the authors, including those unnamed ones who helped. Putting practice, and the evidence to support it, to paper can be daunting, especially when doing so means late nights rewriting drafts, long weekends in the library and asking your family to be patient for "just a little longer." Although we are considered a "small niche," Springer saw the importance of providing such a reference and we are grateful for the work they did to bring this to publication.

The editors would also like to acknowledge the University of Missouri Health Care and Barrow Neurological Institute for providing the atmosphere of learning and support that allows us to care for our patients.

Most of all, this book is for our patients and their families. Thank you for letting us be a part of your lives in the midst of crisis and when you are most vulnerable. We recognize that having a child with a neurosurgical disorder can be a life-changing event and we are honored that you "let us in." It is our hope that his book will inform, teach and guide those who have accepted the responsibility to care for these children.

**Cathy C. Cartwright**        **Donna C. Wallace**
Columbia 2007        Phoenix 2007

# Contents

# Contributors

Laurie Baker, MS, RN, ANP, BC
Barrow Neurosurgical Associates Ltd
2910 N. 3rd Ave.
Phoenix, AZ 85013, USA

Patti Batchelder, MSN, APRN, BC, PNP
Department of Neurosurgery
University of Colorado
The Children's Hospital
Denver, CO 80218, USA

Diane Baudendistel, MSN, CNP, RN
Cincinnati Children's Hospital Medical Center
3333 Burnet Avenue
Cincinnati, OH 45229-3039, USA

Jennifer Berlin, RN, MSN, CPNP
Hutzel Women's Hospital/Progressive Nursery
3980 John R
Detroit, MI 48201, USA

Karen W. Burkett, MS, CNP, RN
Center for Professional Excellence
Cincinnati Children's Hospital Medical Center
3333 Burnet Avenue
Cincinnati, OH 45229, USA

Cathy C. Cartwright, RN, MSN, PCNS
Pediatric Clinical Nurse Specialist
Neurosurgery
University of Missouri Health Care
Columbia, MO 65212, USA

Patricia Chibbaro, RN, MS, CPNP
Pediatric Nurse Practitioner
Craniofacial Program
Institute of Reconstructive Plastic Surgery
New York University Medical Center
560 First Avenue, H169
New York, NY 10016, USA

Jennifer A. Disabato, MS, RN, CPNP
Pain Consultation Service
The Children's Hospital
1056 E. 19th Avenue, B-090
Denver, CO 80218, USA

Angela Enix, MS, RN, CPNP-AC
The Children's Medical Center
One Children's Plaza
Dayton, OH 45404, USA

George Marcus Galvan, BSN, MS, MD
The University of Texas Health
Science Center at San Antonio
7703 Floyd Curl Drive
San Antonio, TX 78229, USA

Carol Green, RNC, MSN, CNS/NNP
Neonatal Intensive Care Unit
The Children's Medical Center
One Children's Plaza
Dayton, OH 45404, USA

Sherry Kahn, MS, RN, CPNP
The Children's Medical Center
One Children's Plaza
Dayton, OH 45404, USA

Amy Kolwaite, RN, MS, PNP, NPH, Cand.
Barrow Neurological Institute
Phoenix, AZ 85013, USA

Shona S. Lenss, MS, FNP-C
University of Wisconsin Children's Hospital
Department of Neurosurgery
600 Highland Avenue
Madison, WI 53792, USA

Trisha Leonard, RN, MSN, CPNP
Children's Hospital of Michigan
Department of Neurosurgery
3901 Beaubien
Detroit, MI 48201, USA

Elizabeth Limbacher, MN, ARNP
Department of Neurosurgery
Children's Hospital and Regional Medical Center
4800 Sand Point Way N.E.
P.O. Box 5371/6E-1
Seattle, WA 98105, USA

Arbelle Manicat-Emo, RN, MS, ACNP
Division of Neurosurgery
The Hospital for Sick Children
555 University Ave.
Toronto, Ontario M5G 1X8, Canada

Susan McGee, MSN, CNP, RN
Cincinnati Children's Hospital Medical Center
3333 Burnet Avenue
Cincinnati, OH 45229-3039, USA

Suzan R. Miller-Hoover, MS, RN, CCNS
Banner Children's Hospital
at Banner Desert Medical Center
4937 E. 12th Ave.
Apache Junction, AZ 85219, USA

Jodi Mullen, MS, RN, BC, CCRN, CCNS
Pediatric Intensive Care Unit
The Children's Medical Center
One Children's Plaza
Dayton, OH 45404, USA

Nadine Nielsen, MN, ARNP
Department of Neurosurgery
Children's Hospital and Regional Medical Center
4800 Sand Point Way N.E.
P.O. Box 5371/6E-1
Seattle, WA 98105, USA

Katherine Pearce, MN, ARNP
Children's Hospital and Regional Medical Center
Department of Neurological Surgery
8244 39th Avenue NE
Seattle, WA 98115, USA

Tina Popov, RN, MN, ACNP
Division of Neurosurgery
The Hospital for Sick Children
555 University Ave.
Toronto, Ontario M5G 1X8, Canada

Patricia Rowe, RN, MN, ACNP
Division of Neurosurgery
The Hospital for Sick Children
555 University Ave.
Toronto, Ontario M5G 1X8, Canada

Cheri Salazar, RN, MS, CPNP
Children's Hospital of Michigan
Department of Neurosurgery
3901 Beaubien,
Detroit, MI 48201, USA

Mary Szatkowski, MSN, NNP, CPNP
Phoenix Children's Hospital
1919 E. Thomas Road
Phoenix, AZ 85019, USA

Tania Shiminski-Maher, MS, CPNP
Pediatric Neurosurgery
The Children's Hospital at Montefiore
111 East 210th Street
Bronx, NY 10467, USA

Mary Smellie-Decker, RN, MSN, NP-BC
Children's Hospital of Michigan
Department of Neurosurgery
3901 Beaubien
Detroit, MI 48201, USA

Donna C. Wallace, RN, MS, CPNP
Pediatric Nurse Practitioner
Barrow Neurological Institute
St. Joseph's Hospital and Medical Center
500 West Thomas Road
Phoenix, AZ 85013, USA

Kristin Wall Strother, RN, MSN, NP-BC
Children's Hospital of Michigan
Sickle Cell Center
3901 Beaubien
Detroit, MI 48201, USA

Herta Yu, RN, MN-ACNP, CNN(c)
Department of Neurosurgery
Hospital for Sick Children
555 University Ave.
Toronto, Ontario M5G 1X8, Canada

Maria Zak, RN, MN, ACNP
Division of Neurology
The Hospital for Sick Children
555 University Ave.
Toronto, Ontario M5G 1X8, Canada

# Neurological Assessment of the Neonate, Infant, Child, and Adolescent

*Jennifer A. Disabato and Karen W. Burkett*

## Contents

## ■ Introduction

### ■ Importance of Neurological Assessment

Serial, consistent, and well-documented neurological assessments are the most important aspect of nursing care for the pediatric neurosurgical patient. Subtle changes in the neurological assessment may first be noted by a bedside nurse. Keen observation skills and the ability to extract information about a patient's baseline level of neurological function from the parents or primary caregivers are essential. The nurse's response to assessment changes is essential to the prevention of secondary neurological sequelae and other complications associated with neurological disorders [11]. These potential complications include, among others, inability to protect the airway, immobility, endocrine disorders related to central hormonal dysregulation, impaired communication, and behavioral issues [20].

It is understood that children are not always under the care and custody of their parents. In this book, however, the term "*parent(s)*" is intended to include family members who have custody of a child, foster parents, guardians, and other primary caregivers.

### ■ Nursing Approach to Neurological Assessment

Neurological assessment should be an integral part of the entire physical assessment. The approach to neurological assessment should be systematic and include pertinent health history, for example coexisting conditions, the developmental status of the child, the nature and extent of the injury or surgery performed, and potential complications [9]. Sources of this information include the verbal report or patient record and the neurosurgeon, neurologist, or other medical providers. Nurses must be aware that other physical and developmental disorders not directly associated with the neurological condition, such as renal, cardiac, or pulmonary, may also affect the patient's long-term prognosis and ultimate quality of life. Care planning should be a team approach that involves the parents and the multidisciplinary team to assure optimal outcomes. Factors that impact the assessment will be the age of the child, the family dynamics, the nature of the child's illness, the setting in which the assessment takes place, and input from other member of the multidisciplinary team.

## Diagnostic Imaging and Testing in Neurological Assessment

Diagnostic imaging and other diagnostic tests play an important role in understanding the nature of neurological disorders. Advances in medicine, technology, and pharmacology have contributed to safer outcomes for children who may need sedation for diagnostic tests. Imaging or other tests may be performed to obtain a baseline for future studies.

In general, radiographic or digital imaging is looking at brain structure, while other diagnostic tests like electroencephalogram (EEG), single photon emission computed tomography scanning (SPECT), nuclear medicine scans, and Wada tests are evaluating specific functions of the brain. Positron emission tomography (PET) scans look at metabolic function and utilization of glucose by the brain. Newer technologies allow for the evaluation of cerebral blood flow and brain perfusion. Some tests serve both diagnostic and therapeutic outcomes (Table 1.1) [19].

## Developmental Assessment: Growth and Developmental Tasks by Age

Knowledge of human growth parameters and normal developmental landmarks is critical to the assessment of each age group. Growth is defined as changes in the values given certain measurements of maturity; where as development may encompass other aspects of differentiation of form or function, including those emotional or social changes preeminently shaped by interaction with the environment [4].

Serial measurements can indicate the normal or abnormal dynamics of the child's growth. One key growth measurement important to the neurological assessment of the child is the head circumference. The measurement is taken around the most prominent frontal and occipital bones which offer the maximal circumference. How rapidly the head circumference accelerates or decelerates away from the percentile curve can determine whether the underlying cause of the growth change is more benign or serious. An example of a benign finding is the presence of extra-axial fluid collections of infancy, which often present with an accelerating head circumference. Generally, the infant with this finding is observed over time, but no intervention is warranted. On the other hand, an accelerating head circumference can also be a sign of increasing intracranial pressure in uncompensated hydrocephalus, which would require immediate evaluation and treatment.

Development is the essential distinguishing feature of pediatric nursing. Normal development is a function of the integrity and maturation of the nervous system. Only with a working knowledge of age-related developmental standards can the examiner be sensitive to the deviations that indicate slight or early impairment of development and an abnormal neurological assessment. An abnormality in development from birth suggests an intrauterine or perinatal cause. Slowing of the rate of acquisition of skills later in infancy or childhood may imply an acquired abnormality of the nervous system. A loss of skills (regression) over time strongly suggests an underlying degenerative disease of the central nervous system [4].

Voluntary motor skills generally develop in a cephalocaudal and proximodistal progression, as it parallels the process of myelination. First the head, then the trunk, arms, hands, pelvis, legs, bowel, and bladder are brought under voluntary control. Early in life, motor activity is largely reflexive, and generalized movements predominate. Patterns emerge from the general to the specific; for example, a newborn's total-body response to a stimulus is contrasted with the older child, who responds through simply a smile or words. So, as the neuromuscular system matures, movement gradually becomes more purposeful and coordinated [33]. The sequence of development is the same for all children, but the rate of development varies from child to child.

Finally, also important to a complete neurological exam is an assessment of the child's cognitive and

**Table 1.1.** Neurological diagnostic and imaging modalities. Adapted from Disabato and Wulf (1994) [9] and Barker (2005) [3]. *MRI* Magnetic resonance imaging, *MRA* magnetic resonance angiography, *MRV* magnetic resonance venography, *SPECT* single photon emission computerized tomography, *SISCOM* subtracted ictal spectroscopy coregistered with MRI, *PET* positron emission tomography, *EEG* electroencephalogram, *SSER* somatosensory evoked potentials, *VEP* visual evoked potentials, *BAER* brainstem auditory evoked potentials, *CNS* central nervous system

| Diagnostic or imaging modality | Technology utilized | Nursing and patient considerations |
|---|---|---|
| X-rays of the skull and vertebral column | X-rays to look at boney structures of the skull and spine, fractures, integrity of the spinal column, presence of calcium intra-cranially. | Patient should be immobilized in a collar for transport if there is a question of spinal fracture. |
| Cranial ultrasound | Doppler sound waves to image through soft tissue. In infants can only be used if fontanel is open. | No sedation or intravenous access needed. Used to follow ventricle size/bleeding in neonates/infants. |
| Computerized tomography with/without contrast | Differentiates tissues by density relative to water with computer averaging and mathematical reconstruction of absorption coefficient measurements. | Non-invasive unless contrast is used or sedation needed. Complications include reaction to contrast material or extravasation at injection site. |
| Computerized tomography - bone windows and/or three-dimensional reconstruction | Same as above with software capabilities to subtract intracranial contents to look specifically at bone and reconstruct the skull or vertebral column in a three-dimensional model. | No changes in study for patient. Used for complex skull and vertebral anomalies to guide surgical decision-making. |
| Cerebral angiography | Intra-arterial injection of contrast medium to visualize blood vessels; transfemoral approach most common; occasionally brachial or direct carotid is used. | Done under deep sedation or anesthesia; local reaction or hematoma may occur; systemic reactions to contrast or dysrhythmias; transient ischemia or vasospasm; patient needs to lie flat after and CMS checks of extremity where injection was done are required. |
| MRI with or without contrast (gadolinium) | Differentiates tissues by their response to radio frequency pulses in a magnetic field; used to visualize structures near bone, infarction, demyelination and cortical dysplasias. | No radiation exposure; screened prior to study for indwelling metal, pacemakers, braces, electronic implants; sedation required for young children because of sounds and claustrophobia; contrast risks include allergic reaction and injection site extravasation. |
| MRA MRV | Same technology as above used to study flow in vessels; radiofrequency signals emitted by moving protons can be manipulated to create the image of vascular contrast. | In some cases can replace the need for cerebral angiography; new technologies are making this less invasive study more useful in children with vascular abnormalities. |
| Functional MRI | Technique for imaging activity of the brain using rapid scanning to detect changes in oxygen consumption of the brain; changes can reflect increased activity in certain cells. | Used in patients who are potential candidates for epilepsy surgery to determine areas of cortical abnormality and their relationship to important cortex responsible for motor and speech functions. |
| **Physiologic imaging techniques - nuclear medicine imaging** | | |
| SPECT | Nuclear medicine study utilizing injection of isotopes and imaging of brain to determine if there is increased activity in an area of abnormality; three-dimensional measurements of regional blood flow. | Often used in epilepsy patients to diagnoses areas of cerebral uptake during a seizure (ictal SPECT) or between seizures (intraictal SPECT). |
| SISCOM | Utilizing the technology of SPECT with MRI to look at areas of increased uptake in conjunction with MRI images of the cortex and cortical surface. | No significant difference for patient; software as well as expertise of radiologist is used to evaluate study. |
| PET | Nuclear medicine study that assesses perfusion and level of metabolic activity of both glucose and oxygen in the brain; radiopharmaceuticals are injected for the study. | Patient should avoid chemicals that depress or stimulate the CNS and alter glucose metabolism (e.g., caffeine); patient may be asked to perform certain tasks during study. |

**Table 1.1.** (Continued)

| Electrical studies | | |
| --- | --- | --- |
| EEG<br>Routine<br>Ambulatory<br>Video | Records gross electrical activity across surface of brain; ambulatory EEG used may be used for 24–48 h with data downloaded after study; video combines EEG recording with simultaneous videotaping. | Success of study dependent on placement and stability of electrodes and ability to keep them on in children; routine studies often miss actual seizures but background activity can be useful information. |
| Evoked responses<br><br>SSER<br><br>VER<br><br>BAER | Measure electrical activity in specific sensory pathways in response to external stimuli; signal average produces waveforms that have anatomic correlates according to the latency of wave peaks. | Results can vary depending on body size, age and characteristics of stimuli; sensation for each test will be different for patient – auditory clicks (BAER), strobe light (VER), or electrical current on skin – somatosensory (SSER). |

emotional development. These abilities impact directly on expectations of the child's behavioral, social, and functional capabilities. The younger the child, the more developmental history is needed from the parents. Accurate identification of the child's mastery of cognitive and emotional developmental milestones, as it relates to chronological age, is necessary for a comprehensive neurological assessment.

### Neonate

Aside from head shape and size and assessment of the fontanels, there are other aspects unique to the neurological exam of the neonate and/or infant. These are important to understanding the integrity of the nervous system early in life and are detailed in this section (Fig. 1.1).

### Maternal and Pregnancy/Labor and Delivery History

An interview with the biological mother, or another familiar with the pregnancy, should include questions about any maternal illness, nutrition status, drug and/or alcohol use, chronic diseases, and any medications taken routinely, including prescription, over-the-counter, and herbal supplements. Important factors to know about the delivery include the administration of anesthesia or drugs, difficulties with the delivery such as the need for forceps or vacuum devices, and Apgar scores. A need for supplemental oxygen, glucose, and abnormalities of bilirubin levels are also important. A history of postbirth infections, a need for medications and/or seizures may also indicate underlying problems.

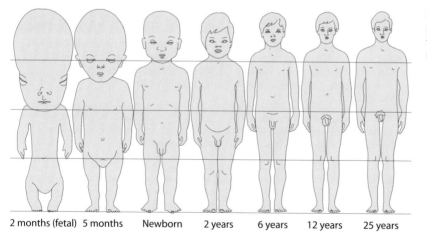

**Fig. 1.1.** Changes in body proportions from second fetal month to adulthood. Obtained from Robbins et al. [31]

2 months (fetal)   5 months    Newborn    2 years    6 years    12 years    25 years

### Physical Appearance

The neonatal period is often defined as the first 4 weeks of life. The neonate may be term or premature and the physical characteristics of neonates vary with their gestational age. Inspection of the shape, symmetry, and mobility of the head of the neonate is critical for evaluating cranial abnormalities or soft tissue injuries. Head circumference at term will range from 34 to 36 cm, within the 25–75% range. Neonates outside this range should be accurately plotted on the appropriate growth chart and serially measured [29]. Further examination of the neonate's head for a patent fontanel, and tautness and approximation of the cranial sutures is vital. Fontanels are best palpated when the neonate is in the upright position and quiet. The cranial sutures should be well approximated, especially the coronal, squamosal, and lambdoidal sutures, and should not admit a fingertip. The sagittal suture may be wider in normal newborns, especially if the baby is premature. The posterior fontanel may be palpated up to 4 weeks of age. More detailed information and illustrations regarding cranial sutures and related abnormalities can be found later in this textbook in Chap. 3 (Craniosynostosis).

Spine assessments include evaluation for abnormal midline lumps, dimples, hairy patches, and palpation for vertebral anomalies. Skin markings such as petechiae, hemangiomas, and hypopigmented or hyperpigmented spots may be present at birth and indicative of neurological congenital conditions. In addition, congenital anomalies of the heart, lungs, and gastrointestinal tract may suggest abnormalities of brain development. However, optic or facial dysmorphisms more accurately predict a brain anomaly [8, 25].

### Functional Capabilities

Neonatal function is primarily reflex activity and necessitates the assessment of infantile automatisms (i. e., those specific reflex movements that appear in normal newborns and disappear at specific periods of time in infancy; Table 1.2) [25]. Functional examination may begin by observation of the neonate in the supine and prone positions, noting spontaneous activity in each position and the presence of primitive reflexes. The posture of the neonate is one of partial flexion, with diminishing flexion of the legs as the neonate ages. Look for random movements of the extremities and attempt to distinguish single myoclonic twitches, which are normal, from the repetitive movement seen with seizures. Some neonates have an excessive response to arousal with "jitteriness" or tremulousness. This is a low-amplitude, rapid shaking of the limbs and jaw. It may appear spontaneously and look like a seizure. However, unlike seizures, jitteriness usually follows some stimulus, can be stopped by holding the limb or jaw, and does not have associated eye movements or respiratory change. When prominent, slow, and coarse, it may be related to central nervous system stress or metabolic abnormalities, but otherwise it is often a normal finding [30]. Strength is assessed by observing the newborn's spontaneous and evoked movements and by eliciting specific newborn reflexes. Neonates with neuromuscular conditions may manifest with abnormally low muscle tone (hypotonia), paradoxical breathing, or contractures. The neonate is capable of reacting to moving persons or objects within sight or grasp, both for large and small objects. Neonates can visually fixate on a face or light in their line of vision [4]. The quality of the cry can suggest neurological involvement. A term newborn's cry is usually loud and vigorous. A weak or sedated neonate will cry only briefly and softly, or may just whimper. A high-pitched cry is often associated with a neurological abnormality or increased intracranial pressure (IICP) [27].

Functional capabilities of the preterm infant will vary by gestational age. Premature infants demonstrate less strength and decreased muscle tone compared to a term infant (Table 1.2).

### Vulnerabilities

The most critical need of both the term and premature neonate is for the establishment of adequate respiratory activity. Respiratory immaturity added to the neurological insults from seizures, congenital conditions (such as spina bifida and genetically linked syndromes), intraventricular hemorrhage, and hydrocephalus all have the capability to severely limit the neonates' ability to buffer these conditions. Infections and gastrointestinal deficiencies also can severely compromise the neonate's ability to dampen the physiological effects of neurological conditions. For the preterm neonate with a neurological disorder, dampening the effects becomes even more crucial and makes the preterm infant vulnerable to multisystem failures. Developmental care teams can be mobilized to augment the neonate's capacity for optimal growth and interaction with their environment.

**Table 1.2.** Interpreting the neurologic examination in the young child. Obtained from McGee and Burkett (2000) [25]

| Reflexes | Methods of Testing | Responses/Comments |
|---|---|---|
| Palmar grasp<br>P* - birth<br>D** - 3–4 months | Press index finger against palmar surface; Compare grasp of both hands. | Infant will grasp finger firmly. Sucking facilitates grasp. Meaningful grasp occurs after three month. |
| Plantar grasp<br>P - birth<br>D - 8–10 months | Press index finger to sole of foot. | Toes will flex in an attempt to grasp finger. |
| Acoustic - cochleopalpebral | Create loud noise. | Both eyes blink. This reflex may be difficult to elicit in first few days of life. |
| Rooting<br>P - birth<br>D - 3–4 months when awake<br>D - 3–8 months when asleep | Stroke perioral skin or cheek. | Mouth will open and infant will turn to stimutated side. |
| Sucking<br>P - birth<br>D - 10–12 months | Touch lips of infant | Infant will suck with lips and tongue. |
| Trunk incurvation (Galants)<br>P - birth<br>D - 2 months | Hold infant prone in one hand and stimulate one side of back about three centimeters from midline. | Trunk will curve to stimulated side. |
| Vertical suspension positioning<br>P - birth<br>D - 4 months | Support baby uppright with hands under axillae. | Legs flex at hips and knees. Legs extend after four months. Scissoring of legs indicates spastic paraplegia. |
| Placing response<br>P - few days after birth<br>D - 10–12 months | Hold baby upright with hands under axillae and allow dorsal surface of foot to touch undersurface of table without plantar-flexing foot. | Infant will flex hip and knee and place foot on table with stepping movement. |
| Stepping response<br>P - birth<br>D - 3 months | Hold infant upright with hands under axillae and feet flat on table. | Infant will pace forward alternating feet. |
| Tonic neck reflex<br>P - birth- 6 weeks<br>D - 4–6 months | Turn head to one side. | Arm and leg on same side extend and others flex. |
| Traction response<br>P - birth | Pull infant from supine position to sitting with his hands. | Shoulder muscle movement will be noted. |
| Perez reflex<br>P - birth<br>D - 3 months | Hold in prone position with one hand and move thumb from sacrum to head. | Infant will extend head and spine, flex knees on chest, cry, and urinate. |
| Moro reflex<br>P - birth<br>D - 4–6 months | Create loud noise or sudden movement such as extension of the infant`s neck. | Infant stiffens, extremities extend, index finger and thumb form C shape, and fingers and toes fan. |

*P - present  **D - disappears

## Tips in Approach to Child/Family

Observation of the neonate at rest is the first step in a comprehensive approach to neurological assessment of the neonate. Usually, the head can be inspected and palpated before awakening the neonate and measuring the head circumference. Most neonates arouse as they are unwrapped and responses to stimulus are best assessed when the neonate is quietly awake. As the neonate arouses further, the strength of his spontaneous and active movement can be observed and cranial nerves assessed. Stimulation of selected reflexes, like the Moro reflex, and eye exam are reserved for last, since they usually elicit vigorous crying. The typical cry of an infant is usually loud and angry. Abnormal cries can be weak, shrill, high-pitched, or cat-like. Crying usually peaks at 6 weeks of age, when healthy infants cry up to 3 h/day, and then decreases to 1 h or less by 3 months [4]. Consolability, including the sucking response, can be evaluated whenever the neonate is agitated. The sequence of the examination can always be altered in accordance with the newborn's state or situation. Excessive stimulation or cooling may cause apnea or bradycardia in the preterm neonate, and components of the exam may need to be postponed until the neonate is stabilized.

### Infant

### Physical Appearance

Infancy is defined as 30 days to 12 months of age. An infant's head grows at an average rate of 1 cm/month over the 1st year. Palpation of the head should reveal soft and sunken fontanels when quiet and in the upright position. A bulging fontanel in a quiet infant can be a reliable indicator of IICP. However, vigorous crying of an infant can cause transient bulging of the fontanel. The posterior fontanels will close by 1–2 months of age, with wider variability in the anterior fontanel, often closing between 6 and 18 months of age. If the sutures close prematurely, evaluate for craniosynostosis. Delayed closure of the sutures may indicate IICP or hydrocephalus, warranting further evaluation. Inspection of the scalp should include observation of the venous pattern, because IICP and thrombosis of the superior sagittal sinus can produce marked venous distention [4].

Observation of the spine should include an examination for lumps, bumps, dimples, and midline hemangiomas and hair. Examination of rectal tone for an anal wink should be performed, especially when suspicion is present for a spinal dysraphism. Absence of an anal wink is noted if the anal sphincter does not contract when stimulated. Identification of a sensory level of function in an infant with a spinal abnormality can be very difficult. If decreased movement of the extremities is noted, observe the lower extremities for differences in color, temperature, or perspiration, with the area below the level of spinal abnormality usually noted to be cooler to touch and without perspiration [25].

### Functional Capabilities

Assessment of the infant's function requires knowledge of normal developmental landmarks (Table 1.3).

### Vulnerabilities

When typical ages for maturation of selected milestones are not reached and/or primitive reflexes persist beyond their expected disappearance, neurological problems may be implicated. Most primitive reflexes have disappeared by the age of 4–6 months, with reflexes of sucking, rooting during sleep, and placing responses lingering until later in infancy. Specifically, if there is persistent rigid extension or flexion of the extremities, opisthotonos positioning (hyperextension of the neck with stiffness and extended arms and legs), scissoring of the legs, persistent low tone of all or selected extremities, asymmetry of movement or reflexes, and asymmetrical head rotation to one side, these behaviors alone can suggest central nervous system disease or insult during this rapid period of growth and development [21].

### Tips in Approach to Child/Family

A comprehensive review of the infant's developmental milestones, activity level, and personality is critical when obtaining a history from the parent. Pictures of the infant at birth and baby book recordings may trigger additional input to supplement the history. Approach to the physical exam in early infancy (before infant sits alone) at 4–6 months, differs from the older infant. During early infancy, they can be placed on the examining table assessing for positioning abilities in prone and supine. Reflexes can be elicited as extremities are examined. The entrance of stranger anxiety at 6–8 months of age presents new challenges and can result in clinging and crying behaviors for the infant. Reducing separations from the parent by completing most of the exam on the parent's lap can diminish these responses. This is a time to gain cooperation with distraction, bright objects, smiling faces, and soft voices [35]. Use of picture books between infant and parent can provide an environment to demonstrate language abilities. The assessment should proceed from the least to the most painful or intrusive to maximize the infant's cooperation, and are often performed in a toe-to-head fashion [21]. Evaluation of muscle strength and tone, and cerebellar function should precede the cranial nerve examination with palpation, auscultation, and measurement of the head reserved for last.

**Table 1.3.** Age-appropriate neuroassessment table. A brief guide to developmental milestones in children from infancy to age 12 years as a guide when performing a neurological assessment (Phoenix Children's Hospital)

| Age | Gross Motor | Fine Motor | Personal/social | Language |
|---|---|---|---|---|
| Newborn | Head down with ventral suspension Flexion Posture Knees under abdomen-pelvis high Head lag complete Head to one side prone | Hands closed Cortical Thumbing (CT) | With sounds, quiets if crying; cries if quiet; startles; blinks | Crying only monotone |
| 4 weeks | Lifts chin briefly (prone) Rounded back sitting head up momentarily Almost complete head lag | Hands closed (CT) | Indefinite stare at surroundings Briefly regards toy only if brought in front of eyes and follows only to midline Bell sound decreases activity | Small, throaty noises |
| 6 weeks | In ventral suspension head up momentarily in same plane as body Prone: pelvis high but knees no longer under abdomen | Hands open 25% of time | Smiles | Social smile (1st cortical input) |
| 2 months | Ventral suspension; head in same plane as body Lifts head 45° (prone) on flexed forearms Sitting, back less rounded, head bobs forward Energetic arm movements | Hands open most of the time (75%) Active grasp of toy | Alert expression Smiles back Vocalizes when talked to Follows dangled toy beyond midline Follows moving person | Cooing Single vowel sounds (ah. eh, uh) |
| 3 months | Ventral suspension; head in same plane as body Lifts head 45° (prone) on flexed forearms Sitting, back less rounded, head bobs forward Energetic arm movements | Hands open most of the time (75%) Active grasp of toy | Smiles spontaneously Hand regard Follows dangled toy 180° Promptly looks at object in midline Glances at toy put in hand | Chuckles "Talk back" if examiner nods head and talks Vocalizes with two different syllables (a-a. oo-oo) |
| 4 months | Head to 90° on extended forearms Only slightly head lag at beginning of movement Bears weight some of time on extended legs if held standing Rolls prone to supine Downward parachute | Active play with rattles Crude extended reach and grasp Hands together Plays with fingers Toys to mouth when supine | Body activity increased at sight of toy Recognizes bottle and opens mouth For nipple (anticipates feeding with excitement) | Laughs out loud increasing inflection No tongue thrust |
| 6 months | Bears full weight on legs if held standing Sits alone with minimal support Pivots in prone Rolls easily both ways Anterior proppers | Reaches for toy Palmar grasp of cube Lifts cup by handle Plays with toes | Displeasure at removal of toy Puts toy in mouth if sitting | Shy with strangers Imitates cough and protrusion of tongue Smiles at mirror image |
| 7 months | Bears weight on one hand prone Held standing, bounces Sit on hard surface leaning on hands | | Stretches arms to be taken Keeps mouth closed if offered more food than wants Smiles and pats at mirror | Murmurs "mom" especially if crying Babbles easily (M's, D's, B's, L's) Lateralizes sound |

**Table 1.3.** (*Continued*)

| Age | Gross Motor | Fine Motor | Personal/social | Language |
|---|---|---|---|---|
| 9 months | Sits steadily for 15 min on hard surface<br>Reciprocally crawls<br>Forward parachute | Picks up small objects with index finger and thumb (Pincer grasp) | Feeds cracker neatly<br>Drinks from cup with help | Listens to conversation<br>Shouts for attention<br>Reacts to "strangers" |
| 10 months | Pulls to stand<br>Sits erect and steadily (indefinitely)<br>Sitting to prone<br>Standing: collapses and creeps on hands knees easily<br>Prone to sitting easily<br>Cruises – laterally<br>Squats and stoops – does not recover to standing position | Pokes with index finger, prefers small to large objects | Nursery games (i.e., pat-a-cake), picks up dropped bottle, waves bye-bye | Will play peek-a-boo and pat-a-cake to verbal command<br>Says Mama, Dada appropriately, finds the hidden toy (onset visual memory) |
| 12 months | Sitting; pivots to pick up object<br>Walks, hands at shoulder height<br>Bears weight alone easily momentarily | Easy pinch grasp with arm off table<br>Independent release (ex: cube into cup)<br>Shows preference for one hand | Finds hidden toy under cup<br>Cooperated with dressing<br>Drinks from cup with two hands<br>Marks with crayon on paper<br>Insists on feeding self | One other word (noun) besides Mama, Dada (e.g., hi, bye, cookie) |
| 13 months | Walks with one hand | Mouthing very little<br>Explores objects with fingers<br>Unwraps small cube<br>Imitates pellet bottle | Helps with dressing<br>Offers toy to mirror image<br>Gives toy to examiner<br>Holds cup to drink, tilting head<br>Affectionate<br>Points with index finger<br>Plays with washcloth, bathing<br>Finger-feeds well, but throws dishes on floor<br>Appetite decreases | Three words besides Mama, Dada<br>Larger receptive language than expressive |
| 14 months | Few steps without support | Deliberately picks up two small blocks in one hand<br>Peg out and in<br>Opens small square box | Should be off bottle<br>Puts toy in container if asked<br>Throws and plays ball | Three to four words expressively minimum |
| 15 months | Creeps up stairs<br>Kneels without support<br>Gets to standing without support<br>Stoop and recover<br>Cannot stop on round corners suddenly<br>Collapses and catches self | Tower of two cubes<br>"Helps" turn pages of book<br>Scribbles in imitation<br>Completes round peg board with urging | Feeds self fully leaving dishes on tray<br>Uses spoon turning upside down, spills much<br>Tilts cup to drink, spilling some<br>Helps pull clothes off<br>Pats at picture in book | Four to six words<br>Jargoning<br>Points consistently to indicate wants |
| 18 months | Runs stiffly<br>Rarely falls when walking<br>Walks upstairs (one hand held-one step at a time)<br>Climbs easily<br>Walks, pulling toy or carrying doll<br>Throws ball without falling<br>Knee flexion seen in gait | Tower of three to four cubes<br>Turns pages two to three at a time<br>Scribbles spontaneously<br>Completes round peg board easily | Uses spoon without rotation but still spills<br>May indicate wet pants<br>Mugs doll<br>Likes to take off shoes and socks<br>Knows one body part<br>Very negative oppositions | One-step commands<br>10-15 words<br>Knows "hello" and "thank you"<br>More complex 'jargon' rag<br>Attention span 1 min<br>Points to one picture |

**Table 1.3.** (Continued)

| Age | Gross Motor | Fine Motor | Personal/social | Language |
|-----|-------------|------------|-----------------|----------|
| 21 months | Runs well, falling some tires<br>Walks downstairs with one hand held, one step at a time<br>Kicks large ball with demonstration<br>Squats in play<br>Walks upstairs alternating feet with rail held | Tower of five to six cubes<br>Opens and closes small square box<br>Completes square peg board | May briefly resist bathing Pulls person to show something Handles cup will Removes some clothing purposefully Asks for food and drink Communicates toilet needs helps wit h simple household tasks 3 body parts | Knows 15–20 words and combines 2–3 words<br>Echoes 2 or more<br>Knows own name<br>Follows associate commands |
| 24 months | Rarely falls when running<br>Walks up and down stairs alone one-step-at-a time<br>Kicks large ball without demonstration<br>Claps hands<br>Overthrow hand | Tower of six to seven cubes<br>Turns book pages singly<br>Turns door knob<br>Unscrews lid<br>Replaces all cubes in small box<br>Holds glass securely with one hand | Uses spoon, spilling little<br>Dry at night<br>Puts on simple garment<br>Parallel play<br>Assists bathing<br>Likes to wash 6 dry hands<br>Plays with food<br>+ body parts<br>Tower of 8. Helps put things away | Attention span 2 min<br>Jargon discarded<br>Sentences of two to three words<br>Knows 50 words<br>Can follow two-step commands (ain't)<br>Refers to self by name<br>Understands and asks for "more"<br>Asks for food by name<br>Inappropriately uses personal pronouns (e.g., me want)<br>Identifies three pictures |
| 3–5 years | Pedals tricycle<br>Walks up stairs alternating feet<br>Tip toe<br>Jump with both feet | Copies circles<br>Uses overhand throw | Group play<br>Can take turns | Uses three-word sentences |
| 5–12 years | Activities of daily living | Printing and cursive writing | Group Sports | Reads and understands content<br>Spells words |

## Toddler

### Physical Appearance

During the toddler years of age 1–3 years, brain growth continues at a more gradual rate. Head growth measurements for boys average 2.5 cm/year and girls slightly less with a 2 cm/year increase. From age 24–36 months, boys and girls both slow to only l cm/year. The toddler's head size is only one-quarter the total body length. The toddler walks with a wide-based gait at first, knees bent as feet strike the floor flat. After several months of practice, the center of gravity shifts back and trunk stability increases, while knees extend and arms swing at the sides for balance. Improvements in balance and agility emerge with mastery of skills such as running and stair climbing. Inspection of the toddler's head and spine are aimed at recognition of subtle neurological abnormalities like new-onset torticollis, abnormal gait patterns, and loss of previously achieved milestones.

### Functional Capabilities

Cortical development is 75% complete by the age of 2 years; therefore, the neurological response of the child over 2 years old is similar to that of the adult. Most toddlers are walking by the 1st year, although some do not walk until 15 months. Assessment of language close to the age of 3 years is the first true opportunity for a cognitive assessment (Table 1.3).

### Vulnerabilities

Greater mobility of the toddler gives them access to a larger number of objects, and, as exploration increases, this makes them more at risk for injury. Physical limits on their explorations become less effective; words become increasingly important for behavior control as well as cognition. Delayed language acquisition can be identified at this age and may represent previously unrecognized developmental issues.

### Tips in Approach to Child/Family

The neurological exam is approached systematically, beginning with an assessment of mental/emotional status and following with evaluation of cranial nerves, motor and sensory responses, and reflexes. The toddler may interact better on the parent's lap or floor of the exam room. Initially, minimal physical contact is urged. Later inspection of the body areas through play with "counting toes" and "tickling fingers" can enhance the outcomes of the exam. Exam equipment should be introduced slowly and inspection of equipment permitted. Auscultate and palpate the head whenever quiet. Traumatic procedures such as head measurements should be performed last. Critical portions of the exam may require patient cooperation, and consideration should be given to completing those components first (e.g., walking and stooping abilities).

### Preschooler

### Physical Appearance

This period is defined as ages 3–5 years. Visual acuity reaches 20/30 by age 3 years and 20/20 by age 4 years. Handedness is usually established after age 3 years. If handedness is noted much earlier, spasticity or hemiparesis should be suspected. Bowel and bladder control emerge during this period. Daytime bladder control typically precedes bowel control, and girls precede boys. Bed-wetting is normal up to age 4 years in girls and 5 years in boys [4].

### Functional Capabilities

Although the brain reaches 75% of its adult size by the age of 2 years, cortical development is not complete until the age of 4 years (Table 1.3).

### Vulnerabilities

Highly active children face increased risks of injury. Helmet and bike safety programs are essential ingredients to reducing such risks. Given the escalating language abilities of the preschooler, speech and language delays can be detected with a greater assurance

than in the toddler period. Persistent bowel or bladder incontinence may indicate a neurogenic bladder, which can be a sign of spine anomalies.

Preschoolers can control very little of their environment. When they lose their internal controls, tantrums result. Tantrums normally peak in prevalence between 2 and 4 years of age. Tantrums that last more than 15 min, or if they are regularly occurring more than three times a day, may reflect underlying medical, emotional, or social problems.

### Tips in Approach to Child/Family

To maximize the preschooler's cooperation during the neurological assessment, many approaches can be offered. The presence of a reassuring parent can be more comforting to a preschooler than words. The older preschooler may be willing to stand or sit on the exam table, while the younger preschooler may be content to remain in the parent's lap. If the preschooler is cooperative, the exam can proceed from head to toe; if uncooperative, the approach should be as for the toddler exam. Equipment can be offered for inspection and a brief demonstration of its use. Formulating a story about components of the assessment, such as "I'm checking the color of your eyes," can maximize the child's cooperation. The examiner can make games out of selected portions. Using positive statements that expect cooperation can also be helpful (e.g., "Show me your pretty teeth").

### School-Age Child

### Physical Appearance

This is the phase of the middle childhood years aged 5–12 years. The head grows only 2–3 cm throughout the entire phase. This is a reflection of slower brain growth with myelination complete by 7 years of age. Muscular strength, coordination, and endurance increase progressively throughout this growth period. School children's skills at performing physical challenges like dribbling soccer balls and playing a musical instrument become more refined with age and practice.

### Functional Capabilities

School-aged children are able to take care of their own immediate needs and are generally proficient in the activities of daily living. Motor skills are continuing to be refined. Children at this age participate in extracurricular and competitive activities outside of school in arenas such as academic clubs, sports, art, and music. Their world is expanding and accomplishments progress at an individual pace.

School makes increasing cognitive demands. Mastery of the elementary curriculum requires that a large number of perceptual, cognitive, and language processes work efficiently. By third grade, children need to be able to sustain attention through a 45-min period. The goal of reading becomes not only sounding out the words, but also understanding the content, and the goal of writing is no longer spelling but composition. By the third or fourth grade, the curriculum requires that children use these fundamentals to learn increasingly complex materials. If this critical leap in educational capabilities is not made, then what appear as subtle deficits in academic performance in the third or fourth grade can translate into insurmountable academic challenges in the fifth and sixth grades.

### Vulnerabilities

The most significant vulnerabilities of children this age are to injury. They are now mobile, in neighborhoods, playing without supervision. Children with physical disabilities may face special stresses because of their visible differences, whereas those children with silent handicaps (e.g., traumatic brain injury, seizure disorders) may experience acute and daily stressors as differences surface in peer relationships and school performance.

### Tips in Approach to Child/Family

For the neurological exam of school-age children, they usually prefer sitting and are cooperative in most positions. Most children this age still prefer a parent's presence. The assessment usually can proceed in a head-to-toe direction. Explaining the purpose of the equipment and significance of the procedure, such as the optic exam, can further reduce anxiety and maximize consistent findings.

### Adolescent

### Physical Appearance

Adolescence is generally considered the time when children undergo rapid changes in body size, shape, physiology, and psychological and social functioning. For both sexes, acceleration in stature begins in early adolescence, but peak growth velocities are not reached until middle adolescence. Boys typically peak 2–3 years later than girls and continue their growth in height for 2–3 years after girls have stopped. The development of secondary sex characteristics are usually classified by Tanner's stages of sexual maturity (or sexual maturity ratings), and define sequential changes in pubic hair, breast changes, and testicular and penile growth [4].

### Functional Capabilities

Motor skills are refined into an adult pattern. The functional development of this age group is marked by pubertal changes, which can affect self-esteem. They are able to construct a reasonable evaluation of consequences for risk-taking behaviors.

### Vulnerabilities

Adolescents are vulnerable to traumatic brain and spinal cord injuries due to frequent engagement in risk-taking behaviors. Injury prevention programs are geared to reduce teens' participation in risk-taking behaviors like drinking and driving, but knowledge does not consistently control behavior. As an age group, adolescents sustain the highest number of traumatic brain injuries from motor vehicle collisions as unbelted passengers and inexperienced drivers. The growth of competitive sports has also contributed to increasing injuries. Teenagers are also vulnerable to the onset of a seizure disorder in the presence of a previously known or unknown low seizure threshold, compounded by the major hormonal changes that occur during this developmental phase.

### Tips in Approach to Child/Family

The assessment of an adolescent can proceed in the same position and sequence as for a school-aged child. Offering the option of a parent's presence is important when developmentally appropriate. If the parent is interviewed alone, it should be done first, before the interview with the child to avoid undermining the adolescent's trust. For many neurosurgical conditions, the teenager may be anxious about the outcome of the assessment and will want the parent(s) present. It remains important to continue to respect the need for privacy during the spine assessment, along with ongoing explanations of the findings.

## Developmental Assessment Tools

With the diagnosis of a neurosurgical condition, often comes the awareness of potential or realized developmental delays. A comprehensive approach to assessment includes a family history, developmental observations, comprehensive neurological assessment, and developmental screening. Selected screening tools can aid in early identification of developmental delays.

There are few currently available screening tools that are equally accurate in detecting developmental delays in speech, language, fine and gross motor activities, and emotional and intellectual development [13]. It is recommended that developmental skill attainment not be based on any one assessment tool (Table 1.4).

When administering a developmental assessment tool, knowledge of the child's neurological condition is important for interpreting the results. For instance, a child that shows language delays may also have a hearing impairment, which will skew the language assessment. Obtaining a standardized score may also depict the child's developmental abilities, and guide the nurse in describing to the family developmental strengths and weaknesses. Tools should be used as only a component of developmental surveillance and part of a continuous comprehensive approach that includes the parent(s) as partners with professionals [13].

The goal of a comprehensive developmental approach in the hospital or outpatient setting is to determine the most appropriate developmentally based neurosurgical care for the patient. Treatment for identified needs can be better directed toward the developmental age of the child, which, if different from the chronological age, will impact the assessment and patient care of the child. This developmental information can guide the nurse in planning for the child's home care, including targeted resources such as early intervention services, adapted educational plans, rehabilitation and therapy services.

## Hands-On Neurological Assessment

The importance of the well-documented neurological assessment on a child with a neurological diagnosis cannot be understated. Keen observation can give the nurse information regarding a child's level of neurological irritability and motor abilities, including the presence of any asymmetry of movements. The need for a systematic approach cannot be overstated. Repeating the assessment in the same order each time

**Table 1.4.** Developmental screening tools commonly used to assess child development. Data from references: Behrman et al. (2004) [4] and Wong et al. (2000) [35]

| Tool name | Revised Denver developmental screening test (Denver II) | Prescreening developmental questionnaire R-PDQ | Developmental profile II | Draw a person (DAP) test |
|---|---|---|---|---|
| Author | Frankenburg [13] | Frankenburg et al. [14] | Alpern et al. [1] | Goodenough [15] |
| Items scored | Gross motor Fine motor Language Personal-social | Parent answered prescreen of items on Denver II | Physical Self-help Social Academic Communication | Score for body parts |
| Age range | Birth–6 years | Birth–6 years | Birth–7 years | 5–17 years |
| Interview | Parent/child | Parent only | Parent/child | Child only |
| Testing time | 30–40 minutes | 15–20 min | 20–40 min | As needed |
| Training/certified | Yes | Self-instruction | Self-instruction | Self-instruction |
| Pros/cons | Range of items Identify child's strengths/weakness Validity tested Cultural bias Teaching tool | Parent report Can rescreen If delays administer Denver II | Range of items Low rate of sensitivity | Nonverbal Nonthreatening Cultural unbias Few items to score Gives IQ score |

avoids the pitfall of missed information. Bedside assessment should be done when changing caregivers to give the nurse a framework on which to base her description of changes in the assessment [9, 18, 22]. The order of the pediatric neurological assessment in the acute care setting is as follows:

1. Appearance and observation
2. Level of consciousness
3. Cranial nerve assessment
4. Vital signs
5. Motor sensory function
6. Assessment of reflexes
7. Gait and balance
8. Assessment of external monitoring apparatus

## Appearance and Observation

### Head Size, Shape, and Fontanels

Accurate measurement of occipital-frontal circumference is vital. If the child is unconscious, careful placement of the tape while the patient is supine is important. In children under the age of 2 years with a normally shaped skull, this measurement is taken just above the eyes and over the occipital ridge.

Palpation of the scalp is done to look for any alteration in the skin integrity of the scalp and to feel for any abnormal suture ridges or splitting of the sutures. In the injured child, care should be taken to both visually examine and palpate the entire scalp to look and feel for open lacerations and/or subgaleal hematomas. In children with thick hair, adequate light and assistance with alignment while moving the child is important. Pressure sores can develop in the posterior scalp in the area of the occipital protuberance from swelling and prolonged dependent position of the scalp.

Microcephaly is the term used to describe infants whose head does not grow secondary to lack of brain growth. Causes include acquired factors occurring during pregnancy (intrauterine infection, radiation exposure, alcohol or drug teratogenic effects) and familial syndromes, such as familial microcephaly, which is an autosomal recessive disorder. The definition is a head circumference that falls more than two standard deviations below the mean for age and sex. The head appears disproportionately small and many of these children have significant neurological disabilities, including mental retardation and seizures, among others.

Megalencephaly or macrocephaly refers to an unusually large head and skull with a circumference that is greater than two standard deviations above the mean for age and sex. There are many causes for this including hydrocephalus, expanding cysts or tumors, endocrine disorders, congenital syndromes or chromosomal abnormalities. Asymptomatic familial megalencephaly is when the head is large but follows the shape of the growth curve, appears to be genetically determined and does not result in IICP or other neurological or developmental problems [9].

## Level of Consciousness

### Arousal and Content (Awareness)

Level of consciousness (LOC) is comprised of both arousal and content. The assessment of LOC is the most important task that the nurse will perform as part of the overall assessment. The primary goal is to identify changes that may indicate deterioration so that early intervention can prevent complications that may influence overall outcome. Most institutions will use a standardized tool for serial assessments of LOC. In pediatrics, the most commonly used tool is the Modified Glasgow Coma Scale for Infants and Children (Table 1.5). There are many variants of this scale in use currently. Although these scales were initially used for children who had been injured, they are now used for assessing LOC in inpatient pediatric settings for all diagnoses.

Neuroanatomic correlates of consciousness specific to arousal are located in the reticular activating system of the brainstem, just above the midbrain. The assessment of consciousness is closely tied to the assessment of eye findings because of the anatomic proximity of the midbrain to the nuclei of cranial nerves III, IV, and VI – which together control pupillary responses and eye mobility. Anatomic correlates of the level of awareness (mentation) once the child is aroused are located in the cerebral cortex. If a patient has an altered LOC, the first step will be to assess arousal [18].

The nurse should first attempt to arouse the child from sleep using the least amount of stimulation necessary to evoke the best response from the child. Visual stimuli should be first, followed by auditory stimuli like saying the child's name, and finally tactile, by touching the child. Each of these should be applied in increasing levels of intensity with a soft voice, dim light, and gentle touch first, followed by a louder voice, brighter light, and firmer tactile stimulation. In cases where this level of stimulus does not cause arousal, noxious stimuli, which would be considered painful to a child who is fully aware, are used.

Noxious stimuli should be forceful, yet not injure the child. Central stimulus should be applied before peripheral stimulus. A response to central stimulus indicates that the movement is a result of a cortical response, rather than a spinal or reflex response. Three commonly used central stimuli are the trapezius squeeze, mandibular pressure, and sternal rub. The sternal rub is the most common central stimulus used in pediatrics. A single fisted hand is used with the knuckles lightly applied to the child's sternum. Pressure should be for a minimum of 15 s or until a response is obtained, and no longer than 30 s. If there is no response to central stimulus or the response indicates that one or two limbs are not responding as the others are, peripheral stimulus to the affected limbs should be applied; for example, place a pencil between two fingers and squeeze the fingers together [23].

With any stimulus in the less than fully conscious patient, observation of how the child responds is thought of in terms of either a generalized or localized response. A generalized response is one where the child shows general agitation or has increased movement to the stimulus. A localized response is one where the child shows evidence of awareness of where the stimulus is coming from, perhaps reaching to push the examiner away or trying to pull the limb away from the examiner.

The level of the response to stimulus is assessed once it has been determined that the child is arousable. Determining whether a child is oriented to person, place, and time is more challenging because of developmental influences. The pediatric nurse is more likely to report that the child is oriented to the presence of known caregivers, favorite objects (toys or stuffed animals), and other developmentally appropriate stimuli. The ability to follow commands may rely more on the examiner's knowledge of what commands a certain age child would be likely to follow. This assessment distinguishes between simple and more complex commands. Examples of simple commands are "stick out your tongue" and "squeeze my hand." More complex commands involve two or three steps and require a higher level of processing. An example would be, "can you kiss your bear and give it to your mommy." Parents and others who know the child well are often helpful in assessing subtle changes in awareness.

With a fully awake child, awareness is assessed by asking the child more questions related to orientation to place and time, assessing memory by giving them three simple words to remember and asking them to repeat them several minutes later. Children are more likely to be engaged if the examiner is utilizing cur-

**Table 1.5.** Modified Glasgow Coma Scale for infants and children. Coma scoring system appropriate for pediatric patients. Obtained from Marcoux (2005) [24]

| Activity | Score | Infant/non-verbal child (<2 years) | Verbal child/adult (>2 years) | |
|----------|-------|-----------------------------------|-------------------------------|---|
| Eye Opening | 4 | Spontaneous | Spontaneous | |
| | 3 | To Speech | To verbal stimuli | |
| | 2 | To Pain Only | To pain only | |
| | 1 | No Response | No response | |
| Motor Response | 6 | Normal/ spontaneous movement | Obeys commands | |
| | 5 | Withdraws to touch | Localizes pain | |
| | 4 | Withdraws to pain | Flexion withdrawal | |
| | 3 | Abnormal flexion (decorticate) | Abnormal flexion | |
| | 2 | Extension (decerebrate) | Extension (decerebrate) | |
| | 1 | No response | No response | |
| | | | **2–5 years** | **> 5 years** |
| Verbal Response | 5 | Cries appropriately, coos | Appropriate words | Oriented |
| | 4 | Irritable crying | Inappropriate words | Confused |
| | 3 | Inappropriate screaming / crying | Screams | Inappropriate |
| | 2 | Grunts | Grunts | Incomprehensible |
| | 1 | No Response | No response | No Response |

rent events, holidays or school routines, questions about pets or other topics that are familiar to the child [9].

### Cranial Nerve Assessment – Brainstem Function

Cranial nerve assessment is basically an assessment of brainstem function because nuclei of 10 of the 12 cranial nerves are located in the brainstem. The proximity of these nuclei to the reticular activating system (arousal center) located in the midbrain is the anatomic rationale for assessing cranial nerves in conjunction with LOC. Important neurological functions and protective reflexes are mediated by the cranial nerves and many functions are dependent on more than one nerve. Some of the cranial nerves have both motor and sensory functions (Fig. 1.2, Table 1.6).

The two cranial nerves that do not arise in the brainstem are the olfactory nerve (CN I) and the optic nerve (CN II). CN I is located in the medial frontal lobe and is responsible for the sense of smell. This can be difficult to assess in the younger child, so is often omitted unless there is specific concern that there has been damage in that area. Taste may also be affected with injuries to CN I. CN II is assessed by determining a child's visual acuity. This may be done more formally with visual screening or more generally by noting if the child's vision appears normal in routine activities [22].

Pupil size and response to direct light are mediated by CN II and the oculomotor nerve (CN III) as well as the sympathetic nervous system. Many things can affect the pupillary response in a child, including damage to the eye or the cranial nerves, pressure on the upper brainstem, local and systemic effects of certain drugs, anoxia, and seizures. Pupillary size varies with age and is determined by the amount of sympathetic input, which dilates the pupil and is balanced by the parasympathetic input on CN III, which constricts the pupil. Pupillary response in the eye that is being checked with direct light as well as the other pupil (consensual response) are significant in that they can

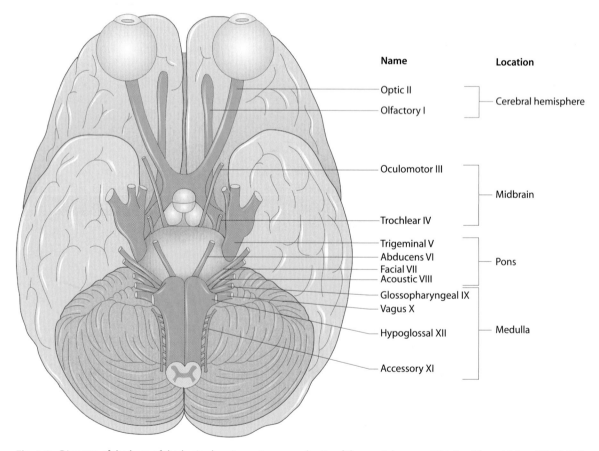

**Fig. 1.2.** Diagram of the base of the brain showing entrance and exits of the cranial nerves. Obtained from Hickey (2003) [20]

**Table 1.6.** Assessment of cranial nerves in the child. Obtained from Hadley (1994) [17]. *S* Sensory, *M* motor, *EOM* extraocular movement

| Cranial | Test for function |
|---|---|
| **I Olfactory (S)** | |
| Olfactory nerve, mucous membrane of nasal passages and turbinates | With eyes closed child is asked to identify familiar odors such as peanut butter, orange, and peppermint. Test each nostril separately |
| **II Optic (S)** | |
| Optic nerve, retinal rods and cones | Check visual acuity, peripheral vision, color vision, perception of light in infants, fundoscopic examination for normal optic disk |
| **III Oculomotor (M)** | |
| Muscles of the eyes (superior rectus, inferior rectus, medial rectus, inferior oblique) | Have child follow an object or light with the eyes (EOM) while head remains stationary. Check symmetry of corneal light reflex. Check for nystagamus (direction elicited, vertical, horizontal, rotary). Check cover-uncover test. |
| Muscles of iris and ciliary body | Reaction of pupils so light, both direct and consensual, accommodation |
| Levator palpebral muscle | Check for symmetric movement of upper eyelids. Note ptosis |
| **IV Trochlear (M)** | |
| Muscles of eye (superior oblique) | Check the range of motion of the eyes downward (EOM). Check for nystagmus |
| **V Trigeminal (M, S)** | |
| Muscles of mastication (M) | Palpate the child's jaws, jaw muscles, and temporal muscles for strength and symmetry. Ask child to move lower jaw from side to side against resistance of the examiner's hand |
| Sensory innervation of face (S) | Test child for sensation using a wisp of cotton, warm and cold water in test tubes, and a sharp object on the forehead, cheeks, and jaw. Check corneal reflex by touching a wisp of cotton to each cornea. The normal response is blink |
| **VI Abducens (M)** | |
| Muscles of eye (lateral rectus) | Have child look to each side (EOM) |
| **VII Facial (M, S)** | |
| Muscles for facial expression | Have child make faces: look at the ceiling, frown, wrinkle forehead, blow out cheeks, smile. Check for strength, asymmetry, paralysis |
| Sense of taste on anterior two-thirds of tongue. Sensation of external ear canal, lachrymal, submaxillary, and sublingual glands | Have a child identify salt, sugar, bitter (flavoring extract), and sour substances by placing substance on anterior sides of tongue. Keep tongue out until substance is identified. Rinse mouth between substances |
| **VIII Acoustic (S)** | |
| Equilibrium (vestibular nerve) | Note equilibrium or presence of vertigo (Romberg sign) |
| Auditory acuity (cochlear nerve) | Test hearing. Use a tuning fork for the Weber and Rinne tests. Test by whispering and use of a watch |
| **IX Glossopharyngeal (M, S)** | |
| Pharynx, tongue (M) | Check elevation of palate with "ah" or crying. Check for movement and symmetry. Stimulate posterior pharynx for gag reflex |
| Sense of taste posterior third of the tongue | Test sense of taste on posterior portion of tongue |
| **X Vagus (M, S)** | |
| Mucous membrane of pharynx, larynx, bronchi, lungs, heart, esophagus, stomach, and kidneys<br><br>Posterior surface of external ear and external auditory meatus | Note same as for glossopharyngeal. Note any hoarseness or stridor. Check uvula for midline position and movement with phonation. Stimulate uvula on each side with tongue depressor – should rise and deviate to stimulated side. Check gag reflex. Observe ability to swallow |

**Table 1.6.** *(Continued)*

| Cranial | Test for function |
|---|---|
| **XI Accessory (M)** | |
| Sternocleidomastoid and upper trapezius muscles | Have child shrug shoulders against mild resistance. Have child turn head to one side against resistance of examiner's hand. Repeat on the other side. Inspect and palpate muscle strength, symmetry for both maneuvers |
| **XII Hypoglossal (M)** | |
| Muscle of tongue | Have child move the tongue in all directions, then stick out tongue as far as possible: check for tremors or deviations. Test strength by having child push tongue against inside cheek against resistance on outer cheek. Note strength, movement, symmetry |

point to where damage to nerves exists and are an objective clinical sign that can be followed over time [9].

## Visual Field Testing and Fundoscopic Examination

Visual field testing and fundoscopic examination are usually not performed by the bedside nurse, but they are important to the assessment of the function of CN II. If the child is awake and able to cooperate, the examiner will position themselves about 2–3 feet (6–9 m) in front of the patient and have the patient look directly at their nose while bringing a brightly colored object from the periphery (right, left, upper, and lower) into the central visual area. The child is asked to indicate when they see the object and this is compared with the examiner's ability to determine if there is a gross defect in the visual field. In the nonacute setting, formal visual field testing is done by a pediatric ophthalmologist and generates a computerized report showing whether the visual field is full or has areas where vision is absent. This baseline determination is required in patients undergoing epilepsy surgery, where cortical resection in the area of the temporal lobe is often proximate to, or overlaps with, the optic nerves as they project from the retina in a posterior fashion to the occipital lobe [28].

Fundoscopic examination in the acute setting is utilized to look for evidence of papilledema and/or retinal hemorrhages. The former is a sign of IICP, generally of a gradual and long-standing nature. The latter is a sign of traumatic injury to the retina as a result of infant shaking in cases of nonaccidental trauma or child abuse.

Extraocular eye movements (EOM's) are mediated by three cranial nerves (III, IV, and VI) as well as the medial longitudinal fascicules tract of the midbrain and pons, and the vestibular system. Eye movements are observed using an object, toy, or just by having the child follow the examiner's finger. The primary descriptors used to describe EOM's are "intact" or "conjugate" if they are normal, indicating that the eyes move together, and "dysconjugate" when they do not move together. Fixed eye movements, a gaze preference (eyes returning to right or left gaze, even if briefly tracking), or roving eye movements indicate damage to nerves and other brain structures. Nystagmus is defined as involuntary back and forth or cyclical movements of the eyes. The movements may be rotatory, horizontal, or vertical, and are often most noticeable when the child gazes at objects in the periphery or that are moving by rapidly. The presence of nystagmus indicates structural lesions or changes in the brainstem, cerebellum, or vestibular system, but can also be present as a result of drug intoxications, notably phenytoin [3, 20].

The motor component of the trigeminal nerve (CN V) supplies innervation to the chewing muscles, and the sensory component has three branches that supply sensation to the eye, face, and jaw. Trigeminal nerve function is evaluated in comatose patients when corneal sensation is tested with a wisp of cotton (referred to as the corneal reflex). A lack of response indicates pressure on or damage to CN V.

The facial nerve (CN VII) innervates the muscles of the face, as well as supplying the anterior two-thirds of the tongue with sensory input allowing for taste of sweet, sour, and salty foods. This is tested by looking closely for symmetry while asking the child to smile, frown, make a face, or "blow-up" their cheeks. Formal testing of taste is usually deferred in the acute care setting.

The acoustic nerve (CN VIII) has a cochlear division, which is responsible for hearing, and a vestibular division, which is responsible for balance. A quick, albeit gross, method of testing hearing is to hold a ticking watch or rubbing strands of hair together near the child's ear and ask if they can hear the sound and describe what it is they are hearing.

Three of the lower cranial nerves, the glossopharyngeal, vagus, and hypoglossal nerves (CNs IX, X, and XII, respectively), are often referred to as a whole in the clinical setting because of their roles in swallowing and the ability to gag and cough, which ultimately support the integrity of the airway. These nerves are especially important in pediatrics because the airway structures are less stable and more at risk for dysfunction and slow recovery if damaged. Damage to these nerves results in impaired swallowing, a decrease in tongue mobility, and speech articulation problems. These problems lead to excessive drooling, frequent aspiration, and nutritional deficits related to poor oral intake. The usual method of assessing these three nerves is to observe for excessive drooling (indicating inability to swallow secretions), cough and gag with suctioning, and/or use a tongue blade to illicit the gag reflex.

The spinal accessory nerve (CN XI) is responsible for innervation of the sternocleidomastoid and trapezius muscles. It can only be tested in the child who is conscious. Assessment is done by having the child shrug their shoulders and push their head against the examiners hand in both directions. If the child is supine in bed, it can be tested by having them raise their head from the bed and flex forward against the force of the examiner's hand [3, 10, 20, 22, 27, 32].

### Assessment of Vital Signs

Neurological alterations can affect vital signs. Vital sign assessment is usually done in conjunction with neurological assessment, so that the child is disturbed once and the information obtained can be evaluated as a whole to determine if changes are occurring that could indicate pending deterioration. Fluid balance, intake, and output are also assessed at this time. Awareness of the relationships between neurological assessment findings, fluid balance, and vital signs in the postoperative neurosurgery patient is essential to avoiding an ominous slide from an alteration in LOC to brainstem herniation and death [3, 24].

Changes in vital signs are a late sign of IICP and require immediate response from the bedside nurse and medical team. Vital signs changes, including a widening pulse pressure, bradycardia, and altered respiratory patterns including central hyperventilation are referred to as Cushing's Triad. This triad of vital sign changes occurs before the more ominous signs of pressure affecting the lower medulla, which manifest as a very deep coma (evidenced by flaccid muscles, absent reflexes, and fixed and dilated pupils). At this point, vital signs display a low blood pressure, a low pulse, and cessation of spontaneous respirations. Herniation of the brainstem has occurred and resulted in brain death [24]. Concepts related to IICP are covered in greater detail in Chap. 7 (Traumatic Brain Injury).

Temperature dysregulation in the form of hyperthermia occurs because of damage to or pressure around the hypothalamus where the regulation of body temperature occurs. Fever without accompanying signs of infection is often referred to as "central," meaning that it has a neurological origin rather than an infectious cause. In the acutely ill child it is important that all diagnostic testing (laboratory tests, x-rays, and cultures including cerebrospinal fluid) have been done to rule out infectious causes of elevated temperature prior to calling a fever central in origin.

Fluid balance, in particular the signs and symptoms of the syndrome of inappropriate antidiuretic hormone (SIADH) and diabetes insipidus, should be assessed and carefully documented in the acutely ill child with a neurological disorder. Frequent measurements of urine output via an indwelling catheter and laboratory tests, including serum sodium and osmolality, are essential to a determination whether these are occurring. Factors such as the administration of diuretics, fluid restrictions in place to decrease the risk of IICP, and recent serum electrolyte and osmolality values should be considered when reviewing intake and output records. Pressure on, or damage to, the anterior pituitary gland can lead to SIADH or diabetes insipidus and may have a significant impact on recovery and outcomes [9].

### Assessment of Motor Function

Motor function is assessed in all children with a neurosurgical diagnosis. Those with a depressed LOC will be observed for the type and quality of movement that occurs in response to noxious stimuli. The nursing assessment of motor function over time will be integral to the determination of long-term outcome for the child. Motor movements that indicate more significant damage to the neurological system are called abnormal motor reflex posturing, or pathological posturing.

In the child without a depressed LOC, assessment of motor function involves observation of the patient's spontaneous movements, as well as responses to direct commands and to tactile stimuli. Key things to observe are the presence of any asymmetries of movement or unusual postures of either the upper or lower extremities. The overall bulk of the muscles and tone is important, especially if there is any question of limb atrophy. In infants, testing of primitive reflexes like the Babinski, Moro, and grasp reflexes assist in the identification of any asymmetries.

Toddlers and preschool-age children respond to the examiner engaging them in play activities. Assessment of spontaneous motor function is done by observation after the child is given objects, toys, or other items to manipulate. Strategies include asking them to give a "high five" with both hands, and having them push their feet against your hands. School-age children will enjoy games of strength and are easily encouraged to cooperate. In the ambulatory, clinic, or school setting, having the child run after a tennis ball, climb onto an exam table, draw a picture or write their name, heel and toe walk, hop, skip, gallop and/or walk a few stairs while observing is the best way to get an accurate functional motor assessment. Asking the child to hold both hands upright in front of their body for several seconds with their eyes closed will give the examiner the opportunity to look for a drifting down ("drift") of one extremity, which can indicate subtle weakness on one side that may not be noted when testing hand grasp strength [9].

### Assessment of Sensory Function

Sensory function is usually assessed in conjunction with motor function. Certain populations of children with neurological abnormalities are more likely to undergo routine assessment of sensory function. These populations include those with spina bifida, spinal cord lesions, or injuries as well as those with indwelling epidural analgesia for postoperative pain management.

The response to superficial tactile stimulation is the most common technique used to assess sensation. More complex testing involves using objects that are both sharp and/or dull to determine if the child can discriminate between them. Assessment of the child's ability to feel a vibration can be done with a tuning fork. Proprioception (awareness of the body in space) is tested by having the child identify flexion or extension of their toe while blocking their visualization of the motion ("Is your toe going up or down?").

Like motor function, any asymmetries of sensory function should be noted. In cases of brain or spinal cord injury or after spinal cord surgery, sensation may be asymmetric and should be documented as such. A baseline exam should be documented so that accurate comparisons can be made. The accepted tool for documentation of the spinal level where sensation is felt is the dermatome chart, which is shown in Fig. 1.3. [7]. A nurse should identify the spinal level at which sensation is present by utilizing either a sharp object or crushed ice in a glove. The examiner first confirms the sensation of the chosen stimulus on a part of the body with normal sensation, then uses the stimulus on the affected area and asks the child to compare with what they have confirmed is "normal." Both anterior and posterior levels are pictured on the chart, which should be readily accessible to nurses who care for these patients. Dermatome levels are also routinely assessed and documented on children with epidural catheters in place to deliver regional analgesia for pain relief in the postoperative period [33].

### Assessment of Reflexes

Both superficial and deep tendon reflexes will be assessed as part of a comprehensive neurological exam. The bedside nurse may not be directly testing the reflexes, but is often present during the exam. Superficial reflexes include the abdominal, cremasteric, and gluteal (anal wink) reflex. Deep tendon reflexes include tapping a reflex hammer on the respective tendons in the bicep, tricep, brachioradialus, patella, and Achilles. Deep tendon reflexes are usually documented using the following scoring system: 0 = absent; +1 = sluggish; +2 = active; + 3 = hyperactive; +4 = transient clonus; +5 = permanent clonus.

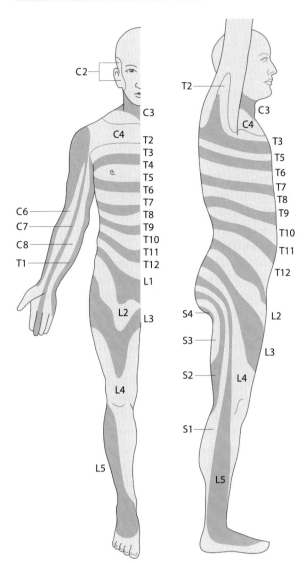

**Fig. 1.3.** Dermatome chart used to assess sensation. Cutaneous distribution of the spinal nerves (dermatomes). Obtained from Conn (1995) [7]

The Babinski reflex is a neurological sign elicited by stimulating the lateral aspect of the sole of the foot with a blunt point or fingernail. A positive response is when the toes fan and the great toe dorsiflexes (goes up). The child can usually dorsiflex the foot and flex the knee and hip. A positive Babinski is normal in an infant and child up to about 18 months of age, around the time a child begins ambulating. After then, the response is considered abnormal and should be documented, and any asymmetry noted [33].

### Assessment of Gait and Balance

Gait and balance are controlled in part by the cerebellum. Assessment of cerebellar function includes the ability to move limbs smoothly in space and the steadiness of the gait. The extent of the assessment of a child's gait and balance will depend on the ability of the child to cooperate with the assessment. Children who are seen in the acute care setting may be too critically ill or sedated to fully assess, although as the child arouses, some simple tests can be done at the bedside for the child who will cooperate.

Ataxia is the term to describe a lack of muscular coordination, and can be termed truncal, appendicular (relating to an appendage), or gait ataxia. It often occurs when voluntary muscle movements are attempted. Cerebellar lesions and drug intoxications can be etiologies of ataxia. Children may exhibit ataxia after a seizure in the postictal phase. Some children will exhibit ataxia as a result of a high serum level of an anticonvulsant [28, 33].

Ataxia is tested by having the child walk in their usual casual gait, both forward and backward. Having the child walk heel-to-toe on a straight line will require that the child put their hands out for balance. Standing balanced on one foot and then the other is also a way to challenge the child's balance. Testing for appendicular ataxia can be done while seated by having the child touch their finger to your finger held about 12–18 inches (30–45 cm) in front of them and then touch their nose and go back and forth. This is often more appealing to the child when a stuffed animal is used as a prop. Ask the child to touch the nose several times while moving the animal.

It is normal for the child to be slightly less coordinated in their nondominant hand, but movements should be smooth. A coarse tremor while doing this finger to nose testing is called "dysmetria," which refers to the inability to control the range of a movement. Often the tremor will worsen when the child is near the target, which is referred to as an "intentional" tremor.

Ataxia may be more noticeable when a child is fatigued, or late in the day, especially if the child is recovering from a neurological trauma. Comparisons used to measure progress should be done by the same individual at the same time of the day so as to not confound the exam findings and to more accurately assess progress in recovery.

### Assessment of Brain Death: Herniation Syndromes and Brainstem Reflexes

Progression of brain insult without appropriate identification and treatment will continue to manifest down the brainstem, affecting the cranial nerves in succession. As noted above, the vital signs are the last to demonstrate signs of progressive neurological deterioration. Children with brain injuries, traumatic or otherwise, are at risk for brain herniation from the primary or secondary effects of their injury.

Herniation can be defined as displacement of brain structures resulting in a sequence of neurological signs and symptoms related to compression of brain structures and to compromised blood flow [2]. Herniation syndromes are categorized by supratentorial and infratentorial locations. Supratentorial herniation includes cingulate herniation, central herniation, and uncal herniation. These types of herniation syndromes result from expanding lesions in one hemisphere of the brain causing pressure medially, downward, or displacement against bone. Infratentorial herniation results from displacement of the cerebellar tonsils below the foramen magnum or, in rare cases, upward herniation of the brain across the tentorium from an expanding lesion in the posterior fossa. Herniation can be reversed with early identification and treatment of the signs and symptoms of IICP, but ends in brain death if the rapid progression of events is not reversed.

Brain death occurs when there is no discernible evidence of cerebral hemispheric and brainstem function for a sustained period due to structural damage or known metabolic insult, and lack of evidence of depressant drugs, poisonings, or hypothermia [2]. The brain death exam requires documentation of the absence of response to stimulation, absence of motor responses, absence of brainstem reflexes, and the absence of spontaneous respirations. Criteria for determination of brain death further requires a relatively normal body temperature and absence of any drugs that might impair consciousness. All of the aforementioned criteria must be met and documented for determination of brain death in the adult. Documentation and the sequencing of the exam to confer brain death is age specific and different for children and adults. All of the criteria listed below are needed for children and adult brain death exams, but in addition, children younger than 5 years of age must show evidence that coma and apnea coexist and that no brainstem function is elicited. The brain death exam according to age includes:

1. Age 7 days to 2 months: two examinations and two EEGs, 48 h apart.
2. Age 2–12 months: two examinations and two EEGs, 48 h apart or one exam and an initial EEG showing no activity combined with a radionucleotide angiogram showing no cerebral blood flow, or both.
3. Age older than 12 months: if irreversible conditions exists, laboratory testing is optional and two exams 12–24 hours apart is sufficient [2].

### Brainstem Reflexes

One commonly used test for the determination of brainstem function in the unconscious child in a comatose state is the assessment of the oculocephalic reflex or "doll's eyes." This maneuver can only be done if a patient is unconscious and is performed by holding the patient's eyelids open and briskly rotating the head laterally in one direction, then the other. This is not done if there is a possibility of cervical spine injury. A normal response is conjugate eye deviation to the opposite side of the head position with return to midline. This is usually documented as "doll eyes present." An abnormal response is the eyes moving in the same direction as the head and/or dysconjugate movements and is documented as "doll eyes absent." The latter indicates damage to the brainstem [20].

Another commonly used test for brainstem function in the comatose child is the assessment of the oculovestibular reflex, also called ice water calorics. This test assesses the function of the vestibular branch of CN X, the vagus nerve. The test is done by irrigating each ear canal with iced water. The child's head is elevated to about 30 degrees. Approximately 5 ml of ice water is drawn into a syringe and attached to a butterfly catheter with the needle cut off. Another individual holds the child's eyes open during the rapid injection of the water into the ear canal. A normal response is nystagmus to the opposite side of the ear being irrigated, then return to midline [20].

Other brainstem reflexes include the corneal reflex, which tests the sensory branch of the trigeminal nerve (CN V) using stimulation of the cornea (using a cotton swab) and the gag reflex (using a tongue blade), which tests the sensory branch of CN X using stimulation of the palate and pharynx.

Testing of these brainstem reflexes is part of the exam performed to assess whether brain death has occurred. They may be repeated over a period of 24 h to confirm that the clinical exam is consistent with other electrical and radiographic findings, and a decision can be made to take the child off life support and declare death. The possibility of organ harvest and donation should have been discussed with the family prior to this and can proceed if medically appropriate and consent has been given by the child's family or legal guardians.

## Assessment of External Monitoring Apparatus

Any equipment related to the neurological monitoring of the child should be assessed by the bedside nurse at regular intervals. This is usually done at the same time as vital sign and neurological assessment. Any concern regarding malfunction of or leakage around a monitoring device should be addressed immediately, following the specific institutional protocol, so that patient safety is assured. Biomedical technicians should be available for routine equipment evaluation so that equipment is ready and in working order.

An important rule in dealing with equipment, or any other technology, is to always look at the patient first, rather than the machine, as the definitive answer in the determination of patient status. This is an important lesson as machines can malfunction. If something doesn't "make sense," the nurse should seek opinions from others and not always assume that the equipment is correct. Monitors used in these patients including intracranial pressure monitors, external ventricular drains, cerebral perfusion monitors and other devices that are covered in more detail in Chap. 7.

## Pain Assessment in the Child with a Neurological Diagnosis

Children with neurological abnormalities may suffer pain from either their primary diagnosis, in the postoperative period after neurological surgery, or during procedures that must be performed in the course of medical care (e.g., lumbar punctures, intravenous starts, shunt taps, dressing changes). Some children will unfortunately suffer chronic pain related to actual nerve injury or a defect in the ability of the ner-

vous system to "turn off" the pain impulses. The last 10 years have been a significant period of change and progress in terms of the overall understanding of pain and how it is manifested, physiologically understood, and treated in the pediatric population. These advances have led to the availability of comprehensive pain management programs available at most of the pediatric tertiary care centers in the United States and abroad [6].

Neurologically impaired children may present the most challenging dilemmas to healthcare providers who are entrusted to assess and manage their pain. These dilemmas relate to issues of how to assess pain in a developmentally delayed child and the desire to not "oversedate" the child so that an accurate neurological assessment is not affected by medications chosen to treat pain. Confounding the issue is the relationship of anxiety to pain and how to determine which is having more of an impact on the child's overall level of comfort. Another important factor in the neurologically impaired child is the input of the parents and other primary care providers, who may have specific experiences and insights that impact their ability to "speak" for the child. Pain in this population of children is very likely undertreated.

Despite the fact that many children suffer pain needlessly, there are still many barriers that exist to providing adequate pain relief to children. These barriers include personal family beliefs, institutional cultures, and individual nurse, physician, and other healthcare provider beliefs. A child's perception of pain is related to both anatomic and physiologic factors, as well as cognitive and behavioral factors. Many involved in pain research agree that a child's response to pain is in part a learned response. Infants and young children may have more atypical responses, whereas older children's pain behaviors are more likely to produce actions from others that lead to pain relief [12].

Pain assessment should be done using validated, age-appropriate scales when the child is able to participate. For those who cannot report their pain, because of age and/or injury, physiologic parameters, observation, and response to ordered pain relief measures should be carefully documented and communicated to promote optimal pain relief. Parent report may also be a reliable indicator when the child is unable to participate or is uncooperative.

Although there are many tools now available for the assessment of pain in infants and children, be-

**Table 1.7.** FLACC (Face, Legs, Activity, Cry, and Consolability) pain assessment tool. From Merkel et al. (1997) [26]. The FLACC is a behavioral observational tool for acute pain that can be used for infants, toddlers, and preschool children. It may also be useful for cognitively impaired children and adolescents. The patient is observed and the score noted for each category (i.e., face, legs, activity, cry, and consolability). The sum of all categories will give score out of maximum 10

| Categories | 0 | 1 | 2 |
| --- | --- | --- | --- |
| Face | No particular expression or smile | Occasional grimace or frown, withdrawn, disinterested | Frequent-to-constant quivering chin, clenched jaw |
| Legs | Normal position or relaxed | Uneasy, restless, tense | Kicking or legs drawn up |
| Activity | Lying quietly, normal position, moves easily | Squirming, shifting back and forth, tense | Arched, rigid or jerking |
| Cry | No cry (awake or asleep) | Moans or whimpers, occasional complaint | Crying steadily, screams or sobs, frequent complaints |
| Consolability | Content, relaxed | Reassured by occasional touching, hugging or being talked to, distracted | Difficult to console or comfort |
| Total score: | | | |

cause of space constraints, only a few will be highlighted in this text as examples. Institutional approaches should utilize published evidence and input from specialists from multiple disciplines (e.g., nurses, physicians, child-life specialists, psychologists) to determine the best tools for each setting. Educating nurses and medical staff regarding the use of pain tools is an ongoing endeavor. The use of a validated pain tool does not necessarily correlate with improved outcomes for children in pain. The use of these tools must be tied to protocols for pain management so that evaluation of pain relief measures, both pharmacological and nonpharmacological, can occur [16]. As complementary and alternative approaches to disease become more widely accepted, many centers have access to therapists skilled in hypnosis, biofeedback, guided imagery, relaxation techniques, acupuncture, and music and art therapy, among others.

Tables 1.7–1.9 display three pain assessment tools that are commonly used in clinical practice: the FLACC (face, legs, activity, cry, and consolability), NCCPC-R (NonCommunicating Children's Pain Checklist-Revised) and the PIPP (Premature Infant Pain Profile) [5, 26, 34].

Management of pain in children undergoing neurosurgical procedures includes the use of nonsteroidal anti-inflammatory drugs, Cox-2 inhibitors, opioids, local anesthetics, antispasmodics, and other drugs that are continually being developed and trialed in the clinical arena. For children with chronic or neuropathic pain, tricyclic antidepressants like amitriptyline, and γ-aminobutyric acid agonists like gabapentin and pregabalin may be used. Administration of medications can be oral, intravenous via intermittent dosing, or patient-controlled analgesia, regional via epidural catheters, transcutaneous (dermal patches), transmucosal (oralettes), and rectal [12].

Whatever pain medications are chosen, the nurse plays the most important role of any caregiver in assessing, evaluating, documenting, preventing, and educating about pain in the ill child. No medication can ever replace a caring, comforting confident, reassuring, and truly present nurse to both the child and family in improving the overall comfort and recovery of the hospitalized child experiencing pain for any reason.

## ■ Conclusion

The last quarter of the 20th century witnessed rapid advancements in technology and successful treatments in the field of pediatric neurosurgery. That coincided with the evolution of the expanded roles and responsibilities of nurses. As the members of the healthcare team with the most direct patient contact, nurses generally have the best opportunity to note signs of neurological problems or subtle changes in a child's condition. Thorough and accurate neurological assessments can make the difference between recovery or complication, and even life or death. Therefore, nurses who have accepted the responsibility of caring for children should strive to develop and consistently apply their assessment skills.

**Table 1.8.** *NCCPC-R* (NonCommunicating Children's Pain Checklist-Revised): a tool for assessing pain in children who are non-communicating

| NCCPC-R |
|---|

Name: _____ Unit/ File#: _____ Date: _____ (dd/mm/yy)

Observer: _____ Start Time: _____ AM/ PM    Stop Time: _____ AM/ PM

How often has this child shown these behaviors in the last 2 hours? Please circle a number for each item. If an item does not apply to this child (for example, this child does not eat solid food or cannot reach with his/her hand), then indicate "not applicable" for that item.

| 0 = not at all | 1 = just a little | 2 = fairly often | 3 = very often | NA = not applicable |
|---|---|---|---|---|

**I    Vocal**

| | | | | | | |
|---|---|---|---|---|---|---|
| 1. | Moaning, whining, whimpering (fairly soft) | 0 | 1 | 2 | 3 | NA |
| 2. | Crying (moderately loud) | 0 | 1 | 2 | 3 | NA |
| 3. | Screaming/yelling (very loud) | 0 | 1 | 2 | 3 | NA |
| 4. | A specific sound or word for pain (e.g., a word, cry or type of laugh) | 0 | 1 | 2 | 3 | NA |

**II    Social**

| | | | | | | |
|---|---|---|---|---|---|---|
| 5. | Not cooperating, cranky, irritable, unhappy | 0 | 1 | 2 | 3 | NA |
| 6. | Less interactive with others, withdrawn | 0 | 1 | 2 | 3 | NA |
| 7. | Seeking comfort or physical closeness | 0 | 1 | 2 | 3 | NA |
| 8. | Being difficult to distract, not able to satisfy or pacify | 0 | 1 | 2 | 3 | NA |

**III    Facial**

| | | | | | | |
|---|---|---|---|---|---|---|
| 9. | A furrowed brow | 0 | 1 | 2 | 3 | NA |
| 10. | A change in eyes, including: squinting of eyes, eyes opened wide, eyes frowning | 0 | 1 | 2 | 3 | NA |
| 11. | Turning down of mouth, not smiling | 0 | 1 | 2 | 3 | NA |
| 12. | Lips puckering up, tight, pouting, or quivering | 0 | 1 | 2 | 3 | NA |
| 13. | Clenching or grinding teeth, chewing or thrusting tongue out | 0 | 1 | 2 | 3 | NA |

**IV    Activity**

| | | | | | | |
|---|---|---|---|---|---|---|
| 14. | Not moving, less active, quiet | 0 | 1 | 2 | 3 | NA |
| 15. | Jumping around, agitated, fidgety | 0 | 1 | 2 | 3 | NA |

**V    Body and Limbs**

| | | | | | | |
|---|---|---|---|---|---|---|
| 16. | Floppy | 0 | 1 | 2 | 3 | NA |
| 17. | Stiff, spastic, tense, rigid | 0 | 1 | 2 | 3 | NA |
| 18. | Gesturing to or touching part of the body that hurts | 0 | 1 | 2 | 3 | NA |
| 19. | Protecting, favoring or guarding part of the body that hurts | 0 | 1 | 2 | 3 | NA |
| 20. | Flinching or moving the body part away, being sensitive to touch | 0 | 1 | 2 | 3 | NA |
| 21. | Moving the body in a specific way to show pain (e.g., head back, arms down, curls up) | 0 | 1 | 2 | 3 | NA |

**VI    Physiological**

| | | | | | | |
|---|---|---|---|---|---|---|
| 22. | Shivering | 0 | 1 | 2 | 3 | NA |
| 23. | Change in color, pallor | 0 | 1 | 2 | 3 | NA |
| 24. | Sweating, perspiring | 0 | 1 | 2 | 3 | NA |
| 25. | Tears | 0 | 1 | 2 | 3 | NA |
| 26. | Sharp intake of breath, gasping | 0 | 1 | 2 | 3 | NA |
| 27. | Breath holding | 0 | 1 | 2 | 3 | NA |

**VII    Eating/Sleeping**

| | | | | | | |
|---|---|---|---|---|---|---|
| 28. | Eating less, not interested in food | 0 | 1 | 2 | 3 | NA |
| 29. | Increase in sleep | 0 | 1 | 2 | 3 | NA |
| 30. | Decrease in sleep | 0 | 1 | 2 | 3 | NA |

**Score Summary**

| Category | I | II | III | IV | V | VI | VII | Total |
|---|---|---|---|---|---|---|---|---|
| Score: | | | | | | | | |

Version 01.2004 © 2004 Lynn Breau, Patrick McGrath, Allen Finley, Carol Camfield

**Table 1.9.** Premature infant pain profile (PIPP) assessment tool. The PIPP is a biobehavioral observational tool for acute and procedural pain. It can be used to assess full- and preterm neonates. The infant is observed as indicated and their score noted. The sum of all categories will give a score out of a maximum of 21. From Stevens et al. 1996 [34]. *O₂ sat* Oxygen saturation, *Min* minimal, *Mod* moderate, *Max* maximal

| Procedure | Indicator | 0 | 1 | 2 | 3 | Score |
|---|---|---|---|---|---|---|
| | Gestational age | >36 weeks | 32–36 weeks | 28–32 weeks | <28 weeks | |
| Observe infant or 15 s for baseline, heart rate, and $O_2$ sat | Behavioral state | Active awake (eyes open, facial movements) | Quiet awake (eyes open, no facial movements) | Active sleep (eyes closed, facial movements) | Quiet sleep (eyes closed, no facial movements) | |
| Observe infant for 30 s | Heart rate | 0–4 bpm increase | 5–14 bpm increase | 15–24 bpm increase | >25 bpm increase | |
| | $O_2$ Sat | 0–2.4% decrease | 2.5–4.9% decrease | 5.0–7.4% decrease | >7.5% decrease | |
| | Brow bulge | None (0–9% of the time) | Min (10–39% of the time) | Mod (40–69% of the time) | Max (>70% of the time) | |
| | Eye squeeze | None (0–9% of the time) | Min (10–39% of the time) | Mod (40–69% of the time) | Max (>70% of the time) | |
| | Nasolabial furrow | None (0–9% of the time) | Min (10–39% of the time) | Mod (40–69% of the time) | Max (>70% of the time) | |
| | | | | | Total | |

## Pediatric Practice Pearls
## Pediatric Neurological Assessment Tools 1

One useful and inexpensive tool for neurological assessment of both infants and young children is a small retracting tape measure with a brightly colored push button for tape retrieval.

This simple tool can be used for the following:

- Assessment of occipital frontal circumference.
- Gross assessment of hearing by watching the response of the child when you pull the tape out close to their ears prior to measurement of their occipital frontal circumference.
- Assessment of EOMs by moving the tape in all visual fields while holding the child's head steady.
- Assessment of cerebellar function by looking for tremor or dysmetria when asking the child to take their "pointer finger" and touch the button and then touch their nose. You can test both hands individually. Children do not usually notice if you put your free hand gently on the hand you don't want them to use.
- Assessment of dexterity when you ask them to pull the tape out and then push the button to let it go back in – see if you can get them to do it with both hands.
- Assessment of cognitive skills by asking them to put it back into your bag or pocket – hint: young children do not like to give things back, but often will put an item back into something as they are used to "emptying and filling" in many of their routine play activities.

## Pediatric Practice Pearls
## Pediatric Neurological Assessment Tools 2

One often useful and inexpensive tool for both neurological assessment of infants and younger children are small wooden blocks with colors, letters, and numbers on them.

These blocks can be disinfected between patients and used for the following:

- The ability to grasp the block(s), bring them to the mouth, transfer them from hand to hand, and clap them together (infants, toddlers).
- The ability to stack or clap two blocks together (manual dexterity), count, and name colors, letters, and numbers (cognitive skills).
- The ability to throw the block to the examiner or into the exam bag (coordination, following directions).

## References

1. Alpern G, Boll T, Shearer M (1986) Developmental Profile II Manual, Los Angeles, Western Psychological Services
2. Bader MK, Littlejohns LR (eds) (2004) AANN Core Curriculum for Neuroscience Nursing, 4th edn. Saunders, St. Louis
3. Barker E (2005) Neuroscience Nursing: A Spectrum of Care, 2nd edn. Mosby, St. Louis
4. Behrman RE, Kliegman RM, Jenson HB (eds) (2004) Nelson's Textbook of Pediatrics, 17th edn. Saunders, Philadelphia
5. Breau L, McGrath P, Finley A, Camfield C (2002) Psychometric properties of the non-communicating children's pain checklist-revised. Pain 99 (1–2) 349–357.
6. Brislin RP, Rose JB (2005) Pediatric acute pain management. Anesthesiol Clin North America 23:789–814
7. Conn PM (1995) Neuroscience in Medicine. Lippincott, Philadelphia
8. DeMeyer W, Zeman W, Palmer CG (1964) The face predicts the brain: diagnostic significance of median facial anomalies for holoprosencephaly. Pediatrics 34:256–263
9. Disabato J, Wulf J (1994) Altered neurologic function. In: Betz C, Hunsberger M, Wright S (eds) Family Centered Nursing Care of Children, 2nd edn. by. Saunders, Philadelphia, pp 1717–1840
10. Engel J (1989) Pocket Guide to Pediatric Assessment, Nervous System. Mosby, St. Louis, pp 188–203
11. Ferguson-Clark L, Williams C (1998) Neurological assessment in children. Paediatr Nurs 10:29–33
12. Foster R, Stevens B (1994) Nursing Management of Pain in Children. In: Betz C, Hunsberger M, Wright S (eds) Family Centered Nursing Care of Children, 2nd edn. Saunders, Philadelphia, pp 882–914
13. Frankenburg WK (1994) Preventing developmental delays: is developmental screening sufficient? I. Developmental screening and the Denver II. Pediatrics 93:586–589
14. Frankenburg WK, Fandal LA, Thornton S (1987) Revision of the Denver Prescreening Developmental Questionnaire. J Pediatr 110:653–657
15. Goodenough FL (1926) Measurement of Intelligence by Drawings. World Book, New York
16. Greco C, Berde C (2005) Pain management for the hospitalized pediatric patient. Pediatr Clin North America 52:995–1027
17. Hadley J (1994) Assessing child health. In: Betz C, Hunsberger M, Wright S (eds) Family Centered Nursing Care of Children, 2nd edn. Saunders, Philadelphia, pp 458–512
18. Haymore J (2004) A neuron in a haystack: advanced neurologic assessment. AACN Clin Issues 15:568–581
19. Hedlund G (2002) Neuroradiology of the central nervous system in childhood. Neurol Clin 20:965–981
20. Hickey J (2003) The Clinical Practice of Neurological and Neurosurgical Nursing, 5th edn. Lippincott, Williams and Wilkins, Philadelphia
21. Hobdell E (2001) Infant neurological assessment. J Neurosci Nurs 33:190–193
22. Kaufman J (1990) Nurse's guide to assessing the 12 cranial nerves. Nursing 20:56–58
23. Lower J (2002) Facing neuro assessment fearlessly. Nursing 32:58–65
24. Marcoux K (2005) Management of increased intracranial pressure in the critically ill child with an acute neurological injury. AACN Clin Issues 16:212–231
25. McGee S, Burkett KW (2000) Identifying common pediatric neurosurgical conditions in the primary care setting. Nurs Clin North Am 35:61–85
26. Merkel SL, Voepel-Lewis T, Shayeviz JR, Malviya S (1997) The FLACC: a behavioral scale for scoring postoperative pain in young children. Pediatr Nurs 23:293–297
27. Murray TA, Kelly NR, Jenkins S (2002) The complete neurological examination: what every nurse practitioner should know. Adv Nurse Pract 10:24–30
28. Neatherlin J (1999) Neuroassessment for neuroscience nurses. Nurs Clin North Am 34:573–592
29. Nellhaus G (1968) Head circumference from birth to eighteen years: practical composite international and interracial graphs. Pediatrics 41:106–114
30. Parker S (1990) Jitteriness in full term neonates: prevalence and correlates. Pediatrics 85:17–23
31. Robbins CT et al Growth. Yale University Press, New Haven
32. Slota MC (1983) Neurological assessment of the infant and toddler. Crit Care Nurse 3:87–92
33. Slota MC (1983) Pediatric neurological assessment. Crit Care Nurse 3:106–112
34. Stevens B, Johnston C, Petryshen P, Taddio A (1996) Premature infant pain profile (PIPP): development and initial validation. Clin J Pain 12:13–22
35. Wong DL, Hockenberry-Eaton M, Winkelstein ML, Wilson D, Ahmann E, DiVito-Thomas PA (eds) (2000) Whaley and Wong's Nursing Care of Infants and Children, 6th edn. Mosby, St. Louis

# Hydrocephalus

*Nadine Nielsen, Katherine Pearce,*
*Elizabeth Limbacher, and Donna C. Wallace*

**2**

## Contents

## Introduction

Hydrocephalus is a condition resulting from an imbalance between the production and absorption of cerebral spinal fluid (CSF). This imbalance results in an increased volume of spinal fluid, dilation of the ventricular system, and often increased intracranial pressure. Hydrocephalus can be acute and occur over hours or days. It may also be chronic and occur over months or years. Hydrocephalus can occur as an isolated condition or one associated with numerous other neurological conditions and diseases.

## History of Hydrocephalus

The term hydrocephalus is derived from the Greek words "hydro" meaning water, and "cephalus" meaning head. The description and treatment of hydrocephalus dates back to the era of Hippocrates and Galen. Galen (AD 130–200) identified the ventricles. He believed that the soul was purified through the pituitary gland, and that waste was discharged via the nose as "pituita." During the Renaissance, Vesalius (1514–1564) described the ventricular system in his original text on human anatomy. A century later, Franciscus Sylvius (1614–1672) described the cerebral aqueduct. Morgagni (1682–1771) described the pathology of hydrocephalus, and Monro (1733–1817) named the intraventricular foramen. In 1786, Whytt distinguished the internal and external hydrocephalus.

Early treatments included bleeding, purging, surgical release of the fluid, puncturing the ventricles to drain the fluid, injection of iodine or potassium hydriodate into the ventricles, binding of the head, application of a plaster of herbs to the head, application cold wraps to the head, lumbar puncture, and diuretics. Confusion about hydrocephalus persisted into the 1800s. It was thought to be caused by fevers, rheumatism, pulmonary consumption, and worms; however, treatment did not change.

The earliest attempts at surgery occurred during the late 1800s. The first shunts diverted CSF from the ventricles to the subcutaneous or subdural spaces. During the early 1900s, other surgical procedures were attempted to treat the condition. These procedures included surgical removal of the choroid plexus, diversion of spinal fluid through a third ventriculostomy, and continued attempts at shunting, including attempts to shunt into the vascular space. Most of these patients did poorly, and either suffered the consequences of prolonged increased intracranial pressure or died. Many institutions cared for these disabled children with very large heads, small bodies, and severe mental retardation.

Modern shunting procedures began in the 1950s with the introduction of the antireflux valve. The first valves developed by Nulson and Spitz in 1952, used a spring and steel ball valve. Holter then developed the first slit valve. He was particularly interested in shunt development, as he had a son with a myelomeningocele and hydrocephalus. These first modernized shunts diverted CSF from the ventricles to the right atrium of the heart. The ventricular-to-peritoneal shunt became the preferred shunt in the 1970s because it allowed for the child to grow, and not outgrow the length of the shunt tubing. This has remained the preferred shunt procedure among modern neurosurgeons. Neurosurgeons have also placed shunts leading from the ventricle to the pleural space, gall bladder, ureter, or fallopian tube if the abdominal cavity is not an appropriate place to terminate the shunt. Numerous improvements in shunt hardware have occurred in the last four decades.

A genetic understanding of hydrocephalus and the diseases associated with hydrocephalus has occurred in the last decade. Such knowledge of genetics has allowed for improved prenatal diagnosis and genetic counseling.

## Incidence of Hydrocephalus

Hydrocephalus is the most common neurosurgical problem encountered by pediatric neurosurgeons. The overall incidence is difficult to determine, as hydrocephalus can occur as an isolated condition or in conjunction with many other neurological diseases and conditions. The overall incidence of hydrocephalus at birth is between 0.5 and 4 per 1000 live births. As an isolated congenital disorder, the incidence of hydrocephalus is 0.5–1.5 per 1000 live births. Hydrocephalus occurs in about 80–85% of such infants born with a myelomeningocele. Because hydrocephalus is associated with so many other diseases and conditions, it is impossible to know how many such children actually exist in the general population. The Hydrocephalus Association (www.hydrocephalus.org) reports that about 25,000 shunt operations are preformed annually in the United States [13]. Other sources quote figures as high as 50,000 shunt surgeries annually in the United States (including adults). Surgeries to place and revise shunts comprise approximately half of a pediatric neurosurgeon's annual operative cases [21].

## Prognosis

The prognosis for children with hydrocephalus has markedly improved with modern shunting. The natural history of unshunted hydrocephalus was studied, and it revealed a 46% 10-year survival rate [18]. Of the surviving population, 62% suffered from intellectual impairment [18]. Children who are adequately treated for hydrocephalus have a considerably better outcome. Their survival rate after 10 years is 95%, and only 30% have impaired intellectual function [37].

The prognosis of an infant or child with hydrocephalus is mostly dependent on the underlying cause of the hydrocephalus. Prognosis may also be related to the complications that occur, such as shunt malfunctions and infections. The best predictors of a good outcome are the prompt treatment of the hydrocephalus and the ability of the brain to grow in the newborn once a functioning shunt is placed. Shunt dependency is associated with a 1% mortality rate per year [12].

## Classifications of Types of Hydrocephalus

Hydrocephalus is subdivided into several different categories. Communicating and noncommunicating are the most common categories. These terms

**Table 2.1.** Classifications of hydrocephalus

| Communicating |
| --- |
| **Congenital** |
| Achondroplasia |
| Arachnoid cyst |
| Dandy-Walker malformation |
| Associated with craniofacial syndromes |
| **Acquired** |
| Posthemorrhagic: intraventricular or subarachnoid |
| Choroid plexus papilloma or choroid plexus carcinoma |
| Venous obstruction as in superior vena cava syndrome |
| Postinfectious |

| Noncommunicating |
| --- |
| **Congenital** |
| Aqueductal stenosis |
| Congenital lesions |
|    (vein of Galen malformation, congenital tumors) |
| Arachnoid cyst |
| Chiari malformations either with |
|   or without myelomeningocele |
| X-linked hydrocephalus |
| Dandy-Walker malformation |
| **Acquired** |
| Aqueductal gliosis (posthemorrhagic or postinfectious) |
| Space-occupying lesions such as tumors or cysts |
| Head injuries |

were previously used interchangeably with obstructive and nonobstructive. The latter terms have fallen from use, as it is believed that in almost all cases of hydrocephalus there is some obstruction of CSF reabsorption; the exception is the rare state of overproduction of CSF. Hydrocephalus is also subdivided into congenital versus acquired, and internal versus external (Table 2.1). Other categories include normal pressure hydrocephalus and ex vacuo hydrocephalus.

### Communicating Hydrocephalus

Communicating hydrocephalus is a condition that results when the arachnoid villi are unable to adequately reabsorb CSF. Intraventricular or subarachnoid hemorrhage may cause the arachnoid villi to become unable to function adequately, either temporarily or permanently. This is a consequence of the effect of the end products of red blood cell breakdown on the arachnoid villi. Infectious processes such as meningitis may also render the arachnoid villi to be nonfunctional due to, for example, toxins or scarring. Com-

municating hydrocephalus may also be due to the overproduction of CSF. This is rare and is usually associated with a choroid plexus papilloma or a choroid plexus carcinoma.

### Noncommunicating Hydrocephalus

Noncommunicating hydrocephalus is a condition that results when the ventricular system does not communicate with the arachnoid villi due to some obstruction in the normal pathways of CSF flow. Consequently, CSF is produced in the ventricular system but cannot flow to the arachnoid villa to be reabsorbed. Such obstruction can occur when pathways are blocked by a tumor, congenital abnormalities of the brain, cysts, inflammation from infection, or any other condition that interferes with the patency of these pathways. Some consider the failure of the arachnoid villi to reabsorb CSF to be an obstruction at the level of the arachnoid villi.

### Congenital Hydrocephalus

Congenital hydrocephalus is caused by any condition that existed before birth. The hydrocephalus may or may not be present at birth. Examples include aqueductal stenosis, Dandy-Walker malformation, and X-linked hydrocephalus. Hydrocephalus is also associated with myelomeningocele, Chiari malformations, and encephalocele, and with prenatal infections such as cytomegalo inclusion virus (CMV) or rubella.

### Acquired Hydrocephalus

Acquired hydrocephalus is hydrocephalus resulting from a condition that did not previously exist in the patient. The condition either obstructs normal spinal fluid flow, causes overproduction of CSF, or prevents reabsorption of CSF. Examples include tumors that obstruct CSF flow and other space-occupying lesions that were not congenital. Infection in the brain may also occlude small passageways. Overproduction of CSF may be caused by a choroid plexus tumor. Acquired conditions that interfere with reabsorption of CSF include intraventricular hemorrhage (IVH) and subarachnoid hemorrhage.

## Internal Hydrocephalus

Internal hydrocephalus refers to ventricular dilation and the associated pathophysiology. The term hydrocephalus is used most commonly to refer to internal hydrocephalus.

## External hydrocephalus

External hydrocephalus refers to the accumulation of CSF in either the subarachnoid or subdural spaces. CSF collection in the subarachnoid space may be a benign condition in infancy, which is called benign subdural hygromas of infancy. CSF mixed with blood in the subdural space may not be benign and usually requires further investigation and treatment. It may be related to trauma. If these fluid collections exert pressure on the brain and cause symptoms or cause accelerated head growth, surgical treatment may be necessary.

## Ex Vacuo Hydrocephalus

Ex vacuo hydrocephalus refers to a condition of brain volume loss. The condition may be present at birth. It may be the result of failure of the fetal development of the brain as in schizencephaly or hydranencephaly. The brain may also undergo destruction or atrophy from infections, very poor nutrition, or unknown causes. The ventricles become large to "fill the space" where there is an absence of brain tissue, and may or may not be under increased pressure. There is technically not an imbalance of CSF production and absorption, but rather there is a loss of brain matter.

## Normal Pressure Hydrocephalus

Normal pressure hydrocephalus is a condition that occurs without increased intracranial pressure. There is ventricular dilation with compression of the cerebral tissue, but the intraventricular pressure is normal. Patients develop symptoms slowly over time. The classic symptoms include dementia, gait difficulties, and urinary incontinence. This is primarily a condition of the elderly.

## Pathophysiology of Hydrocephalus

## Overview of CSF Production and Flow Dynamics

Most of the CSF (approximately 60%) is produced in the choroid plexus; the rest is produced in the ependyma of the cerebral ventricles, the aqueduct of Sylvius, and the subarachnoid space. Studies by Milhorat looking at CSF production after choroid plexectomy demonstrated that the total amount of produced CSF was reduced by only one-third, thus suggesting that other sites can produce larger amounts of CSF [22]. He proposed that CSF is also produced as the result of cellular metabolism of periventricular cortical gray matter. These other areas account for 20% to 50% of CSF production. CSF production requires the expenditure of energy [2].

## CSF Pathways

CSF flows from the ventricles, passes through a series of channels, and exits the ventricular system via the fourth ventricle. There are two lateral foraminae on the lateral aspect of the fourth ventricle, named the foramina of Luschka, and a medially located opening called the foramina of Magendie. After exiting the fourth ventricle, the CSF flows into the subarachnoid space and up over the convexities of the brain, to be absorbed into the large intracranial sinuses [2]. Alternative pathways for CSF have been scientifically supported, and include lymphatic drainage into the cervical lymphatic chain and paranasal sinuses. After being absorbed, the CSF is returned to the right atrium via the superior vena cava [2].

## Intracranial Pressure

A study of rabbits by Dr. McComb found that CSF flows passively, and absorption of CSF does not require the expenditure of energy [2]. For each drop of CSF that is produced, the same amount should be absorbed. Several factors affect the flow of CSF, including resistance, which may result from an obstruction or constriction of a pathway. Other considerations include the plasticity of the brain itself, as well as the flexibility of intracranial venous structures.

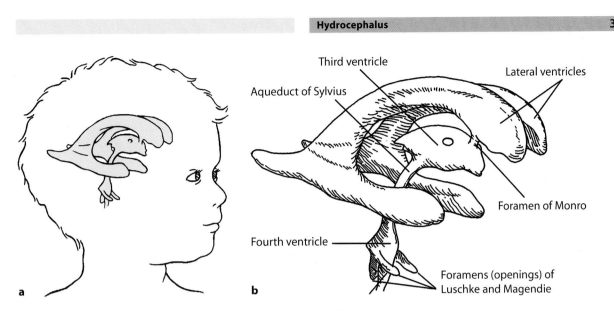

Third ventricle

Aqueduct of Sylvius

Lateral ventricles

Foramen of Monro

Fourth ventricle

Foramens (openings) of Luschke and Magendie

a     b

**Fig. 2.1.** Illustration of position and configuration of intracranial ventricles

Plasticity refers to the brain's ability to change shape. For example, an increase in intraventricular volume will enlarge the ventricles, causing distortion of the cerebral cortex. As we age, our brains may become stiffer. Neonatal brains are very elastic. Anoxic injury can change the brain's ability to be maintain its normal stiffness, and can also be hypoplastic.

The intracranial venous system includes the dural sinuses, which are more rigid than the cortical veins. Cortical veins join the dural sinuses at such an angle that a valvular mechanism is created and a pressure gradient is maintained. The jugular veins, returning the blood to the heart, have no valves. When we stand, negative pressure produced in the jugular veins causes them to collapse, and assists humans in maintaining normal intracranial pressure. Shunting systems are used when the CSF pathways are somehow obstructed. The valves that are used to regulate the flow, attempt to mimic normal flow.

The normal rate of CSF production in infants and children is about 0.33 ml/kg/h. Normal newborns have about 5 ml total volume of CSF. Adults have about 125 ml of total CSF, with about 20 ml located within the ventricles. CSF is produced continually by the choroid plexus, which is located within the ventricles. It is continually reabsorbed by the arachnoid villi (Figs. 2.1 and 2.2).

The pathophysiology of hydrocephalus is much more complex than the radiographic picture. The computed tomography (CT) or magnetic resonance imaging (MRI) scan may reveal many structural changes, including enlarged ventricles, thinning of the cortical mantle, distortion of structures, and possible transependymal flow of CSF. These visible changes may also affect the biochemistry, metabolism, and maturation of the brain. Adequate treatment and resolution of the dilated ventricles does not always reverse the other injuries that have occurred to the brain.

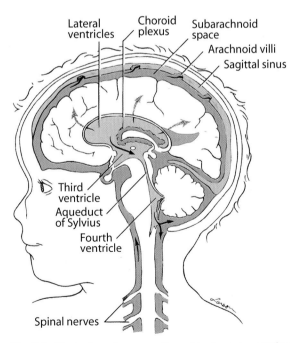

Lateral ventricles

Choroid plexus

Subarachnoid space

Arachnoid villi

Sagittal sinus

Third ventricle

Aqueduct of Sylvius

Fourth ventricle

Spinal nerves

**Fig. 2.2.** Illustration of cross-section of brain and ventricles shows pathways of cerebrospinal fluid (CSF) flow

Three factors are critical in determining the severity of injury caused by hydrocephalus. They are age at onset, and the underlying cause (etiology) and duration of the hydrocephalus. Age is a salient factor because hydrocephalus may affect the normal maturation processes of the brain in addition to the other expected effects of increased intracranial pressure. Furthermore, the underlying disease process responsible for the hydrocephalus may have its own destructive effects on maturation and brain function. Examples of such diseases are encephalitis, meningitis, tuberous sclerosis, and tumors. Treatment of these diseases may also have destructive effects on the brain and brain maturation. An example of this is radiation treatment of brain tumors in very young children. The interruption of normal maturation may be permanent, and normal development does not always follow, even after the resolution of the hydrocephalus. The duration of the hydrocephalus plays has a critical role in determining the long-term recovery. Long-standing ventricular dilation and increased intracranial pressure tend to lead to poor recovery of function, even after ventricular size normalizes.

## Structural Changes

Ventricular dilation seen on the CT or MRI is the hallmark of hydrocephalus. The temporal and frontal horns of the lateral ventricles usually dilate first and are sometimes asymmetrical. This is due to the accumulation of spinal fluid and leads to distortion of the adjacent structures, compression of the nearby white matter, reduction of the cerebral cortex, and thinning of the cortical mantle. The ependymal cells lining the ventricles may become damaged and allow transependymal flow of CSF. The septum pellucidum may become damaged, leading to its disappearance and the formation of one large ventricular cavity.

## Vascular Changes

The distortion of the brain tissue that occurs with hydrocephalus also affects the arteries, veins, and capillaries. Deep vessels are affected the most as they may be directly compressed from the increased ventricular size. Peripheral vessels are also affected as they try to supply the brain tissue that is suffering from the insult of increased intracranial pressure. Blood flow

has been shown to be globally decreased to the brain in acute hydrocephalus [10]. Blood flow is primarily decreased to the periventricular white matter in chronic hydrocephalus [10]. Hypoperfusion may cause damage to neurons and glia and interfere with the normal maturation of all brain structures.

## Metabolic Changes

The brain of a child consumes 50% of total body oxygen; infants consume more than 50% and the adult brain consumes only 20% [38]. The brain uses glucose as its primary source of energy, with few exceptions. Therefore, any decrease in cerebral blood flow that decreases the amount of oxygen and glucose available can markedly alter metabolism. This impairment of metabolism may lead to damage to the brain. Furthermore, during infancy and childhood, a significant portion of the energy used by the brain is used in maturational activities such as myelination, neuronal maturation, and protein production. Normal maturation is disturbed, and possibly permanently altered, due to these metabolic alterations.

## CSF Changes

Abnormal amounts of CSF in the brain may lead to changes in the CSF itself. Metabolites may accumulate in the CSF during hydrocephalus. Protein levels in the CSF may be altered by the underlying cause of the hydrocephalus. For example, after an IVH, protein levels may be very elevated. If the hydrocephalus damages the ependymal cells lining the ventricles, the CSF may flow out of the ventricles into the periventricular white matter. CSF production may or may not decrease as intracranial pressure increases. As intracranial pressure increases reabsorption of CSF increases, assuming that the arachnoid villa are functional.

## Brain Tissue Changes

The white matter surrounding the enlarged ventricles is called the periventricular white matter. As the ventricles dilate, the white matter may become compressed, saturated with CSF, and possibly damaged. Periventricular leukomalacia may result from ischemia to affected white matter. The corpus callosum may also become thinned.

The myelination process may also be delayed in children with hydrocephalus. Myelination occurs at specific times in the development in a stepwise fashion. If one step is interrupted, it can not occur at a later time, and this prevents subsequent steps in the overall process.

The cerebral cortex is also markedly affected by hydrocephalus. The cortex is thinned as it is pushed out by the ventricles and restricted by the skull. Histological changes within the cortex are usually subtle, but damage to cells occurs and results in a change in function.

The goal of treatment is to prevent further damage and to restore function. Treatment usually reverses the acute symptoms of acute hydrocephalus. However, timing is critical and treatment should occur before vascular, metabolic, and other changes described interfere with normal maturation and brain function. Without prompt treatment, acute hydrocephalus and increased intracranial pressure can lead to brainstem herniation and death.

## Etiologies of Hydrocephalus

Hydrocephalus is primarily a condition of obstructed CSF circulation or absorption. In infants and children, it may be congenital or associated with other congenital abnormalities. It may also be associated with central nervous system (CNS) infection, hemorrhage, tumors, cysts, or other diseases.

## Aqueductal Stenosis

The most common cause of hydrocephalus in children is aqueductal stenosis, which accounts for 70% of cases [14]. In 1900, Bourneville and Noir noted an association between hydrocephalus and stenosis of the aqueduct of Sylvius [7]. The aqueduct of Sylvius is a narrow passageway connecting the third and fourth ventricles. Hydrocephalus due to aqueductal stenosis is characterized by enlargement of the lateral and third ventricles with a normal fourth ventricle. This constriction of the aqueduct of Sylvius may also be seen on MRI scan.

Stenosis of this passageway may be congenital or acquired, although in 50-75% of cases, the cause may be unknown. It may be associated with Chiari I malformation, vein of Galen malformation or Dandy-Walker malformation. Aqueductal stenosis may also be due to a x-linked recessive gene occurring only in males. This is rare and is associated with characteristic adducted thumbs, spastic paraparesis, and mental retardation. Acquired cases of aqueductal stenosis may be the result of hemorrhage, inflammation from infection, or obstruction from a nearby tumor or cyst.

## Myelomeningocele and Chiari II Malformation

Myelomeningocele is a neural tube defect that occurs during embryonic development, resulting in failure of the neural tube to close. This malformation involves the entire CNS. At the level of the spinal defect there is a midline lesion containing meninges, spinal cord, nerves, and CSF. The bony structures of the spine may be abnormal or absent. Associated abnormalities in the brain include Chiari II malformation, hydrocephalus, and possibly other structural abnormalities.

Chiari II malformation occurs in almost all infants born with myelomeningocele. It is a malformation of the hindbrain, fourth ventricle, and brainstem and includes herniation of these structures into the cervical spinal canal. Herniation of the brainstem and fourth ventricle may result in obstruction of CSF flow. The development of the hydrocephalus is related to the Chiari II malformation, aqueductal stenosis, venous hypertension in the posterior fossa, and closure of the myelomeningocele [35]. Myelomeningocele is discussed in detail in Chap. 4, and Chiari II in Chap. 5.

Hydrocephalus develops in about 85% of children with myelomeningocele. Approximately 50% have significant hydrocephalus at birth [41]. About 80–90% will eventually require a CSF shunt [11] or an endoscopic third ventriculostomy. Before modern shunting of these infants in the 1960s, only about 20% of nonshunted children lived into adulthood. Today the hydrocephalus can usually be adequately treated. Infants and children who die from this complex condition usually die from the Chiari II malformation and brainstem dysfunction.

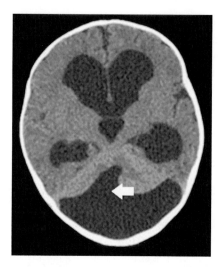

**Fig. 2.3.** Two-month-old female with Dandy-Walker malformation. Magnetic resonance imaging (MRI) shows a posterior fossa cyst of the fourth ventricle and subsequent development of severe hydrocephalus (*arrow*)

## Chiari I Malformation

Chiari I malformation is one of the four types of Chiari malformations. In Chiari I, the cerebellar tonsils are elongated and herniated into the cervical spinal canal. Chiari I is not associated with myelomeningocele, and may be acquired from increased intracranial pressure or occur as an isolated condition. Chiari malformations are discussed in detail in Chap. 5.

Hydrocephalus occurs in 10% of children with Chiari I malformation, most likely due to blockage of CSF flow at the craniovertebral junction. A small posterior fossa may also alter CSF flow. Treatment for patients with symptomatic Chiari I malformation is often a posterior fossa decompression. A small percentage of children develop hydrocephalus after the decompression.

## Dandy-Walker Malformation

Dandy-Walker malformation is a continuum of posterior fossa abnormalities, including Dandy-Walker malformation and Dandy-Walker variants. The abnormalities associated with these conditions include: cystic dilation of the fourth ventricle, partial or complete absence of the cerebellar vermis, upward displacement of the tentorium, and usually hydrocephalus. Dandy-Walker may be differentiated from a pos-

terior fossa cyst by the atrophy or agenesis of the vermis seen on MRI scan. Dandy-Walker malformation/variant may also be associated with other intracranial abnormalities in 70% of patients. These include agenesis of the corpus callosum, aqueductal stenosis, schizencephaly, holoprosencephaly, neural tube defect, and occipital encephalocele. Dandy-Walker is found in 2–4% of all children with hydrocephalus [14]. Other abnormalities associated with Dandy-Walker malformation/variant include congenital heart defects, renal malformations, polydactyly/syndactyly, cleft palate, perineal malformations, Klieppel-Feil malformation, and facial hemangiomas.

Hydrocephalus occurs in 90% of children with Dandy-Walker malformation/variant [14]. Initially, it was believed that the hydrocephalus was caused by obstruction of the foramina of Luschka and Magendie. Dandy and Blackfan (1914) believed that the foramina failed to develop or were obstructed due to a prenatal inflammatory process. However, in some cases the foramina are found to be patent. Also, about 80% of infants with Dandy-Walker malformation do not have hydrocephalus at birth [7]. The pathophysiology of the hydrocephalus is now felt to be multifactorial. Contributing factors include aqueductal stenosis, basal arachnoiditis from an inflammatory process, abnormally developed subarachnoid space, and venous hypertension from direct pressure from the posterior fossa cyst (Fig. 2.3) [7].

## Vein of Galen Malformation

A vein of Galen malformation is a rare vascular malformation (Fig. 2.4). It is a venous aneurysm of the vein of Galen fed by numerous aberrant branches of the carotid or vertebrobasilar vessels. In addition, arteriovenous malformations may occur within the feeding vessels.

Infants with a vein of Galen malformation often present at birth with congestive heart failure and hydrocephalus. They may also develop hydrocephalus later. Hydrocephalus may be caused by the venous malformation causing obstruction of the cerebral aqueduct. Elevated intracranial venous pressure may also decrease CSF reabsorption and cause hydrocephalus.

**Fig. 2.4 a, b.** Four-month-old male with vein of Galen malformation. **a** MRI shows the dilated vein of Galen. **b** Cerebral angiogram shows the dilated vein of Galen and the surrounding vasculature

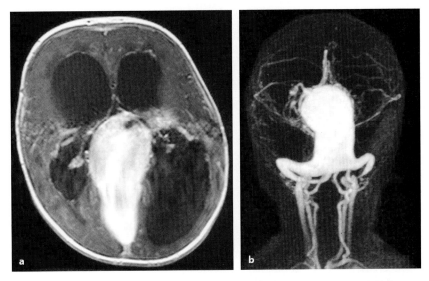

## Arachnoid Cysts

An arachnoid cyst is a benign congenital cyst occurring within the brain (Fig. 2.5). The cyst forms during fetal development with the splitting of the arachnoid membrane [26]. An intra-arachnoid space is created and the cyst develops. Most of these cysts do not change or cause any other problems. Such cysts are often found incidentally when a child has a scan for some other reason (i.e., head injury). If the cyst enlarges, it may compress the surrounding structures and cause symptoms from mass effect. Depending on the location, as the cyst expands, it may compress nearby CSF pathways and cause hydrocephalus. A suprasellar cyst may expand upward, pressing on the floor of the third ventricle and obstructing the foramen of Monro or aqueduct of Sylvius. A cyst in the quadrigeminal cistern or supracollicular region may cause obstruction of the aqueduct of Sylvius. A posterior fossa arachnoid cyst can cause obstruction at the level of the fourth ventricle. A posterior fossa cyst can be differentiated from a Dandy-Walker malformation by the presence of the cerebellar vermis and a normal appearing fourth ventricle on an MRI. The etiology of expansion of the cyst is unknown. Surgical intervention is required if hydrocephalus occurs or there are symptoms of mass effect from the cyst.

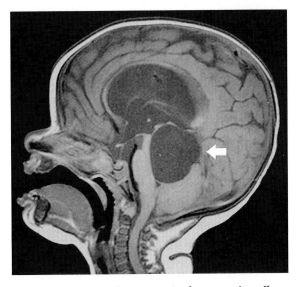

**Fig. 2.5.** MRI shows a large posterior fossa cyst that effaces the aqueduct of Sylvius and fourth ventricle, causing severe hydrocephalus (*arrow*)

## Posthemorrhagic Hydrocephalus of Prematurity

The most common cause of hydrocephalus in the premature infant is a germinal matrix hemorrhage. The germinal matrix is a very vascular area in the fetal brain, in the subependymal region located at the level of the foramen of Monro. It is from the very thin-walled germinal matrix vessels that the bleeding is thought to occur in preterm infants. Bleeding can spread, most often to the adjacent ventricles and into

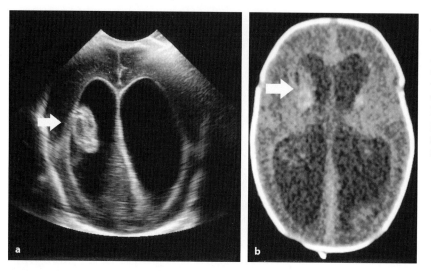

**Fig. 2.6 a, b.** Twenty-five-week premature male with an intraventricular hemorrhage and subsequent development of hydrocephalus. **a** Conventional ultrasound (CUS) shows the right-sided intraventricular hemorrhage (*arrow*). **b** Computed tomography (CT) also shows parenchymal hemorrhage (*arrow*)

the surrounding parenchyma. The germinal matrix gradually involutes after 34 weeks gestation and nearly disappears by 40 weeks. A grading system has been devised to describe the severity of the bleeding – grades I–IV (Table 2.2) [41].

Premature infants of less than 34 weeks gestation with very low birth weight (<1500 g) are at greatest risk for developing IVH. With current management, 20% of these preterm infants will develop an IVH. The risk of developing posthemorrhagic hydrocephalus (PHH) is related directly to the extent of the hemorrhage. Hydrocephalus develops in 20–74% of infants with IVH [3]. Infants with a grade I or II bleed do not have hydrocephalus by definition; 55% of infants with a grade III hemorrhage and 80% of those with a grade IV bleed develop hydrocephalus [3]. PHH may develop as a result of the accumulation of blood and hemorrhagic debris within the ventricles and subarachnoid spaces (Fig. 2.6). Obstruction of the aqueduct of Sylvius or foramen of Monro may occur. The breakdown of blood may also render the arachnoid villi unable to reabsorb the CSF. Multiloculated hydrocephalus may occur after IVH due to ventriculitis. Ventricular septations develop causing isolated compartments of fluid within the ventricles.

Many premature infants require surgical intervention to treat the hydrocephalus until it is resolved. About 20–30% will require permanent shunting [3]. Figure 2.6 illustrates IVH and PHH of prematurity.

**Table 2.2.** Grading of intraventricular hemorrhage [41]. *IVH* Intraventricular hemorrhage

| Grade | Extent of hemorrhage |
|-------|----------------------|
| I | Subependymal germinal matrix hemorrhage |
| II | IVH without ventriculomegaly |
| III | IVH with ventriculomegaly |
| IV | IVH with parenchymal hemorrhage |

### Postinfectious Hydrocephalus

Intracranial infection may be the cause of hydrocephalus throughout the spectrum of life. Hydrocephalus may follow bacterial, fungal, viral, and parasitic infections of the CNS. In utero, CNS infections may cause intracranial injury leading to obstruction of CSF flow. Toxoplasmosis may cause inflammation and blockage of the CSF pathways and blockage within the subarachnoid spaces [8]. During the neonatal period, Gram-negative bacteria are the leading cause of bacterial meningitis [8]. Gram-negative bacteria may cause ventriculitis [8], leading to hydrocephalus.

After the neonatal period, Gram-positive bacteria are the leading cause of meningitis. Meningitis and ventriculitis may lead to multiloculated hydrocephalus, a condition where noncommunicating pockets of CSF occur within the ventricles. Viral infections, including CMV, parainfluenza, and influenza A, affect ependymal cells leading to acquired aqueductal stenosis [8]. Tuberculosis meningitis may cause obstructive hydrocephalus from mass effect of a tuberculoma, or cause a communicating type of hydrocephalus by affecting the basal cisterns. Hydrocephalus may develop in conjunction with the intracranial infection or much later after recovery.

Cysticercosis occurs throughout the world. It is rare in the United States, but is found throughout Latin America. Humans can acquire the pork tapeworm, *Taenia solium*, by eating uncooked pork or by consuming the tapeworm eggs from food contaminated with human feces. The tapeworm larva enter the body and form cystircerci. Neurocysticercosis results when the cysts enter the brain. The cysts can implant in the parenchyma, ventricles, subarachnoid space, or cisterns. Hydrocephalus can occur when cysts are in the ventricles, subarachnoid space, or cisterns, or cause arachnoiditis. In areas such as southern California and Mexico, neurocysticercosis must be considered as an etiology of hydrocephalus.

## CNS Tumors

Hydrocephalus is a complicating factor of pediatric brain tumors. Brain tumors are discussed in detail in Chap. 6. Hydrocephalus can be present at the time of diagnosis of the tumor, may occur during or after tumor treatment, or may develop if the tumor reoccurs. Most of the time, hydrocephalus associated with tumors is due to the obstruction of CSF pathways.

About 60% of brain tumors in children are located infratentorially or in the posterior fossa. These tumors occur in the cerebellum, fourth ventricle, or brainstem. The most common tumors of this region include medulloblastoma, astrocytoma and ependymoma. Hydrocephalus is common with tumors in this area. It results from obstruction of CSF flow, particularly if the tumor is in the fourth ventricle or exerting pressure on the fourth ventricle. A tectal plate tumor is an indolent tumor of the midbrain and results in hydrocephalus. In all of these tumors, hydrocephalus is often a major contributor to symptoms at the time of diagnosis. If the hydrocephalus is severe, urgent treatment is needed to relieve increased intracranial pressure.

Hydrocephalus may also occur from blood and debris in the CSF after tumor resection. Approximately 25–50% of children will require placement of a permanent shunt [41] or endoscopic third ventriculostomy after the tumor resection. Certain factors are associated with the need for permanent CSF diversion, including: age less than 10 years, midline tumors, incomplete tumor resection, CSF infection, and persistent pseudomeningocele [31].

About 40% of pediatric brain tumors occur in the supratentorial area. The most common site is the suprasellar region, followed by the cerebral hemispheres, thalamus and basal ganglia, pineal region, intraventricular spaces, and meninges. Hydrocephalus is associated with some of these tumors and is usually due to obstruction of CSF flow at the aqueduct of Sylvius. Tumors in the suprasellar region most commonly associated with hydrocephalus are craniopharyngioma and optic pathway glioma. Craniopharyngiomas can also form cysts that exert a mass effect that causes symptoms and/or hydrocephalus. Occasionally, germ cell tumors and pituitary adenomas may cause hydrocephalus. Pineal region tumors are commonly associated with hydrocephalus. Tumors that grow within the ventricles may cause hydrocephalus as a result of overproduction of CSF. There are two types of choroid plexus tumors: choroid plexus papilloma and choroid plexus carcinoma. They arise from the choroid plexus, located within the lateral, third, and fourth ventricles. Hydrocephalus may also occur in patients with neurofibromatosis or tuberous sclerosis secondary to obstruction of CSF flow.

Spinal cord tumors are rare in children. They may be associated with hydrocephalus due to arachnoiditis and elevated protein in the CSF (Fig. 2.7).

## Head Trauma

Hydrocephalus may occur after head injury if there is intracranial blood. This is particularly true if there is subarachnoid or IVH. The breakdown of blood may alter the ability of the arachnoid villi to absorb CSF. Debris and blood may also obstruct normal CSF pathways and cause obstructive hydrocephalus.

## Signs and Symptoms of Hydrocephalus

The signs and symptoms of hydrocephalus in infants and children vary depending on their age, the degree of hydrocephalus at presentation, the primary etiology, and the time over which the hydrocephalus develops. Because of the plasticity of the infant brain and the ability of the cranium to expand, ventriculomegaly can progress without obvious signs of increased intracranial pressure. In premature infants, in which

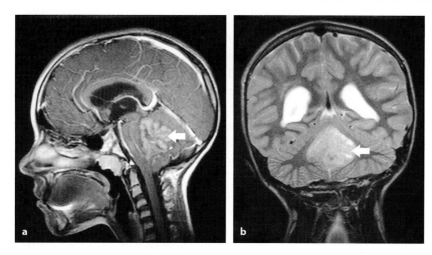

**Fig. 2.7 a, b.** Eight-year-old female with a posterior fossa brain tumor and hydrocephalus

**Table 2.3.** Signs and symptoms of hydrocephalus in children

| Premature infants | Full-term infants | Toddlers and older |
|---|---|---|
| Apnea | Macrocephaly | Headache |
| Bradycardia | Rapid head growth | Nausea |
| Hypotonia | Decreased feeding | Vomiting |
| Acidosis | Increased drowsiness | Irritability |
| Seizures | Tense fontanel | Lethargy |
| Rapid head growth | Vomiting | Delayed development |
| Tense fontanel | Distended scalp veins | Decreased school performance |
| Splayed cranial sutures | Splayed cranial sutures | Behavioral disturbance |
| Vomiting | Poor head control | Papilledema |
| Sunsetting eyes | Parinaud's sign | Parinaud's sign |
| | Sunsetting eyes | Sunsetting eyes |
| | Frontal bossing | Bradycardia |
| | | Hypertension |
| | | Irregular breathing patterns |

hydrocephalus is caused predominately by an IVH, there is a general correlation between the severity of hemorrhage and the degree of hydrocephalus (Table 2.3). Infants with PHH may have minimal symptoms, or may exhibit increasing spells of apnea and bradycardia. They may also have hypotonia, sunsetting eyes, ophthalmoplegia and seizures. As the ventriculomegaly progresses, the fontanel will bulge, become tense and nonpulsatile, and the cranial sutures become splayed. In a healthy premature infant, the head circumference generally increases about 1 cm a week. In premature infants with progressive ventriculomegaly, the head circumference may increase more rapidly than normal (when charted on the head

growth chart), but may not accurately reflect the rate of increase in ventricular size.

In full-term infants, signs often include macrocephaly and progressively increasing occipital frontal head circumference, crossing percentile curves. Normal head circumference for a full-term infant is 33–36 cm at birth. A normal head circumference increases by approximately 2 cm/month during the first 3 months, by 1.5 cm/month during the 4th and 5th months, and by about 0.5 cm/month from months 6–12 (Fig. 2.8).

Other common signs in full-term infants include a bulging, tense anterior fontanel, splayed cranial sutures, irritability, poor feeding, episodes of spitting

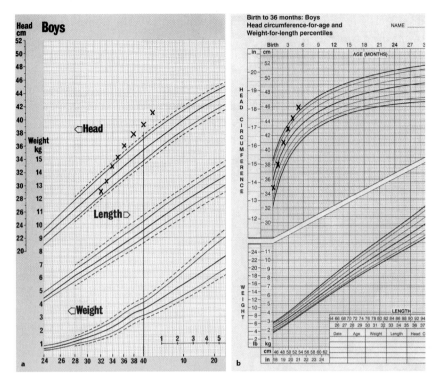

**Fig. 2.8 a, b.** Growth charts show the head circumference rapidly crossing percentile curves. **a** Premature male infant growth chart. **b** Full-term male growth chart

up or vomiting, increased sleeping, distended scalp veins, and, if the head is large relative to body size, poor head control. Visual changes may also be noted and include paralysis of upward gaze (Parinaud's sign) and sunsetting eyes.

Children older than 2 or 3 years may have a more acute presentation of symptoms since the cranial fontanels and sutures are closed, and the skull is no longer able to compensate for the increasing ventricular size. The predominant symptom is usually a persistent headache that typically occurs upon wakening and is often associated with nausea, vomiting, and lethargy. The child is often irritable. A child who has a gradual onset of hydrocephalus may have more subtle signs, such as delayed development in both motor and cognitive function. Older children often present with decreased school performance and behavioral disturbance. Other less common signs may include papilledema and visual complaints. If hydrocephalus is severe, Cushing's triad of bradycardia, systemic hypertension, and irregular breathing patterns may occur. This triad denotes a severe case of increased intracranial pressure and requires emergent treatment.

## Diagnosis of Hydrocephalus by Imaging Studies

The three major techniques used for diagnosis and evaluation of hydrocephalus are ultrasonography (US), CT, and MRI.

### Ultrasonography

Prenatal US can be highly reliable and accurate in diagnosing hydrocephalus. Hydrocephalus can be detected in a fetus as early as the later part of the first trimester of pregnancy, although abnormal dilation of the fetus's ventricles are more clearly detectable after 20–24 weeks gestation [13]. Although prenatal US can detect abnormal CSF collection, it may not show the precise site or cause of the obstruction. Amniocentesis can often detect the presence of open neural tube defects, such as myelomeningocele, chromosome abnormalities, and in-utero infections, and may also help indicate the overall health of the fetus. In general, the first trimester development of significant hydrocephalus can be a poor prognostic sign for infant mortality and developmental progress. In some cases, mild ventricular dilation identified by US will resolve by the third trimester [13].

Cranial US is useful in infants and young children while the anterior fontanel is still open, usually under the age of 18 months (Fig. 2.9). Through the fontanel, it can demonstrate lateral ventricular morphology and intraventricular clots. It is less accurate in its ability to look at the third and fourth ventricles and subarachnoid spaces. For this reason, the precise diagnosis and cause of hydrocephalus is rarely made by US alone. It is particularly useful, however, for follow-up screening of infants with untreated and treated hydrocephalus. The equipment is portable, involves no radiation, does not require sedation, and is considerably less expensive than CT/MRI.

## Computed Tomography

Since the advent of CT scanning in 1976, it continues to be the most commonly used radiologic technique for the diagnosis and follow-up of hydrocephalus. CT images can accurately demonstrate the ventricular size and shape, the presence of blood and calcifications, cysts, and shunt hardware. In hydrocephalus, an enlarged ventricular system is usually seen, and is usually first seen in the lateral ventricles (Fig. 2.10). CT images can also accurately reflect signs of increased intracranial pressure, such as compressed cerebral sulci, absent subarachnoid spaces over the convexity, and transependymal reabsorption of CSF in the white matter. When contrast enhancement is used, tumors, abscesses, and some vascular malformations can be visualized. It is currently the most rapid diagnostic screening tool, taking only a few minutes, and few children need to be sedated for the procedure. Despite the fact that it

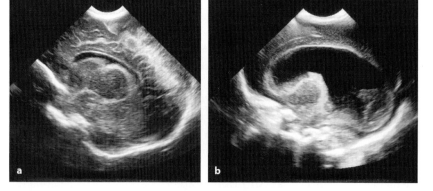

**Fig. 2.9 a, b. a** Normal CUS in a 1-month-old female. **b** Hydrocephalus in a 3-week-old male

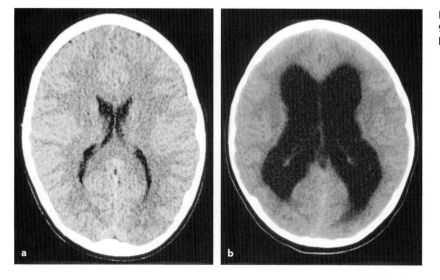

**Fig. 2.10 a, b. a** Normal CT in a 9-year-old male. **b** Hydrocephalus in a 2-week-old male

uses low-level radiation, little is known about the long-term effects of multiple scans. CT scanning has a lower resolution than MRI and is usually only performed in the axial plane.

## Magnetic Resonance Imaging

Commercially available MRI was introduced in 1986 and is the examination of choice for revealing the underlying cause of hydrocephalus. It allows anatomical visualization in the axial, coronal, and sagittal planes, providing detailed information regarding the anatomy, and the position and extent of lesions. Subtle findings, such as white matter pathology, dysmorphic anatomy, and characteristics of lesions can be readily demonstrated. In addition, the aqueduct of Sylvius can be visualized, as well as membranes and loculated ventricular systems. With the addition of gadolinium (an intravenous contrast medium), some neoplasms and vascular lesions can be better visualized. CSF flow dynamics can be visualized through the use of phase-contrast cine MRI. This sequence takes only a few extra seconds and allows for real-time flow measurements that are demonstrated on the sagittal plane of the MRI. Furthermore, constructive interference in the steady state (CISS) sequence MRI may be used. This sequence provides great detail of the ventricular system, basal cisterns, and may show membranes not otherwise seen on conventional MRI. Both phase-contrast cine MRI and CISS sequence MRI can be very helpful in determining the underlying cause of hydrocephalus. They can also provide valuable pre-operative information related to the potential success of endoscopic third ventriculostomy, as well as post-operative information by being able to visualize the CSF flow pattern. MRI takes approximately 45 min or longer and, therefore, young children need to be sedated for the exam. Typically, children with normal development over the age of 5 or 6 years can often do the exam without sedation. Aqueductal stenosis and hydrocephalus are shown in Figs. 2.11, 2.12, and 2.13, along with cine and CISS MRI scans.

## Treatment of Hydrocephalus

## Medical Therapy

There is currently no medical therapy that definitively treats hydrocephalus effectively. Occasionally, in borderline cases of progressive hydrocephalus and in PHH, diuretics may be useful as a temporizing measure to try to avoid the need for a permanent shunt. Acetazolamide, a carbonic anhydrase inhibitor, has been shown to decrease CSF production. The dose may be as high as 100 mg/kg, and in order for it to be effective, more than 99% of carbonic anhydrase must be blocked before CSF production decreases significantly. Furosemide, 1 mg/kg/day, has also been used. The mechanism of action is unknown, but it is thought to decrease brain extracellular fluid. Although these have been used historically as temporizing measures, comprehensive analysis of data from clinical trials on diuretic therapy for PHH by the Cochrane Collaboration concluded that acetazolamide and furosemide were neither effective nor safe for the treatment of PHH [42].

Serial lumbar or ventricular punctures to evacuate CSF as a temporizing measure are also used. The ef-

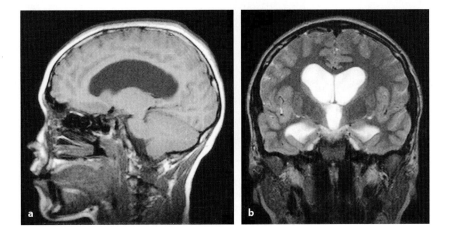

**Fig. 2.11.** Thirteen-year-old male with aqueductal stenosis and hydrocephalus. **a** Sagittal T1 MRI shows enlarged lateral ventricles (CSF appears black). **b** Coronal T2 MRI shows enlarged lateral and third ventricles (CSF appears white)

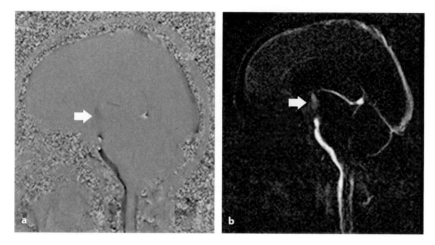

**Fig. 2.12 a, b.** Thirteen-year-old male with hydrocephalus secondary to aqueductal stenosis, status following endoscopic third ventriculostomy. CSF cine flow study demonstrates CSF flow across the fenestration in the anterior third ventricle (*arrows*). **a** Phase-contrast magnitude cine MRI. **b** Phase-contrast directional cine MRI

ficacy of these punctures is controversial, but some centers routinely use them in infants until they are stable enough to tolerate a surgical intervention. The goals are to decrease the intracranial pressure and help clear the CSF of the toxic chemicals produced by the breakdown of blood. If the infant continues to have inadequate CSF reabsorption, a more permanent shunt may be implanted.

## Surgical Intervention

### Shunts

CSF shunting is the most common standard treatment in the long-term management of hydrocephalus. It involves the placement of a ventricular catheter to divert CSF to another body cavity, where it can be absorbed. There are many different shunting devices with different components, all having similar features. The three main components of a shunt are: a proximal (ventricular) catheter, a valve, and a distal catheter (Fig. 2.14). The ventricular catheter is a silastic tube that is placed either through a frontal or parieto-occipital approach, usually in the right nondominant cerebral hemisphere (Fig. 2.15). A burr hole is made in the skull and the catheter tip is generally placed in the frontal horn of the lateral ventricle. This placement is advantageous because there is less cho-

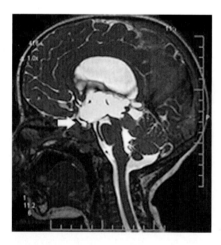

**Fig. 2.13.** Thirteen-year-old male with hydrocephalus secondary to aqueductal stenosis. Preoperative constructive interference in the steady-state MRI demonstrates the floor of the third ventricle and the position of the basilar artery

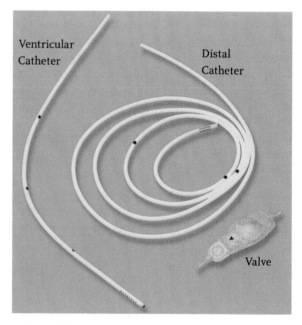

**Fig. 2.14.** Shunt components (courtesy of Medtronic Neurologic Technologies)

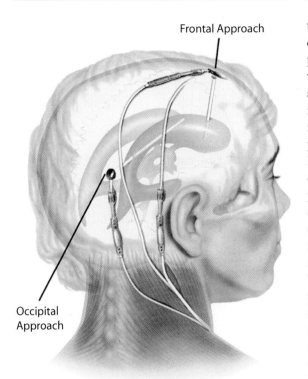

Frontal Approach

Occipital
Approach

**Fig. 2.15.** Illustration demonstrates that proximal catheter placement is generally through a frontal or occipital approach

roid plexus in this area, and therefore less chance for the holes in the catheter to become occluded.

There are many different valves made by many different manufacturers. They all regulate the flow of CSF by means of a one-way valve. The valves most commonly used in the pediatric setting today are differential pressure valves, flow-regulating valves, and siphon-resisting valves. The pressure at which the valves open is termed the opening pressure. Typically,

there are low-, medium-, and high-pressure valves in each category, referring to opening pressures of approximately 5, 10, and 15 cm $H_2O$, respectively. Most valves are differential pressure valves, and are designed to open and allow the drainage of CSF as the intraventricular pressure rises above the valve's opening pressure. Once the pressure falls below the closing pressure, the valve closes and the flow of CSF ceases. Flow-regulating valves attempt to keep the CSF flow constant despite changing pressure differentials and patient position. Siphon-resisting valves are used to avoid siphoning of CSF and the complication of overdrainage. Siphoning is a phenomenon that occurs in some patients in whom there is gravity-enhanced flow of CSF when the patient is in an upright position. The choice of which valve to use is based the personal preference of the neurosurgeon, and is usually based on training and personal experience. No data exist to support a recommendation of one particular shunt design or valve over another. Fixed-pressure valves are shown in Fig. 2.16.

A recent advance in shunt valve technology has been the introduction of programmable valves (Fig. 2.17). Programmable valves can be externally adjusted with the use of a special magnetic device (Figs. 2.18–2.20). The opening pressure of the valve can be adjusted. This avoids the need for an operative procedure should the patient need a valve with a different pressure. This type of valve tends to be well suited for the management of difficult cases of overdrainage or underdrainage, or in children whose pressure needs are expected to change over time. It is not clear that the benefits outweigh the increased cost in all patients. Since the programmable valve contains a magnet, most valves need to be reprogrammed im-

**Fig. 2.16 a, b.** **a** Fixed-pressure valves. **b** Delta valves with siphon control. Courtesy of Medtronic Neurologic Technologies

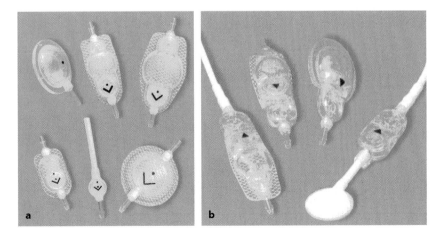

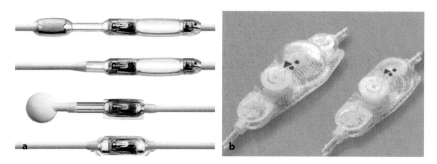

**Fig. 2.17 a, b. a** Codman Hakim programmable valves. **b** Strata programmable valves (courtesy of Medtronic Neurologic Technologies)

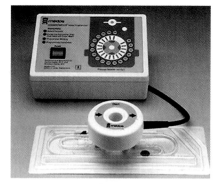

**Fig. 2.18.** Codman Hakim valve programmer

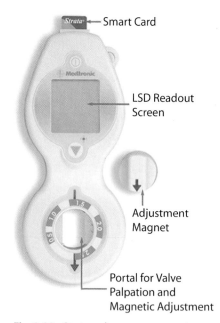

Smart Card

LSD Readout Screen

Adjustment Magnet

Portal for Valve Palpation and Magnetic Adjustment

**Fig. 2.20.** Strata valve programmer (courtesy of Medtronic Neurologic Technologies)

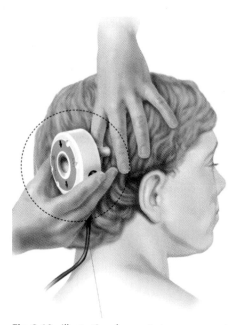

**Fig. 2.19.** Illustration demonstrates programming a Codman Hakim programmable valve

mediately after all MRIs. A programmable valve that is not altered by a magnetic field is also available. It "locks" the setting and can only be changed with the manufacturer's specific magnetic programmer. Com-

mon everyday household equipment like mobile telephones and computers are not strong enough to affect the valve, although special precautions should be taken when the patients are around other strong magnetic sources.

Distal catheters are also made of silastic material. The peritoneal cavity is the preferred and most commonly utilized location for the shunt to terminate. There are two main advantages to placing the distal tubing in the peritoneum. First, if an infection develops, it usually stays localized rather than disseminating, as can happen with shunts placed in the heart. Second, a large amount of tubing can be placed in the peritoneal cavity, to allow for growth of the child and minimize the need for revisions during childhood. In addition, the peritoneal cavity is an extremely efficient site of absorption, and is easily accessible to

**Fig. 2.21 a, b.** Illustration shows placement of ventriculoperitoneal (*VP*) and ventriculoatrial (*VA*) shunts

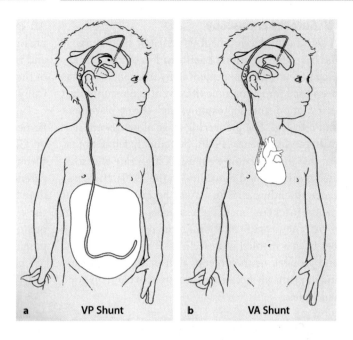

a   VP Shunt      b   VA Shunt

the surgeons. If the peritoneal cavity is not appropriate for placement of the distal tubing, either due to an abdominal malformation, postsurgical adhesions, infection, or inadequate reabsorption, the second and third choices for the distal catheter placement are either the right atrium of the heart or the pleural cavity, respectively.

Ventriculoatrial shunts are placed through the neck, into the jugular vein to the superior vena cava and into the right atrium (Fig. 2.21). The shunt tip should lie just above the tricuspid valve and, on plain chest radiograph, should be at the superior vena cava/right atrial interface. The tip of the catheter can also be evaluated by looking for it at the level of the sixth/seventh thoracic vertebrae. If it above this level a shunt-lengthening procedure may be indicated. Infants should have a chest x-ray every 6 months and older children every year, to make sure the distal placement is in an adequate location.

Ventriculopleural shunts are guided subcutaneously to an area just below the nipple, where an incision is made, and the tube is inserted into the pleural space. There has been some indication that pleural shunting may be poorly tolerated in the young child due to lack of absorptive pleural surface. In addition, the length of time the pleural cavity retains its absorptive capacity varies from individual to individual. Complications may include respiratory compromise secondary to hydrothorax. Other less common distal placements include the gallbladder and ureter.

Less frequently used in the pediatric population, lumboperitoneal shunts are sometimes used in patients with communicating hydrocephalus, slit ventricle syndrome, or benign intracranial hypertension (pseudotumor cerebri). Although classically performed using a limited laminectomy, percutaneous placement using a Touhy needle in children over the age of 2 years is now the preferred method of insertion (Fig. 2.22) [14].

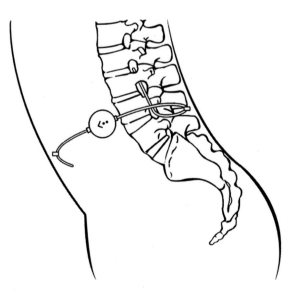

**Fig. 2.22.** Illustration shows lumboperitoneal shunt (LPS) placement

## Surgical Endoscopy

A significant development in pediatric neurosurgery has been the evolution of neuroendoscopy and its application in the management of hydrocephalus. It has been used for endoscopic third ventriculostomy, cyst fenestration and septostomy, and shunt placement and retrieval. The pioneering stage of neuroendoscopy began in the early 1900s, but quickly fell out of favor due to poor equipment and a high rate of associated morbidity and mortality. In the 1970s, there was renewed enthusiasm for its use because of improvements in endoscopes, light sources, camera equipment, and instrumentation. In the past decade, there has been a marked increase in the use of endoscopy, and pediatric neurosurgeons all over the world are using it, primarily because recent studies confirm good outcomes.

## Endoscopic Third Ventriculostomy

Endoscopic third ventriculostomy (ETV) is used as an alternative to shunting in selected patients with noncommunicating hydrocephalus. The success of the procedure depends largely on proper patient selection. The patients most likely to benefit from the procedure are those with significant obstruction of CSF flow between the ventricles and the subarachnoid space, and those with normal CSF absorption between the subarachnoid space and the venous system. An MRI should be done as part of the work-up to confirm that the basilar artery does not sit below the floor of the third ventricle. Such placement of the artery is usually a contraindication for a third ventriculostomy due to the added risk of hemorrhage. Patients with aqueductal stenosis are, in general, excellent candidates for the procedure. It has also been used successfully in patients with posterior fossa tumors. Although controversial, patients under the age of 6 months have not had uniformly good results [6].

The goal of ETV is to bypass the obstruction of CSF by diverting it through the floor of the third ventricle and returning it to the normal subarachnoid space. A rigid endoscope is introduced into the lateral ventricle via a coronal burr hole. The endoscope is advanced through the foramen of Monroe and into the third ventricle. Once the thin translucent floor of the third ventricle is visualized, a rigid probe is used to puncture the membrane and the fenestration is enlarged by balloon catheter dilation. A laser may also be used to fenestrate the floor of the third ventricle.

An external ventricular drain with an intracranial pressure monitor may be placed after the procedure and is usually kept clamped. This allows monitoring of the intracranial pressure and possible diversion of CSF should the ETV be unsuccessful.

Patency of the third ventriculostomy can be confirmed noninvasively using phase-contrast cine MRI, or CISS sequence MRI, to identify the CSF flow through the fenestration. However, the finding of a patent fenestration does not guarantee that the procedure has been successful. If there is an obstruction to the circulation of CSF further downstream or inadequate absorption within the subarachnoid space, it is possible for the procedure to fail, even in the setting of a patent fenestration.

ETV has an overall success rate of approximately 75% after 3 years [40]. Failure of ETV can occur early or late. Early failure may be the result of factors including bleeding around the fenestration site, unnoticed additional arachnoid membranes occluding the flow of CSF, or an inadequate size of the fenestration. Late failure can be caused by subsequent closure of the fenestration by gliotic tissue or arachnoid membrane. Tumor progression and inadequate CSF absorption at the level of the arachnoid villi may result in either early or late failure. Patients with open fenestrations can exhibit deterioration after months of successful ETV, and the problem can be potentially serious because failure can develop over a short period of time and may be unpredictable. The patient develops signs and symptoms of increased intracranial pressure and requires further intervention, either another ETV or a shunt. Patients with an ETV require ongoing neurosurgical follow-up.

## Treatment of Hydrocephalus in Specific Malformations/Diseases

## Posthemorrhagic Hydrocephalus

Infants who develop increasing PHH or become symptomatic need temporizing treatment initially. Some centers will treat these small infants with serial lumbar or ventricular punctures; however, infection is a risk. Repeated ventricular taps may lead to porencephaly.

In infants who have PHH and are able to tolerate a surgical intervention, a ventricular access device (VAD) can be implanted. This is a catheter that is surgically placed in the ventricle with an attached subcutaneous reservoir. The reservoir can be tapped as often as needed through the skin using a 23-gauge butterfly needle. Most infants with a VAD require a tap every 2–3 days, but some may require taps as often as twice daily.

Another procedure that may be used is the placement of a subgaleal shunt. This is similar to a VAD, but the distal limb of the catheter is left to drain into a subgaleal pocket, which is created at the time of the placement of the device. The CSF under pressure drains through the catheter and distends the scalp, which allows absorption of the CSF by the galea. In some cases, CSF production may exceed the absorptive capability of the subgaleal space, and intermittent taps of the pocket may be required. When repeated taps are needed through either the VAD or the subgaleal shunt, there is a high risk of infection. Alternatively, some providers use a temporary external drainage device in the management of PHH. This has the advantage of maintaining a constant intraventricular pressure, whereas with the other aforementioned treatments, intraventricular pressure can alternate between being very high and very low. The disadvantage of all of these devices is that the catheters can become clogged from the blood or its byproducts, or as previously mentioned, infected.

Eventually, over time, it will become clear whether the PHH is resolving or if the infant will need a permanent shunt placed. It has been demonstrated by most of the studies on temporary measures to treat PHH, regardless of the method, 10–35% of infants will show resolution of their hydrocephalus [3]. About 20–30% will require a permanent shunt. In the majority of these infants the shunt dependency is usually lifelong. There is currently some debate as to the most appropriate timing for a permanent shunt placement. A shunt should be considered when the CSF is cleared of posthemorrhagic debris and blood, and the CSF protein is <500 mg/dl [27]. The infant should weigh >1.5 kg (variable), have progressive hydrocephalus, and be otherwise stable [41].

## Myelomeningocele

About 80–90% of children with myelomeningocele will eventually require surgical CSF diversion [11]. The treatment of hydrocephalus in the infant with a myelomeningocele usually involves placement of a ventriculoperitoneal shunt. The timing of the shunt placement depends on the severity of the hydrocephalus, but historically has been deferred until after the myelomeningocele repair. Waiting until the hydrocephalus clearly progresses allows for the proper selection of infants who need permanent shunting. Placing a shunt at the time of the back closure may also be more difficult, since the infant should not be positioned on the newly closed myelomeningocele repair site. The advantages to doing it simultaneously with the myelomeningocele repair include a decreased risk of a CSF leak from the repair site and a decreased risk of CSF infection. Some neurosurgeons perform an endoscopic third ventriculostomy instead of a shunt, although performing an ETV in infants is debated.

The in-utero surgical repair of myelomeningocele is presently being studied at three medical centers in a study funded by the National Insitutes of Health. The purpose of the study is to determine efficacy, safety, and benefit of such closure of the back [39]. Participants are randomized into two groups, in-utero repair at 19–25 weeks gestation, or no in-utero repair with caesarean section after lung maturity is confirmed. The primary results being compared are the need for a ventriculoperitoneal shunt at 1 year and overall fetal/infant mortality [39].

## Vein of Galen Malformation

Initial treatment for the neonate is supportive and includes immediate resuscitative efforts with ventilatory support. The goal is stabilization until a transvenous and/or transarterial endovascular approach for embolization can reduce blood flow through the malformation and feeding vessels. The infant often presents with, or develops, hydrocephalus. However, the placement of a cerebrospinal shunt in an infant or child with a vein of Galen malformation has a very high risk of associated intracranial hemorrhage [33]. Many neurosurgeons will try to avoid placing a shunt by initially treating the malformation with embolization. If the malformation can be embolized successfully, it may shrink and the hydrocephalus may resolve. Although treatment has greatly improved outcome, the mortality and morbidity of infants and children with these malformations remains high.

## Intracranial Cysts

Many types of intracranial cyst may occur, including arachnoid cysts, choroid plexus cysts, neoplastic cysts and mutliloculated cysts associated with infection, tumors, hemorrhage, or trauma. Arachnoid cysts are often diagnosed as an incidental finding when a CT is done for another reason. An MRI is often done at the time of the initial diagnosis of an arachnoid cyst to rule out a tumor. An intracranial cyst may cause no mass effect or symptoms. Conservative treatment of such a cyst, including follow-up scans to verify that there is no change, may be adequate. The cyst can cause a mass effect and symptoms. It can also cause noncommunicating hydrocephalus from obstruction of normal CSF pathways. Surgical intervention is required in these cases.

Neuroendoscopic fenestration of the cyst wall may eliminate the need for a shunt. The surgeon breaks the cyst wall with an endoscope and the fluid in the cyst is allowed to drain into normal CSF passageways. The goal is to reduce the cyst size and avoid placement of a shunt, or if a shunt is necessary, to avoid placing multiple shunts. Some surgeons may decide to shunt the cyst first because of the high rate of cyst reoccurrence after fenestration [1]. The surgeon may also place shunt catheters into the cyst(s) and ventricles. These catheters can be "Y'ed" together into a distal catheter terminating in the peritoneal cavity. The failure rate of multiple shunt catheters is high and it is difficult to determine which catheters are functional and which are not at the time of malfunction. If the lateral ventricles are loculated (isolated) from membranes or cysts, the surgeon may fenestrate the septum pellucidum (septostomy) to eliminate the need for more than one shunt catheter.

### Brain Tumors

Approximately two-thirds of children who present with a posterior fossa tumor will have hydrocephalus. A smaller number of children with supratentorial tumors will have associated hydrocephalus at the time of diagnosis. If the hydrocephalus is severe and the child is very symptomatic, an emergent external ventricular drain or shunt may need to be placed. When the surgeon anticipates a resection of the tumor, an external ventricular drain is usually the most appropriate choice because of the risk of shunt failure after tumor surgery. This is due to blood and debris in the CSF from the surgery. If hydrocephalus is present, most neurosurgeons will place an external ventricular drain immediately before a posterior fossa tumor resection. The CSF is allowed to drain for 48–96 h postoperatively and then the child is gradually weaned from the drainage device over several days. Approximately 25–50% of the children will be unable to tolerate weaning and the removal of the external ventricular drain, and will need a permanent shunt [41]. Those who cannot tolerate the weaning will develop signs and symptoms of hydrocephalus and ventriculomegaly. A shunt or external third ventriculostomy will need to be performed.

## Complications of Shunts and Treatment

Complications of CSF shunts include mechanical failure of the shunt, infection, and overshunting. Depending on the location of the distal catheter of the CSF shunt, risks of other complications are possible.

## Shunt Malfunction

Mechanical failure of the shunt can be due to improper placement, obstruction, disconnection, fracture, and migration of the hardware. Malfunctions may occur in the operating room, soon after surgery, or years later. However, the most common time for a malfunction is within the first 6 months after placement or revision [21].

Obstruction of the shunt hardware comprises 50% of all CSF shunt complications [5]. Most often the obstruction occurs in the proximal portion of the shunt. Total proximal obstruction of the shunt is frequently associated with rapidly increasing intracranial pressure and requires emergent intervention. The proximal catheter may become obstructed in the operating room or shortly thereafter with blood or air. Proximal occlusion may also be the result of the choroid plexus growing around the proximal portion of the catheter, or from blood or other proteinaceous material within the catheter or valve. A further cause may be from the catheter being improperly placed during surgery or slipping out of the ventricle later.

There may be swelling along the shunt tract over the skull and neck, if the proximal catheter is obstructed or partially occluded, with minimal signs of shunt failure. Such swelling may also occur with a functional shunt if there is a large hole in the dura around the shunt, resulting in a CSF leak around the shunt. Obstruction of the distal catheter may be the result of distal infection, scarring, adhesions, or fat occluding the shunt. As the child grows, the distal end of the catheter may slip out of the abdominal cavity. A tract may form allowing CSF to flow beyond the shunt tip, usually failing slowly over time.

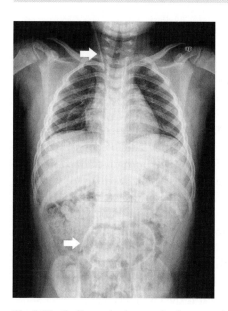

**Fig. 2.23.** Radiograph shows a broken ventriculoperitoneal shunt catheter near the clavicle (*arrow*). The most distal portion of the catheter can be seen in the bottom of the peritoneal cavity

Disconnections happen most often at connection sites between components of the shunt. A disconnection may occur between the ventricular catheter and valve, or between the valve and distal catheter. Tubing that has been in place for a long time may become fixed by the development of scar tissue around the catheter. Over time, calcification may also develop around the catheter and the catheter itself may degrade. Both fixation and calcification may lead to catheter breakage with growth, particularly in the neck where there is constant motion (Fig. 2.23). The patient may also develop pain along an old calcified shunt tract.

Migration of the distal catheter may occur to several sites, including the scrotum, umbilicus, stomach, mouth, intestine, chest, anus, uterus, internal jugular vein, and coronary sinus. When migration occurs, malfunction of the shunt often results from blockage of CSF flow and/or lack of reabsorption of CSF [14]. Infection may also occur in conjunction with migration to another site. Other complications may occur depending on where the distal shunt is located.

### Evaluation and Treatment of Shunt Malfunctions

The initial work-up of the patient with a suspected shunt malfunction includes a thorough history and physical exam. The radiological exam includes shunt series x-rays of the shunt hardware and a CT (without contrast) of the head. Shunt series x-rays include anterior/posterior and lateral films of the skull, neck, abdomen, and pelvis. These are done to evaluate the continuity of the shunt hardware, location of the hardware, valve type and any other abnormalities. There may be areas of the shunt system that seem translucent on the plain films, particularly over the valve and connectors. Comparing the films to previous postoperative films may provide further information about how the shunt appears at baseline. Comparing the films to x-rays of the most common shunt valves and connectors may also be helpful.

The head CT is compared with previous scans. If the ventricles have increased in size, a shunt failure is usually confirmed. It may also be helpful to compare the CT scans with scans associated with previous shunt failures. The CT may also reveal other intracranial complications.

Ventriculomegaly does not always occur with shunt malfunctions. In some patients the ventricles remain small, due to decreased ventricular compliance. The child who does not demonstrate increased ventricle size with shunt failure needs further testing to evaluate shunt function.

Additional information about the shunt may be obtained by tapping the shunt and measuring the intracranial pressure. A 23-gauge butterfly needle connected to a manometer can be used to access the shunt via the reservoir or valve. When the shunt is working, there is usually spontaneous flow of CSF through the catheter into the manometer with good respiratory variation. No flow of CSF from the shunt in the presence of normal or dilated ventricles is suggestive of a proximal obstruction. If the ventricles are slit-like, no flow may be normal. Intracranial pressure is measured manually with the manometer. The pressure is measured with the "0" on the manometer at the level of the external auditory meatus (see section on Nursing Care of the Hydrocephalus Patient After Surgery/External Ventricular Drains). Pressure will vary depending on age and activity of the child (Table 2.4). To obtain a true pressure, the child must be calm. Intracranial pressure measured with a manometer is measured in centimeters of water (cmH$_2$O) and may also be referred to in millimeters of water (mmH$_2$O); intracranial pressure monitoring performed electronically by transducer is measured in millimeters of mercury (mmHg.)

**Table 2.4.** Normal intracranial pressure for infants and children. Adapted from Wang and Avellino [41]

| Age | Pressure (cmH2O)[a] | Pressure (mmHg)[a] |
|---|---|---|
| Neonate | <3 | <2 |
| Newborn | 2–8 | 1.5–6 |
| Young child | 4–9 | 3–7 |

[a]$1.36 \, cmH_2O = 1 \, mmHg$

A nuclear medicine study (shuntogram) is another test that may be useful in the evaluation of shunt function. A 23-gauge butterfly needle is inserted into the shunt reservoir or valve and the opening pressure is measured. A radioisotope is then injected into the shunt and gamma camera images are taken of the head, neck, and abdomen to evaluate movement of the tracer. Normal findings of a shuntogram include an opening pressure of $0–20 \, cmH_2O$ (dependent on the age and activity of the child), and radioisotope flows out of the needle hub, clears out of the reservoir and shunt, and disperses freely into the peritoneal cavity (the half time should be less than 5 min). Both a shunt tap and a nuclear medicine study can sometimes provide confusing results.

If a shunt malfunction is confirmed, the child is taken to the operating room for a shunt revision. Sometimes a very symptomatic patient without clear diagnostic findings during the work-up may be taken to the operating room to explore the shunt. During a shunt revision, all parts of the shunt are evaluated. Shunt hardware parts that are malfunctioning are replaced.

### Shunt Infection

Infection is the second most common complication of CSF shunts. The incidence is greatest in the 1st year after placement, with 80% appearing in the first 6 months. Rates of infection range from 2 to 39%, with an average of 5–10% [15]. Patient characteristics can influence risk. Infants and younger children, those with concurrent infection, those with previous shunt infection, and those with postoperative disruption of the incision exposing the shunt hardware have a higher risk of shunt infection.

The most common infecting organism is staphylococci. *Staphylococcus epidermis* (coagulase-negative staphylococcus) is seen in 50–75% of all shunt infections [15]. *Staphylococcus aureus* (coagulase-positive staphylococcus), Gram-negative organisms (usually *Escherichia coli*, klebsiella, proteus, and pseudomonas), streptococcal species, neisseria, hemophilus influenza, and fungi make up the remainder of most infections. Infections with Gram-positive organisms correlate with a better outcome than those with Gram-negative organisms. The infection usually occurs in one of three ways: (1) via intraoperative contamination, (2) via the bloodstream, or (3) via retrograde travel from a contaminated distal catheter.

### Evaluation and Treatment of a Cerebrospinal Shunt Infection

When a child with a shunt presents with symptoms of infection, one should have a high index of suspicion of a shunt infection if the child has had a recent shunt procedure or a history of infections. If the child is stable and has not had a shunt procedure in the last several months, the most common diseases of childhood should be ruled out. A thorough physical exam and laboratory work (including complete blood count, c reactive protein, erythrocyte sedimentation rate, blood cultures, urinalysis, and chest films) may help locate the source of the infection. Most neurosurgeons are reluctant to tap a shunt unless there is clearly no other source of infection, due to the risk of infecting the shunt with the tap.

The child presenting with a shunt infection may range from minimally to gravely ill. The child may have one or more signs and symptoms of infection, including fever, irritability, redness and/or swelling over the shunt tract, or redness and/or drainage from shunt incisions. The infected shunt may or may not fail. Therefore, the child may or may not have signs and symptoms of a shunt malfunction, including headaches, nausea, vomiting, and lethargy. If the distal portion of the shunt is infected, the child may have abdominal symptoms, including pain, tenderness to palpation, and distension. An abdominal CT or US may reveal an intra-abdominal loculated CSF collection.

Diagnosis of a shunt infection is confirmed by a positive CSF culture from the shunt (or a positive culture from explanted hardware). The shunt reservoir is aspirated via a shunt tap for CSF and sent to the lab for glucose, protein, cell count, Gram stain, and culture. Infection in the tissues surrounding the reservoir is usually a contraindication to tapping the shunt. Even presumed sterile aspiration of the shunt in this setting could lead to contamination and subsequent infection of the shunt.

The treatment of a shunt infection varies, but in general, the principles of treatment of infection in the setting of a foreign body are followed. Cultures are obtained and intravenous broad-spectrum antibiotics are started to cover the most likely organisms. The shunt hardware is either externalized or totally removed, and replaced with an external ventricular drain. Some neurosurgeons may not remove the shunt if it is functional and treat with intravenous antibiotics only. However, this is somewhat controversial.

Once the specific infecting organism sensitivities are known, the antibiotics may be altered. The child is treated with intravenous antibiotics until the CSF has been sterile for several days. There is no consistent agreement about the number of days that the CSF should be sterile before the shunt hardware can be reimplanted. Many neurosurgeons also prefer for the CSF to have less than $50/mm^3$ white blood cells and the protein to be less than 500 mg/dl before replacing the shunt. Most commonly, the child will receive 5–10 days of treatment before the shunt is replaced. There is also no consistent agreement as to the length of antibiotic treatment after the shunt has been replaced. Factors such as the specific organism, the severity of the infection, and previous history of infections may all affect the length of antibiotic treatment.

Preventing infection is the best way to improve outcome. At present, adherence to meticulous intraoperative aseptic technique and perioperative prophylactic systemic antibiotics are accepted procedures. There is no proven drug of choice or length of treatment after a shunt revision. Most neurosurgeons use intravenous cefazolin, nafcillin, vancomycin, ceftriaxone, or methacillin. Length of treatment varies from 24 to 72 h postoperatively.

Antibiotic-impregnated shunts may also be used in an effort to prevent and/or reduce shunt infections, but their efficacy has not been established. These catheters may be impregnated with vancomyin, rifampin, clindamycin, or iodine. They are not used routinely because they carry the risk of inducing bacterial resistance and possibly an adverse reaction to the shunt. They may not be effective against all bacteria. Some studies using these catheters suggest a lower incidence of shunt infections, although longer follow-up and more studies are needed.

## Complications Related to Distal Catheter Location

### Ventriculoperitoneal Shunts

The abdominal cavity is the preferred area to place the distal end of a CSF shunt in most cases. However, the abdomen can frequently be the site of other surgical procedures or diseases. This is particularly an issue in young children with chronic medical conditions. These children may need frequent urological procedures, gastrostomy tube placement and revisions, or other bowel surgeries. Intra-abdominal adhesions and scarring from old procedures or previous shunt infections may decrease the absorptive capability of the peritoneum. Pseudocysts may develop around the tip of the catheter, with or without infection. The presence of an intra-abdominal infection, such as appendicitis, may or may not infect the shunt and make the abdominal cavity unsuitable for another shunt. The distal catheter may erode into the bowel leading to shunt infection and peritonitis. Other complications that may occur from intra-abdominal shunts include a 17% risk of inguinal hernia development (if the shunt is placed in young infants whose process vaginalis is still patent) or the development of a hydrocele.

### Ventriculoatrial Shunts

If the abdomen is not an appropriate site for the distal shunt catheter, it may be placed in the right atrium of the heart. Ventriculoatrial catheters potentially have more serious complications than ventriculoperitoneal catheters. Complications include: migration of the shunt into the superior vena cava (usually with failure of the shunt), pneumothorax, endocarditis, shunt nephritis, pulmonary embolism, septicemia, septic emboli, cardiac arrhythmias, cardiac tamponade, detachment of the catheter with migration into the coronary sinus, and obstruction of the vena cava system. Shunt nephritis is an unusual complication that can cause proteinuria, hematuria, and decreased kidney function, and is often associated with low-grade infection of the shunt. If shunt infection is suspected, blood cultures and a 24-h urine analysis for quantitative protein are obtained in addition to the other labs to rule out shunt nephritis.

Another problem with ventriculoatrial shunts is that extra tubing cannot be placed into the right atrium to allow for growth. Therefore, infants and young children may outgrow these shunts in months, resulting in shunt failure. A ventriculoatrial shunt may require frequent revisions to allow for growth. By examining the chest x-ray, one can diagnose the distal catheter being dislodged from the right atrium.

When examined at autopsy, multiple processes may have occurred around a ventriculoatrial catheter. Fibrinous material may surround the catheter, vegetation may be seen within the wall of the right atrium, and there may be evidence of pulmonary emboli [20].

### Lumboperitoneal Catheter Complications

Historically, several complications have been associated with lumboperitoneal shunts, including frequent shunt failure, scoliosis, arachnoiditis, back stiffness, back pain, sciatica, neurological changes in the lower limbs, and hindbrain herniation [25]. These complications have been reduced with changes in shunt hardware and careful preoperative screening. First, with the introduction of percutaneously implanted shunts and improved shunt catheters, the need to perform a laminectomy for shunt placement is now rare. This has reduced the rate of scoliosis and arachnoiditis. Secondly, preoperative evaluation of patients for hindbrain herniation, including a CSF flow study, can help determine when posterior fossa decompression prior to placement of the lumboperitoneal shunt is appropriate. Thorough preoperative evaluation and the use of a higher-pressure valve may decrease the risk and incidence of hindbrain herniation, and decrease the incidence of lumboperitoneal shunt complications [28].

### Overdrainage Causing Extra-axial Fluid Collection

After a CSF shunt is placed, if the ventricles decompress excessively or too rapidly, extra-axial fluid collections and/or a subdural hematoma may occur. Bridging veins on the brain's surface may tear as the brain falls away from the dura, and bleeding can occur, creating a subdural hematoma (Fig. 2.24). This is a risk when shunts are placed for the first time in older children. Treatment depends on severity, symptoms, and the type of valve used. If the valve is programmable, the pressure may be temporarily increased. If not, the valve may need to be replaced with a higher-pressure valve. By allowing the ventricles to stay dilated, the brain will resume its normal position against the dura and skull. If a subdural hematoma is present, it may need to be drained.

### Special Diagnostic and Treatment Challenge: Slit Ventricle Syndrome

Approximately 75% of patients with slit ventricles on scan have no symptoms. Slit ventricle syndrome usually occurs after the shunt has been in place for many years, making it more common in the older child and adolescent; however, younger children and infants may also be affected. Slit ventricle syndrome has been used in the literature to describe several different situations that include symptomatic small ventricles. This has lead to confusion in choosing the most effective treatment option and evaluating the outcome.

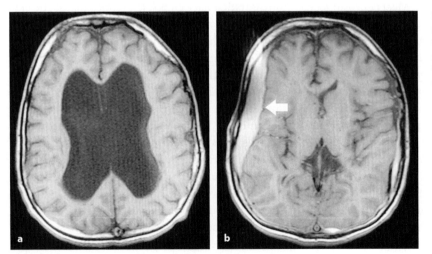

**Fig. 2.24 a, b.** Fifteen-year-old male with achondroplasia and chronic hydrocephalus. **a** Preoperative MRI shows enlarged ventricles. **b** Postoperative MRI shows collapsed ventricles with subsequent development of bilateral (right greater then left) subdural hematomas

In a review of the literature, Olson [25] found at least five different clinical scenarios in which children have radiologically slit ventricles and headaches. Patterns include: an on-off (intermittent) symptom complex, overdrainage and siphoning with negative intracranial pressure (particularly when the patient is upright), recurring proximal ventricular catheter dysfunction, chronic subdural collections due to shunt overdrainage, and headaches unrelated to shunt function. Most authors applied the syndrome to an on-off (intermittent) symptom complex. This has further been defined as "severe intermittent headaches lasting 10–90 min associated with smaller than normal ventricles on imaging studies, and a slow refill on valve pumping devices" [27]. The pathophysiology supporting these symptoms is that with slit ventricles, the catheter becomes intermittently obstructed with surrounding tissue, the pressure rises, and when it is high enough the ventricles minimally dilate, allowing the catheter to function again. To avoid confusion, using the term noncompliant ventricle syndrome instead of slit ventricle syndrome has been recommended. Of children with radiologically slit ventricles and headaches, 6–22% have noncompliant ventricle syndrome [25].

The exact mechanism underlying the syndrome is not known, and may be a combination of proposed theories. First, because there is a relationship between ventricular pressure and intracranial pressure: when CSF pressure drops, there is an increase in venous congestion and brain elasticity. Second, an increased pressure with subependymal flow can cause subependymal gliosis and periventricular gliosis with increased ventricular wall stiffness. Consequently, a higher than normal intracranial pressure is needed to dilate the ventricles. Third, in newborns, overshunting leads to radiologically slit ventricles, and the development of microcephaly and suture synostosis. Because of the small ventricles, catheters easily become plugged. With a small cranial compartment, ventricular dilation is restricted and can lead to increased intracranial pressure.

Symptoms are those associated with shunt malfunction (intermittent headaches, nausea, vomiting, and other signs of increased intracranial pressure). Headaches are the most common complaint. In some patients, being upright worsens the symptoms and lying down improves them.

Evaluation initially involves the typical work-up for shunt malfunction. When the CT is normal, but significant symptoms persist, further studies are warranted. A shuntogram may confirm CSF patency and flow, but can be misleading due to the intermittent nature of the problem. Continuous invasive intracranial pressure monitoring may correlate symptoms with pressure. This may be done via a fiber optic intracranial monitoring device, or via an external ventricular drainage catheter attached to an intracranial monitoring device.

Some patients may benefit from antimigraine therapy using propranolol, dihydroergotamine, or amitriptyline. The mechanism by which these drugs work is probably by reducing venous congestion. Propranolol, a beta blocker, cannot be used in children with asthma, as it will render asthma medications (beta-adrenergic agonist bronchodilators such as albuterol) ineffective.

A revision of the shunt is the most common treatment for noncompliant ventricle syndrome. If headaches occur with low pressure, an anti-\siphon device may be added and the valve may be changed to a higher-pressure or programmable valve. These shunt changes may decrease overdrainage and promote slightly larger ventricles, allowing for more consistent shunt function. Multiple changes in ventricular valve pressure are often needed during the evaluation and treatment of noncompliant syndrome. Programmable valves have made this possible without repeated surgical procedures. Before any such changes in an infant, it is important to rule out craniosynostosis, as increasing the valve pressure in this situation could cause a pathological increase in intracranial pressure. Shunt replacement in the setting of small ventricles can be difficult and may require the use of endoscopy.

Success has recently been reported with the placement of a lumboperitoneal shunt in addition to a ventriculoperitoneal shunt [25]. This may result from an added increase in CSF drainage when an increase in intracranial pressure occurs. A potential risk factor with a lumbar shunt in addition to a ventriculoperitoneal shunt is that if the ventricular catheter fails, hindbrain herniation may occur (acquired Chiari I).

Other surgical procedures have been utilized, including subtemporal decompression, calvarial expansion, and third ventriculostomy. Subtemporal decompression reduces intracranial pressure by removing a portion of the skull. The procedure can be accomplished with low risks, and so some recommend this as a first-line treatment for noncompliant ventricle

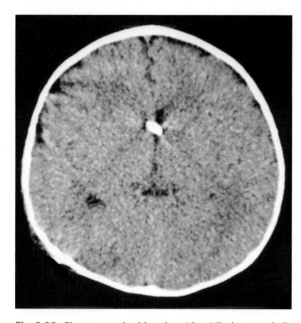

**Fig. 2.25.** Eleven-month-old male with a VP shunt and slit ventricle syndrome. He had many months of irritability and trouble feeding and had several shunt revisions, including the placement of programmable valves and the placement of an LPS. He eventually underwent a cranial expansion procedure and his symptoms improved

syndrome in patients with synostosis and a small calvarium. Calvarial expansion is a much more extensive procedure and bleeding is a significant risk (Fig. 2.25).

## Pseudotumor Cerebri in the Pediatric Population

Another type of CSF absorption problem is a condition known as pseudotumor cerebri (PTC). It is described as elevated intracranial pressure without hydrocephalus, mass lesion, infection, or hypertensive encephalopathy [6]. PTC is the result of CSF malabsorption or obstruction in the intracranial venous system. Sometimes an exact cause can be found, such as a thrombosis, which may be the source of the obstruction. Many times, however, a cause is not found. Thus, PTC is usually a diagnosis of exclusion [4].

In the general population, PTC is found in 0.9 per 100,000, but the incidence increases to 90 per 100,000 of obese adult females. There is a female to male predominance of 8:1–2 in adults, but there is no gender predominance in children. Obesity is less frequently a

cause of PTC in children. There is a peak incidence in the third decade (range 1–55 years), and 37% of cases are in children. Ninety percent of children are diagnosed between 5 and 15 years of age, and PTC is rarely seen in infants [3].

There are three types, or classifications of PTC: primary, secondary, and atypical pseudotumor. The most common form, primary PTC, is idiopathic and the cause unknown. Secondary PTC presents as the result of another illness, or cause. Secondary PTC may be associated with a known neurological disease, the result of a systemic illness (i.e., clotting disorder), or caused by the ingestion or withdrawal of exogenous agents (i.e., vitaminosis A, antibiotics, and others). Finally, atypical PTC presents without papilledema, or may be seen in infants. The most common causes of PTC in children include venous thrombosis, steroid withdrawal, and malnutrition, or exogenous substances. Obesity, as in the general population, is beginning to be seen more frequently as a cause of PTC in children.

## Pathophysiology

CSF is absorbed into the venous system after traveling passively through the arachnoid villi. A failure of CSF absorption may be caused by a blockage somewhere in these veins, such as by a thrombus. Right heart failure in infants sometimes leads to PTC by causing a retrograde elevated intracranial pressure, and thus a CSF absorption problem.

Several exogenous agents have been known to cause PTC. These include vitamin A, chemotherapeutic agents like vincristine, and some antibiotics. Although there are theories as to how these agents cause changes in CSF absorption pathways at the cellular level, the exact cause of PTC from the ingestion of vitamin A or other medicines, remains unclear [1, 6, 7].

## Clinical Evaluation

The examiner should obtain a thorough history and perform a complete physical examination, including an age-appropriate neurological examination (please refer to the Chap. 1 regarding the neurological examination). CT and plain MRI will not aid in diagnosis, but are performed to exclude other causes of increased intracranial pressure such as mass lesions [30]. Magnetic resonance venograms may show an obstruction, or occlusion. A lumbar puncture can demonstrate an elevated opening pressure, and is performed with the patient lying in the lateral position. It is important to position patients on their side, as patients placed on their abdomens may have an artificially elevated opening pressure. Retrograde venography is the measurement of the intracranial venous systems via a catheter threaded upward from the femoral vein. Abnormal readings, including elevation of right-sided heart measurements, demonstrate the exact location of an obstruction; this is known as a "gradient." Ophthalmologic examinations are performed to note any changes in visual fields, papilledema, and other tests of visual acuity. This may be done by a pediatric ophthalmologist. Intracranial pressure monitoring may be done with an intraparenchymal transducer, or similar device. This is helpful to note changes in pressure throughout the day, while awake and asleep. Changes in position may also cause elevations in pressures, such as turning the head from side to side, because of venous obstruction on one side. Psychological evaluations may be performed, as there can be complicated comorbid involvement in some patients who receive secondary gain from having headaches that cannot always be diagnosed.

### Treatment

Sometimes PTC may resolve spontaneously. Serial lumbar punctures to remove CSF have been shown to be beneficial in the resolution of PTC. More permanent CSF diversion may be necessary. This includes the implantation of a lumbar shunt, with the valve system being the choice of the neurosurgeon. The lumbar shunt communicates with the CSF outside the ventricular system at the level of the subarachnoid space [28]. The implantation of a ventricular access device such as a Rickham Reservoir (Codman, Rayham, MA, USA) allows for rapid and accurate measurement of intracranial pressure manometrically with little discomfort to the child. Because the ventricles are small in this condition, the placement of the reservoir is best performed using stereotactic guidance. Shunts from the ventricles to the peritoneum are difficult to maintain because of the small size of the ventricles, and thus the ventricular shunt cannot provide adequate drainage of CSF from the subarachnoid space.

Optic nerve sheath fenestrations are performed to reduce pressure on the optic nerve, as well as drain CSF, because the CSF may communicate with the subarachnoid space.

Medications may helpful by reducing the production of CSF (e.g., acetazolamide, furosemide). This is usually a temporary measure until either a more permanent solution is found or the PTC resolves. Medications are used with caution, as there are side effects that include electrolyte abnormalities.

Obese patients with PTC and stable visual symptoms are best treated with weight loss to avoid shunt placement or optic nerve sheath fenestration [24]. Even a small amount of weight loss can reduce intracranial pressure. Bariatric surgery may be considered for a morbidly obese patient who is in their late teens.

### Nursing Care

Sometimes children are placed in the Pediatric Intensive Care Unit for several days while their intracranial pressure is monitored via an intraparenchymal wire. It is usually inserted in the operating room, under anesthesia, to maintain strict asepsis and to reduce anxiety. The nurse plays an important role in monitoring elevations in pressure, and assisting the family to keep a "headache diary" during their stay. Monitoring of visual changes is also very important.

Patient and family education is needed so that lifestyle changes can be made to prevent loss of vision and the adaptation to the possible shunting systems. There are several web sites that provide education to families, and allow patients to communicate with one another. Patient and family support are provided by nursing, social service, and psychological intervention as needed.

Finally, there is ongoing research for future cures and diagnosis of PTC, including new ways to measure intravenous pressures. The placement of intracranial stenting devices that bypass a venous obstruction have been placed in a small number of adults with some success.

### Nursing Care of the Hydrocephalus Patient after Surgery

The most common operations that children with hydrocephalus undergo are shunt placement, shunt revision, and endoscopic third ventriculostomy. Because these children frequently have other diseases related to the hydrocephalus they often undergo other surgeries to treat a multitude of other problems.

## Neurological Assessment

Neurological assessment is discussed in Chap. 1. The assessment must occur in a developmentally appropriate manner. The nurse must also consider what is developmentally appropriate behavior for the infant or child, based upon his age. It is vital to also consider the individual child and his baseline. Many conditions related to hydrocephalus are also associated with significant delays, and because complications of hydrocephalus may worsen such delays, these children have a wide range of developmental abnormalities. A detailed history of developmental skill and baseline function is a vital part of being able to assess the infant/child.

Parents and families are an excellent resource to provide information about their particular child's developmental level. The signs and symptoms of increasing intracranial pressure may initially be very subtle. Hence, the child's caretaker is a valuable resource in such assessment and may notice subtle changes before nursing and medical staff.

Neurological assessment of the child after surgery to treat the hydrocephalus needs to be done frequently. The surgeon will usually specify the frequency, but assessment should occur every 1–4 h, depending on the condition of the child. An exam that is changing subtly over time may be an indication of a failed surgical treatment or postoperative complication. The first signs of increasing intracranial pressure are usually subtle and related to mildly increasing somnolence, lack of interest in activities (feeding) or play, and subtle behavioral changes. Level of consciousness is the most important single indicator of neurological status. Altered level of consciousness may progress to confusion, disorientation, somnolence, lethargy, obtundation, stupor, and coma.

A thorough neurological assessment starts with watching the child play and interact with those around him. Assessment also includes asking the child if he has a headache. The child should be examined for his ability to answer questions appropriately and follow directions. Asking a child to move his arms and legs will also allow the examiner to assess muscle strength, tone, and movement. Vital signs should also be assessed. Bradycardia can be a sign of increased intracranial pressure. Increased blood pressure is usually not a common finding in children until late in the process of increasing intracranial pressure.

It is important to carefully examine the eyes, noting that checking pupils without further exam is never an adequate exam. The pupils are checked for equality, roundness, and reactivity to light. Dilated and nonreactive pupils are a very late sign of increased intracranial pressure. A "sun-setting" appearance to the eyes or the loss of upward gaze is an abnormal finding. The extraocular movements should be intact.

The infant's head should be examined. The occipital frontal circumference should be measured and documented on a daily basis to determine appropriate head growth. The fontanels should be palpated with the child upright and calm. The anterior fontanel should feel soft and pulsatile. A tense or bulging fontanel is suspicious for increased intracranial pressure. The suture lines of the skull should also be examined. Normal suture lines are palpable and apposed. If they are overriding, the infant may have overdrainage of the system. If the sutures are splayed there is likely increased intracranial pressure.

## Wound and Dressing Care

The child will usually come from the operating room with a dressing over the incision. The dressing is normally removed, or changed, during the first few postoperative days. If a dressing is soiled or saturated with blood, most surgeons agree that it should be replaced. If the child is likely to pick at the incision, a dressing may be left on to prevent infection. Before a child goes home, most surgeons agree the dressing should be changed and the wound inspected for any erythema, drainage, swelling, or infection.

## Medications

A substantial majority of neurosurgeons will order intravenous antibiotics for 24–48 h after the surgery to prevent shunt infection. Cefazolin or nafcillin are the most commonly used antibiotics, as Gram-positive organisms demonstrate a sensitivity to them. Vancomycin may also be used.

Pain management starts with good pain assessment. Age-appropriate pain assessment scales such as CRIES (crying, requires increased oxygen administration, increased vital signs, expression, sleeplessness), the Objective Pain Scale, and Oucher may be used. There is a wide variety of pain experienced by children after surgery for hydrocephalus. Pain may be related to the cranial incision(s), the abdominal incision, the amount of intra-abdominal manipulation, and the tunneling of the distal catheter through the subcutaneous tissue. Other factors influencing pain may include the age of the child, the child and/or family's prior experience with pain, and the child and family's anxiety. Pain is usually managed with medications, although other techniques may be helpful. The first drug of choice is usually acetaminophen. It should be adequately dosed at 15 mg/kg/dose and can be given orally or rectally. Nonsteriodal anti-inflammatory drugs (NSAIDS) may be used, but they can inhibit platelet aggregation and prolong bleeding time. For this reason, some neurosurgeons do not use NSAIDS during the immediate postoperative period.

If the child needs additional medication for pain, the surgeon's beliefs about pain control in neurosurgical patients will be a factor. Some neurosurgeons will order opiates such as morphine sulfate, oxycodone, and codeine. Other surgeons do not want to alter the patient's neurological exam with these drugs. The nurse should not administer these drugs if there is concern that the pain is due to increasing intracranial pressure or the neurological exam is changing. Other modalities to relieve pain may include age-appropriate relaxation techniques, play therapy, music therapy, massage, distraction, and acupuncture or acupressure.

Some children will experience nausea and vomiting from anesthesia that may be worsened by extensive intra-abdominal manipulation during the surgery. Medications to treat this include metoclopramide and ondansetron. The nurse should not administer these drugs repeatedly if there is a possibility that the nausea and vomiting are due to increasing intracranial pressure. Treating the symptoms and ignoring the underlying cause may result in further increased pressure and delay of needed treatment.

Children who are on antiseizure medications preoperatively should have these resumed as soon as possible. Often, because of vomiting before or after the surgery, doses are missed so it is helpful to check blood levels of the drugs to ensure they are therapeutic. If the levels are subtherapeutic, extra doses may be ordered. Children with low levels of their antiseizure medications are at increased risk for seizures.

Infants and children require some intravenous fluids after surgery until they can take adequate fluids orally. Fluid loss from vomiting should be replaced. Electrolytes should also be monitored during periods of vomiting. The nurse should assess the child for symptoms of adequate hydration. Usually the child will receive maintenance fluids postoperatively for at least 12 h. The child with a shunt in place should never have an intravenous line placed into the scalp because of the risk of introducing bacteria to the area around the shunt hardware.

## Other Nursing Care

The surgeon will usually specify the position that the child should assume. Elevating the head of the bed 30–45 degrees will enhance shunt function by gravity aiding the flow of the CSF through the shunt. The surgeon may specify that the infant or child be placed flat if there is concern about overdrainage of the ventricles. If the ventricles are allowed to drain too quickly, the outside of cerebral cortex may pull away from the dura. This may cause tearing of the bridging veins and result in a subdural hematoma. Infants with overriding sutures are usually placed flat to minimize over drainage. If overriding sutures are allowed to occur for a long period of time the sutures may fuse prematurely. The nurse should also position the infant or child off of the incision and shunt hardware. Young infants who are allowed to lie on the hardware may experience skin breakdown, within hours, which can lead to shunt infection.

These children have all the other usual postoperative needs of pediatric surgery patients. Nurses should be concerned with adequate diet, good pulmonary care, mobilization issues, skin care, adequate rest, and emotional care. X-rays of the shunt system are also done during the postoperative period to assure correct placement of the shunt, that the system is intact, and for any other potential complications (i.e., pneumothorax associated with a ventriculoatrial shunt).

## Extraventricular Drainage

CSF can be temporally diverted outside the body using an extraventricular drain (ventriculostomy), and may be used with or without intracranial pressure monitoring. It is commonly used in the treatment of shunt infections, in which the colonized shunt tubing, as well as the infected CSF, needs to be removed in order to completely eradicate the infection. Usually the entire shunt system is removed, although occasionally just the distal portion of the shunt is externalized. In addition, it is commonly used after posterior fossa tumor resections, to help drain blood and surgical debris out of the ventricular system. Other uses may include the administration of intrathecal antibiotics, emergent diversion of CSF in acute hydrocephalus, intracranial pressure monitoring after endoscopic third ventriculostomy, and in association with head injury.

Several different systems are available, but all have similar features (Fig. 2.26). The ventricular catheter is usually put in place in the operating room, which allows for maximal aseptic technique at placement and tunneling of the catheter under the skin before it exits the skin. These two factors may decrease the infection rate with external drains. The ventricular catheter is generally inserted into the frontal horn of the lateral ventricle and is connected to a CSF collection chamber via a closed sterile set-up.

The surgeon should specify the level that the chamber needs to be placed, as well as the level of the head of the bed, in the postoperative orders. The chamber is generally placed in reference to the external auditory meatus, which is at the level of the foramen of Monro. Careful attention needs to be made to assure that the system is set up and measured properly, and that the catheter does not become kinked, dislodged, or disconnected. In addition, it is important to clamp the system before the patient changes position (Fig. 2.26).

The characteristics of CSF drainage need to be monitored regularly: the amount, color, and presence of blood or sediment must be recorded on a frequent basis. The normal amount of CSF that is produced daily is approximately 350–700 ml in adults [4]. Infants and children produce less. Excessive or insufficient CSF drainage is a common complication that may occur. Excessive drainage results when the pressure at which the drainage occurs is too low. This may be caused by the movement of the child above the predetermined ordered level, or increased intracranial pressure secondary to coughing, crying, sneezing, or the Valsalva maneuver. Excessive draining may cause the ventricles to rapidly collapse, leading to a subdural or subarachnoid hemorrhage.

Insufficient CSF drainage causes increased intracranial pressure, with associated symptoms. Inadequate drainage may be caused by patients that have moved lower than the ordered level, by kinks in the catheter, or by occlusion of the catheter from blood or cellular debris. Occlusion should be suspected if there is no fluctuation of CSF in the catheter with respirations, or with lowering of the chamber. If there is no drainage or fluctuation within the tubing, the neurosurgery team should be notified immediately. If the occlusion in the catheter cannot be dislodged by flushing it, the patient may need to return to the operating room and have a new drain placed. If the system is accidentally pulled apart or broken, the proxi-

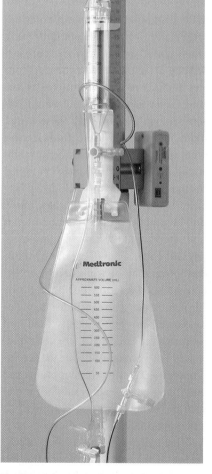

**Fig. 2.26.** An external ventricular drain (courtesy of Medtronic Neurologic Technologies)

mal catheter should be clamped immediately, the open tip placed in a sterile covering, and the neurosurgery team notified.

CSF is generally clear and has the same consistency as water. In the presence of infection, it may become cloudy, darker in color, and more viscous. CSF samples are often drawn on a regular basis to monitor the treatment of infection or to rule out infection. The studies done normally consist of a cell count, levels of glucose and protein, Gram stain, and culture. In the presence of infection, protein and white blood cells are usually elevated and glucose is usually decreased. Blood is often present in posterior fossa tumor resections. The amount of blood present should be noted, as well as any new bleeding.

CSF contains approximately 120 mEq/l of sodium. Therefore, the child's electrolytes should be monitored closely. Some surgeons may want to replace CSF with intravenous fluid normal saline, particularly in younger children.

Other nursing considerations include keeping the head dressing clean, dry, and intact, as well as pain control. Distraction techniques to try to keep the patient from moving or dislodging the catheter, as well as restraining the child may also be necessary.

In patients with posterior fossa tumor resections, there is a chance that the ventricular drain may be weaned and removed completely. This is often done once the cellular debris and blood have cleared. The chamber is raised slowly over 24–96 h and may eventually be clamped. If the patient does not develop signs of increased intracranial pressure and a CT does not show enlargement of the ventricular system, the drain may be removed. If there are symptoms of increased pressure and enlargement of the ventricles, the patient will most likely need a permanent shunt or may be a candidate for endoscopic third ventriculostomy.

## Discharge

Most infants and children can be discharged 24–48 h after a shunt placement or revision. The child undergoing a third ventriculostomy may be in the hospital longer while evaluation of the efficacy of the procedure is carried out. In preparation for discharge, the nurse should discuss with the parents, or other caregiver, wound care, pain management, signs and symptoms of shunt failure and infection, and other issues

that may be relevant. The caregiver should be instructed on how to take care of the dressing and/or wound. The surgeon will usually specify recommendations regarding dressings, bathing, and suture removal. The nurse should know what those specifications are and relay them to the family verbally and in writing. Often, families need to go home with dressing supplies if a dressing is to be kept in place.

Most children can be discharged with acetaminophen or ibuprofen for pain. The nurse should give the care provider the appropriate dose for the child. Some surgeons will prescribe a stronger pain medication such as oxycodone or codeine if it is necessary. Parents should be instructed to use any medication cautiously. If the child's pain is increasing over time, the child may be experiencing another shunt failure or infection. Pain is usually expected to be incisional or related to distal catheter implantation by the time of discharge.

The family needs to be instructed on the signs and symptoms of shunt failure and infection. The signs and symptoms may be subtle and confusing in a child already recovering from surgery. The signs and symptoms of a shunt infection may be subtle, or the child may appear quite ill and toxic. The caregivers should be told that an infected shunt may or may not function. Parents should also be advised that any fever during the 1st month after shunt placement could be related to a shunt infection. The patient's family also needs instruction on what to do if they suspect shunt failure, infection or have other concerns. If the shunt fails at night or on the weekend, the child still needs immediate evaluation. Each surgeon handles this somewhat differently, and the nurse should know the expectations of the particular surgeon. Follow-up appointments should also be scheduled.

## Family Support

Families of children with hydrocephalus are often quite anxious because their child may need to undergo repeated surgeries, because there are often other major illness or conditions associated with hydrocephalus, and because they are concerned about the lifelong implications for the child. These families often worry about shunt failure. Parents always want to know if the infant or young child will be normal, have delays, cerebral palsy, or other conditions related to the hydrocephalus (or it's etiology). The nurse or physician may not be able to adequately answer such questions, and that only further increases parental anxiety.

Families need anticipatory guidance and teaching about hydrocephalus, including what the signs and symptoms are, why they occur and what needs to be done. They need to understand what tests are done to diagnose hydrocephalus and shunt failure. Sometimes these tests are confusing or inconclusive for the provider. This further confuses families and causes more anxiety. Families also need to know the importance of prompt treatment of suspected shunt failure and have a plan as to how that will occur.

A child with a shunt should be encouraged to live as normal a life as is possible. If the child does not have other associated conditions or delays, there will usually be no restrictions. If the child is delayed, in a wheelchair, blind, or otherwise disabled, many restrictions will be needed because of the underlying issues. Parents should still be encouraged to treat the child as normally as possible. Some surgeons do not want children with shunts to play rough contact sports such as football or wrestling, because of the possibility of damaging the shunt hardware and the risk of head injury. There is no contraindication to flying in commercial pressurized aircraft.

Children with shunts need good primary care. The primary care provider as well as the parent can follow head growth in infants. A primary provider or nurse may help the family with all the standard issues that parents face, including discipline, toileting, sleep issues, child care, and schooling. These children need all the regular immunizations. The diphtheria-tetanus-pertussis vaccine should be administered to an infant or child with stable neurological conditions, including controlled seizures [9]. They need good dental care to avoid the possibility of dental caries seeding a shunt infection during a shunt revision. Most neurosurgeons recommend prophylactic antibiotics before dental work if the child has shunt hardware in the heart (ventriculoatrial shunt). Some surgeons also recommend antibiotics before dental work in children who have had repeated shunt infections. Children also need routine vision screening because of the associated visual abnormalities.

Families who have children with hydrocephalus may benefit from a support group. Families may also benefit from information from national organizations such as the following.

## Organizations and Websites

Hydrocephalus Association
870 Market Street, Suite 705
San Francisco, CA 94102, USA
415-732-7040; 888-598-3789
www.hydroassoc.org

Hydrocephalus Foundation
910 Rear Broadway, Rt. 1
Saugus, MA 01906, USA
781-942-1161
www.hydrocephalus.org

National Hydrocephalus Foundation
12413 Centralia Road
Lakewood, CA 90715, USA
562-402-3532; 888-857-3434
www.nhfonline.org

National Information Center for Children and Youth with Disabilities
PO Box 1492
Washington, DC 20013, USA
www.nichcy.org

Spina Bifida Association of America
4590 MacArthur Blvd. NW, Suite 250
Washington, DC 20007-4226, USA
202-944-3285; 800-621-3141
www.sbaa.org

United Cerebral Palsy Association, Inc.
1660 L Street, Suite 700
Washington, DC 20036, USA
www.ucpa.org

## Living with Hydrocephalus

Hydrocephalus is a chronic, lifelong condition. Untreated hydrocephalus has a mortality rate of 50–60%. Surgically treated hydrocephalus in children with minimal or no evidence of irreversible brain damage is associated with a mortality rate of 10% [26]. Some infants have a shunt placed at birth, require few revisions, and grow to be cognitively and physically normal. Others have a shunt placed and require many revisions, experience complications, and are mildly or markedly developmentally delayed. These ongoing issues with the shunt are not usually the only cause of the developmental abnormalities, but they may contribute to them. Some children with hydrocephalus have other chronic diseases that are associated with, or are the cause of the hydrocephalus. Such illnesses include brain tumors, neurofibromatosis, myelomeningocele, craniofacial abnormalities, cerebral palsy, and various brain malformations. The treatment of the hydrocephalus is just one aspect of the complicated care that these children require. Many factors affect the outcome of children with hydrocephalus. Such factors include: the age at onset, the underlying cause, the timing of the surgical intervention, complications such as repeated shunt failures and infections, and the associated comorbidities of other diseases.

All children with hydrocephalus are at risk for certain associated problems, including: cognitive delays, learning disabilities, motor delays, behavioral abnormalities, visual abnormalities, seizures, precocious puberty, and diabetes insipidus. A French study evaluated 129 children with shunts [16]; these children were shunted before age 2 years and followed for 10 years. The study found that 60% had motor disabilities, 25% had visual or auditory abnormalities, and 30% had seizures. Sixty percent were in school, some with special services, and their IQs were highly variable. Thirty percent had IQs that were in the normal range above 90, 30–60% had mild to moderate mental retardation, and 7–20% had severe mental retardation [16]. Many were 1–2 years behind their peers. Behavioral disorders were common.

## ◼ Cognitive Abnormalities

Intellectual function is difficult to predict in the infant and young child. Abnormalities of the CNS and insults to the CNS may both contribute greatly to impaired function. The younger the child at the age of the onset of hydrocephalus, the greater the risk for intellectual abnormalities. Cognitive difficulties can also be caused by the underlying condition and associated treatment. Shunt infections, especially with Gram-negative organisms, can further impair cognitive function. Some infants have extreme hydrocephalus at birth. Once shunted, the brain may grow into the existing space. Some of these children can develop normally. A cortical mantle of less than 5 mm in thickness seems to be predictive of a poor outcome. Cognitive function is also impossible to predict from radiographic studies. Some children are remarkably

functional despite markedly abnormal appearing brains on CT and/or MRI scans. Other children have severe intellectual impairment with relatively normal appearing scans.

A long term French study [15] in which 129 children with shunted hydrocephalus were evaluated over 10 years found that 30% had IQs that were in the normal range (above 90), 30–60% had mild to moderate mental retardation, and that 7–20% had severe mental retardation. Sgouros followed 70 patients with shunts for 16 years [36]. He found that children with IVH and meningitis as the underlying cause of their hydrocephalus did the worst cognitively, and 30–40% of these children had cognitive delays. He also found that two-thirds of these patients were socially independent, but living with their parents.

Among children with spinal defects and hydrocephalus, cognitive abnormalities are more pronounced in those with higher-level spinal defects as compared to those with sacral defects. In children with myelomeningocele, those that require a shunt (80–85%) have overall lower IQ scores than those who do not require shunting [19].

Children with hydrocephalus also have a higher risk of learning disabilities. These children have difficulty with encoding and retrieval in both verbal and nonverbal tasks [34]. In addition, such children may have difficulty with reading comprehension [43]. They also have difficulties with concentration, nonverbal learning, processing complex language, short-term memory, and poor spatial relations. Dysmorphology of the cerebellum may be associated with oral and motor speech deficits [17]. Furthermore, they are at a higher risk of attention deficit hyperactivity disorder than the general population.

Neuropsychological testing of the child will help to better define where the deficits exist. With such knowledge, learning and activities of daily living can be modified to fit the needs of the individual child. Special therapy, such as speech or occupational therapy, may help the child to become more functional.

The importance of social factors must also be considered when evaluating the intellectual function of these children. Those who have access to the most state-of-the art medical care, therapy services and educational services may do better functionally than those who do not. Some of these children also need complex care from their families on a daily basis. While some families are well equipped to deal with these demands, other families seem to be in a continual state of crisis, have several children with special needs, have one or both parents absent, or many other problems that make it difficult to care for these children.

## Motor Disabilities

Sixty percent of children with hydrocephalus have varying degrees of motor abnormalities. The motor deficits are often related to the underlying etiology of the hydrocephalus. Children with hydrocephalus may have global motor delays and achieve milestones, such as sitting and walking late, or not at all. Hydrocephalus may also affect fine motor control. Such fine motor difficulty may be exacerbated by visual impairments. These children may have trouble learning to write, so keyboards and communication boards may be useful. Premature infants with IVH may develop hydrocephalus and cerebral palsy. The cerebral palsy may be mild and affect only the lower extremities (spastic diplegia), or it may be severe and affect the entire body (spastic quadriplegia).

## Ocular Abnormalities

Optic atrophy from chronic papilledema was the leading cause of blindness from congenital malformations before the successful treatment of hydrocephalus. Increased intracranial pressure from hydrocephalus causes pressure on the cranial nerves. The cranial nerves that are involved in eye function are II (optic), III (oculomotor), IV (trochlear), and VI (abducens). As intracranial pressure increases, signs and symptoms become evident as these nerves are affected. Common findings include limited upward gaze, extraocular paresis, decreased vision, and diplopia (Table 2.5).

Papilledema is a less common finding and is very difficult to diagnose in young children. The child is often referred to an ophthalmologist for a complete eye exam, including dilation of the pupil, to correctly diagnose papilledema. Papilledema is not a common finding in children with increased intracranial pressure unless it is chronic. Optic atrophy is more often seen.

Ocular abnormalities are a common finding in infants and children with untreated hydrocephalus and during periods of shunt malfunction. If treatment is not prompt, visual damage is a risk, including blindness. Visual deficits are common in children with hydrocephalus. Refractive and accommodative errors are found in 25–33% of these children. Gaze and movement disorders, such as nystagmus, astigmatism, strabismus, and amblyopia, are found in 25–33% [32]. Abnormalities in vision may be associated with lower IQ scores. These abnormalities may be an easily identifiable factor to assist in diagnosing hydrocephalic children with developmental delays. Correctable vision issues should be identified and treated as early as possible so that they do not add to developmental and learning difficulties.

## Seizures

Hydrocephalus alone is not commonly recognized as a cause of seizures. However, seizures are associated with children with hydrocephalus who have shunts implanted. The incidence of epilepsy in the general population is 1% among children. The incidence of seizures in children with shunted hydrocephalus is 20–50% [32]. Since modern shunting became the

**Table 2.5.** Cranial nerves and eye symptoms

| **II – Optic nerve** |
| --- |
| Responsible for transmitting visual images from the eye to the brain<br>Test: check for light perception, visual acuity, peripheral vision, and normal appearance of the optic disc |
| **III – Oculomotor nerve** |
| Responsible for controlling four of the six muscle groups that move the eye<br>Medial rectus – moves eye inward<br>Superior rectus – moves eye upward and in<br>Inferior rectus – moves eye downward and in<br>Inferior oblique – moves eye upward and out<br>Responsible for constriction and accommodation of the pupil and closing of the eyelid<br>Test: have child follow object in six cardinal positions of gaze, check for pupil reaction to light, check for closing of eyelid |
| **IV – Trochlear nerve** |
| Responsible for controlling the superior oblique muscle, which moves eye inward and down<br>Test: have child look down and in |
| **VI – Abducens nerve** |
| Responsible for the lateral rectus muscle, which moves eye temporally<br>Test: have child look temporally |

standard treatment for hydrocephalus, controversy has existed about shunt procedures and complications of shunts leading to seizures. There are numerous risk factors related to children with hydrocephalus developing epilepsy. These include age at the original shunt placement, the location of the shunt catheter in the brain, the actual placement of the shunt catheter, repeated revisions of the proximal catheter, the presence of the hardware itself in the brain, the location of the burr hole, shunt infections, intracranial hemorrhage at the time of shunt placement or revision, repeated episodes of increased intracranial pressure, the presence of tumors or cysts, the underlying etiology of the hydrocephalus, and any associated developmental delay. When a child has seizures, a work-up is indicated including an electroencephalogram. Seizures are not usually a symptom of shunt malfunction. A very small percentage of patients will present with seizures as the main symptom of shunt malfunction.

## Precocious Puberty

Precocious puberty is defined as the onset of puberty 1–2 years before the expected age. Normal onset of puberty may occur as young as 8 years in girls and 9 years in boys. Precocious puberty is fairly common in children with hydrocephalus, myelomeningocele, cerebral palsy, and microcephaly, and can start as early as 5 years of age.

Precocious puberty is presumed to be caused by chronic or intermittent increased intracranial pressure that affects the hypothalamus and pituitary gland. These two areas deep in the brain are responsible for timing the release of gonadotropins and sex hormones. Children who have had many shunt revisions when they are very young are at greater risk for precocious puberty.

Precocious puberty causes the growth plates to close early in the long bones. This leads to short stature. In addition, precocious puberty is associated with risk of pregnancy in young children with associated cognitive and behavioral difficulties.

## Conclusion

The Nurse's Dictionary of Medical Terms and Nursing Treatment (Morton, circa 1898) stated the following about hydrocephalus: "water on the brain; a disease most common in children, and causing the head to swell to an enormous size. The victim is always idiotic. Nourishing diet –- cod liver oil; as little fluid as possible." As this chapter has shown, nurses today need to know far more about the condition and its treatment. Most importantly, they need to know that many children with hydrocephalus can lead normal lives because of shunts, or even have the underlying cause surgically corrected. Despite advances in technology, and surgical technique, nurses have and will continue to play major roles in achieving the best possible outcomes for these patients.

**Pediatric Practice Pearls**

- If the mother thinks that the child is acting abnormally or that the shunt is not working, there is a high probability that she is right.
- Small ventricles do not assure adequate shunt function.
- Altered mental status is the first and most salient symptom of increased intracranial pressure, thus the child needs to be awakened for assessment.
- Mental status should be assessed over time for changes. Never give patients with altered mental status, or an unstable exam, medications that could mask the exam and symptoms.

## References

1. Abtin K, Walker ML (1999) Congenital arachnoid cysts and the Dandy Walker complex. In: Albright AL, Pollack IF, Adelson PD (eds) Principles and Practice of Pediatric Neurosurgery. Thieme, New York, pp 125–139
2. Albright A, Pollack I, Adelson P (eds) (1999) Principles and Practice of Pediatric Neurosurgery. Thieme, New York
3. Boop F (2004) Posthemorrhagic hydrocephalus of prematurity. In: Cinalli G, Maixner WJ, Sainte-Rose C (eds) Pediatric Hydrocephalus. Springer-Verlag, Milan, pp 121–131
4. Brack M, Taylor AG, Walker ML (1994) Hydrocephalus: etiology, pathologic effects, diagnosis and natural history. In: Cheek WR, Marlin AE, McLone DG, Reigel DH, Walker ML (eds) Pediatric Neurosurgery. Surgery of the Developing Nervous System. WB Saunders, Philadelphia, pp 185–199
5. Choux M, Dirocco C, Hockley AD, Walker ML (1999) Pediatric Neurosurgery. Churchill Livingstone, London

6. Cinalli G, Saint-Rose C, Chumas P, Zerah M, Brunelle G, Lot G, Pierre-Kahn A, Renier D (1999) Failure of third ventriculostomy in the treatment of aqueductal stenosis in children. J Neurosurg 90:448–453

7. Cinalli G, Spennato P, Del Basso De Caro ML, Buonocore MC (2004) Hydrocephalus and the Dandy-Walker malformation. In: Cinalli G, Maixner WJ, Sainte-Rose G (eds) Pediatric Hydrocephalus. Springer-Verlag, Milan, pp 259–277

8. Ciurea AV, Coman TC, Mircea D (2004) Postinfectious hydrocephalus in children. In: Cinalli G, Maixner WJ, Sainte-Rose G (eds) Pediatric Hydrocephalus. Springer-Verlag, Milan, pp 201–218

9. Committee on Infectious Diseases (2000) Report of the committee of infectious diseases (25th edn). The American Academy of Pediatrics, Elk Grove Village, IL

10. Da Silva MD, Michowicz S, Drake JM, et al (1995) Reduced local cerebral blood flow in periventricular white matter in experimental neonatal hydrocephalus – restoration with CSF shunting. J Cereb Blood Flow Metab 15:1057–1065

11. Dias MS (2005) Neurosurgical management of myelomeningocele spina bifida. Pediatr Rev 26:50–58

12. Ditmyer S (2004) Hydrocephalus. In: JacksonPL, Vessey JA (eds) Primary Care of the Child with a Chronic Condition), Mosby, St. Louis pp 543–559

13. Fudge ES (2000) About Hydrocephalus – A Book for Families (Brochure). University of California, San Francisco

14. Greenberg MS (2001) Handbook of Neurosurgery. Thieme, New York

15. Haines SJ (1999) Shunt infections. In: Albright AL, Pollack IF, Adelson PD (eds) Principles and Practice of Pediatric Neurosurgery Thieme, New York, pp 1177–1185

16. Hoppe-Hirsch E, Laroussinie F, Burnett L, Sainte-Rose C, Reiner D, Cinalli G, et al (1998) Late outcome of the surgical treatment of hydrocephalus. Childs Nerv Syst 14:97–97

17. Huber-Okrainec J, Dennis M, Brettschneider J, Spiegler BJ (2002) Neuromotor speech deficits in children and adults with spina bifida and hydrocephalus. Brain Lang 80:592–602

18. Laurance LM, Coates S (1962) The natural history of hydrocephalus. Detailed analysis of 182 unoperated cases. Arch Dis Child 37:345–361

19. Mapstone TB, Rekate HL, Nulson FE (1984) Relationship of CSF shunting and IQ in children with myelomeningocele: a retrospective analysis. Childs Brain 11:112–118

20. Marlin AE, Gaskill ST (1994) Cerebrospinal fluid shunts: complications and results. In: Cheek WR, Marlin AE, McLone DG, Reigel DH, Walker ML (eds) Pediatric Neurosurgery. Surgery of the Developing Nervous System. WB Saunders, Philadelphia, pp 221–231

21. McLone DG (2001) Pediatric Neurosurgery. Surgery of the Developing Nervous System (4th edn). WB Saunders, Philadelphia

22. Milhorat TH (1971) Cerebral spinal fluid production by the choroids plexus. Science 173:330–332

23. Milhorat TH (1982) Hydrocephalus historical notes, etiology, and clinical diagnosis. In: Section of Pediatric Neurosurgery of the American Association of Neurological Surgeons (ed) Pediatric Neurosurgery. Surgery of the Developing Nervous System. Grune and Stratton, New York, pp 192–210

24. Nadkarni T, Rekate H, Wallace D (2004) Resolution of pseudotumor cerebri after bariatric surgery for related obesity. J Neurosurg 101:878–880

25. Olson S (2004) The problematic slit ventricle syndrome. Pediatr Neurosurg 40:264–289

26. Raffel C, McComb JG (1994) Arachnoid cysts. In: Cheek WR, Marlin AE, McLone DG, Reigel DH, Walker ML (eds) Pediatric Neurosurgery. Surgery of the Developing Nervous System. WB Saunders, Philadelphia, pp 104–110

27. Rekate HL (1999) Treatment of hydrocephalus. In: Albright A, Pollack I, Adelson D (eds) Principals and Practice of Pediatric Neurosurgery. Thieme, New York, pp 47–73

28. Rekate HL, Wallace D (2003) Lumboperitoneal shunts in children. Pediatr Neurosurg 38:41–46

29. Rosen S (1998) Educating students who have visual impairments with neurological disabilities. In: Sacks SZ, Silberman RK (eds) Educating Students who have Visual Impairments with Other Disabilities. Paul H. Brooks, Baltimore

30. Said RR, Rosman NP (2004) A negative cranial computed tomographic scan is not adequate to support a diagnosis of pseudotumor cerebri. J Child Neurol 19: 609–613

31. Sainte R (2004) Hydrocephalus in pediatric patients with posterior fossa tumours. In: Cinalli G, Maixner WJ, Sainte-Rose G (eds) Pediatric Hydrocephalus. Springer-Verlag, Milan, pp 155–162

32. Sato O, Yamguchi T, Kettaka M, Toyoma H (2001) Hydrocephalus and epilepsy. Childs Nerv Syst 17:76–86

33. Schneider SJ, Wiscoff JS, Epstein FJ (1992) Complications of ventriculoperitoneal shunt procedures or hydrocephalus associated with vein of Galen malformations in childhood. Neurosurgery 30:906–908

34. Scott MA (1998) Memory functions in children with early hydrocephalus. Neuropsychology 12:578–589

35. Sgouros S (2004) Management of spina bifida, hydrocephalus and shunts. E-Medicine, Retrieved September 9, 2005, from http://www.emedicine.com/ped/topic2976.htm

36. Sgouros S (2004) Hydrocephalus with myelomeningocele. In: Cinalli G, Maixner WJ, Sainte-Rose G (eds) Pediatric Hydrocephalus. Springer-Verlag, Milan, pp 133–144

37. Shurtleff DB, Foltz EL, Loeser JD (1973) Hydrocephalus, a definition of its progression and relationship to intellectual function, diagnosis and complications. Am J Dis Child 125:688–693

38. Sokoloff L (1989) Circulation and energy metabolism of the brain. In: Siegel GJ, Agranoff BW, Albers RW, Molinoff PB (eds) Basic Neurochemistry. Molecular, Cellular and Medical Aspects. Raven, New York, pp 565–590

39. Sutton LN (1994) Spinal dysraphism. In: Rengachary SS, Ellenbogen RG (eds) Principles of Neurosurgery. Elsevier Mosby, New York, pp 100–115

40. Teo C, Mobbs R (2005) Neuroendoscopy. In: Rengachary SS, Ellenbogen RG (eds) Principles of Neurosurgery. Elsevier Mosby, New York, pp 145–156

41. Wang PP, Avellino AM (2005) Hydrocephalus in children In: Rengachary SS, Ellenbogen RG (eds) Principles of Neurosurgery. Elsevier Mosby, New York, pp 117–136

42. Whitelaw A, Kennedy CR, Brion LP (2001) Diuretic therapy for newborn infants with posthemorrhagic ventricular dilation. Cochrane Database Syst Rev 2, CD002270

43. Yamada J (2002) Neurological origins of poor reading comprehension despite fast word decoding. Brain Lang 80:253–259

# Craniosynostosis

**3**

*Cathy C. Cartwright and Patricia Chibbaro*

## Contents

## ■ Introduction

Craniosynostosis is the premature closure of one or more cranial sutures. Sometimes the entire suture is fused, but even a partial fusion can cause a deformity, as the skull growth is restricted. Although the clinical condition of craniosynostosis was described by Hippocrates in BC 400, effective treatments have only been developed in the last century [9]. In 1800, Sömmering described the anatomic structures of calvarial sutures and the results of premature closure [54]. However, the German pathologist Rudolf Virchow first used the term craniostenosis and proposed that "outward growth of the skull is restricted in a direction perpendicular to the prematurely fused suture and compensatory growth occurs in the patent sutures" [58]. This restriction of growth in one direction and compensatory growth in others accounts for the classic skull deformities seen in craniosynostosis.

The most common type of craniosynostosis is nonsyndromic craniosynostosis, which is a congenital disorder. Craniosynostosis also occurs in over 90 syndromes, but these usually involve more than 1 cranial suture and occur far less frequently than nonsyndromic craniosynostosis [10]. Cohen listed the known causes of craniosynostosis as genetic conditions (e.g., mutations in fibroblast growth factor receptors), metabolic disorders (such as hyperthyroidism) mucopolysaccharidoses, ß-glucuronidase deficiency, mucolipidoses, hematological disorders, teratogens, and malformations including microcephaly and encephalocele [9]. Secondary craniosynostosis can result from overshunting hydrocephalus; however, true bony fusion of the suture does not occur in shunt-related craniosynostosis [55].

Most craniosynostosis is recognizable at birth and the parents may suspect that their baby's head "just doesn't look right." Although molding of the skull can occur during the birth process, this usually normalizes by 3 weeks of age, whereas the deformities from craniosynostosis continue to worsen as the child's brain continues to grow. Infants with craniosynostosis have unique characteristics that are not to be confused with birth trauma. Recognizing craniosynostosis early, before 6 months of age, is important so that minimally invasive surgery can be considered instead of the more extensive calvarial vault remodeling required for the older child.

## Nonsyndromic Craniosynostosis

Nonsyndromic craniosynostosis, the predominant type of suture fusion, occurs in 1 out of 2100 children [31]. The sagittal suture is involved in 40–60% of these fusions, the coronal suture in 20–30%, and the metopic suture in 10% [24,31,53]. Lambdoid synostosis, while often mistaken for positional plagiocephaly, is rare, occurring in 1–2% of all craniosynostosis [56]. Multiple-suture synostoses involving two or more cranial sutures occur in 4–8% of nonsyndromic craniosynostosis (Table 3.1) [8,22].

The specific cause of simple nonsyndromic craniosynostosis has not yet been identified. Simple craniosynostosis is usually random in occurrence, but 2–6% of isolated sagittal synostosis and 8–14% of coronal synostosis were found to be familial [9,32]. In utero head restraint has also been named as a cause of cra-

niosynostosis, although it is more commonly seen as positional plagiocephaly [19–21].

The diagnosis is made by physical examination and can be confirmed with radiographs if there is any question about the diagnosis. Plain skull films allow a look at the patency of the suture in question; however, a computed tomography (CT) scan of the head is preferable as the suture can be identified more easily. A CT scan with three-dimensional reconstruction provides further clarity of the skull shape, skull base, and suture patency. Radiodiagnostic testing should be used judiciously, however, because radiation can have deleterious effects on the growing brain [17].

## Pathophysiology

The brain is contained in the neurocranium, which comprises the skull base and cranial vault. Each of these two components of the neurocranium develops in different ways. The calvarial vault develops via intramembranous ossification as fibrous membrane (ectomenix) over the brain, while the skull base develops through endochondral ossification. After the 2nd month of gestation, ossification centers in the ectomenix differentiate into an outer periosteum and inner dura. These ossification centers eventually expand or fuse to form the frontal, parietal, and occipital bones (Fig. 3.1) [35,45]. The edges of these sutures contain special cells called the osteogenic front

**Table 3.1.** Classifications of craniosynostosis

| Type of craniosynostosis | Suture involved | Incidence | Characteristics |
|---|---|---|---|
| Scaphocephaly (dolicocephaly) | Sagittal | 40–60% | Bitemporal narrowing Frontal bossing Occipital cupping Palpable sagittal ridge |
| Anterior plagiocephaly | Coronal | 20–30% | Vertical dystopia Nasional deviation Flattening of frontal bone on affected side |
| Trigonocephaly | Metopic | 10% | Triangular shape Bitemporal narrowing Parietal bossing Hypotelorism Metopic ridge |
| Posterior plagiocephaly | Lambdoid | 1–2% | Trapezoid shape Tilted skull base Occipitomastoid bulge |

[13]. At 16 weeks gestation, sutures form as these osteogenic fronts approach each other [57].

Sutures allow the infant's head to reshape during the birth process and accommodate the expanding brain during rapid growth. Open sutures may also absorb stresses from trauma [12]. The dura (the membrane covering the brain) is essential for suture and calvarial bone growth. The site of suture formation is related to the location of major dural reflections. Dural reflections are bands of dural attachment to the skull base that conform to the early recesses of the brain [55]. In infants with brain malformations, these early recesses may be absent and the suture will not form.

Removing the skull in a neonate with intact dura results in the dura regenerating the skull with sutures placed as dictated by the dura [14,37]. In other words, neonates and young infants can have portions of, or their entire skull removed and an intact dura will regrow the skull bone with appropriate suture locations. This ability to reossify the skull diminishes as the infant ages.

As the brain grows, overall calvarial bone growth occurs from the expanding brain. New bone is deposited at the osteogenic fronts of the open sutures and this bone deposition at the suture margins is driven by the expanding brain [55]. The skull is 35% of adult size at birth and 90% by 7 years of age [43]. The metopic suture closes at approximately 2 years of age, but the other sutures remain open to accommodate brain growth into adulthood. A layer of capsular fibrous tissue surrounding the osteogenic fronts normally keeps the other sutures from fusing [55]. Even partial closure of one or more sutures during the period of rapid cranial growth can cause significant skull deformities (Fig. 3.2).

The following characteristics of each of the four most common suture closures can occur singly or in combination, especially if multiple sutures are involved.

### Sagittal Synostosis

The most common type of craniosynostosis is sagittal, characterized by a scaphocephalic or "boatlike" shape to the skull, various degrees of bitemporal narrowing, frontal bossing, occipital cupping, and a palpable sagittal ridge (Fig. 3.3). Sometimes the scaphocephalic shape, and especially the occipital cupping, is so prominent that when the infant is lying supine with the back of the head on the mattress, the head is flexed in a way that causes the airway to be compromised. The degree of scaphocephaly is determined by measuring cranial index. Using spreading cranial calipers (GPM Instruments, Switzerland) the distance is measured from euryon to euryon, divided by glabella to opistocranion and multiplied by 100 (Fig. 3.4). A cephalic index of 83 would be average, with higher numbers indicating a rounder head and lower numbers indicating a more scaphocephalic shape.

### Coronal Synostosis

Coronal synostosis, or anterior plagiocephaly, is characterized by vertical dystopia, nasional deviation to the ipsilateral (affected or same) side, flattening of the

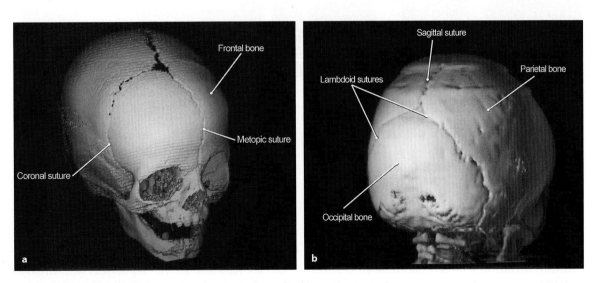

**Fig. 3.1 a, b.** Skull bones and sutures most commonly involved in craniosynostosis

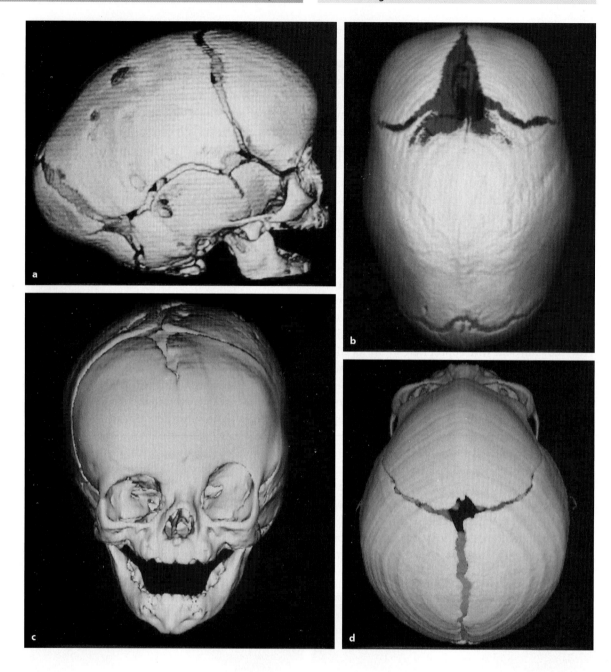

frontal bone on the ipsilateral side and bulging of the frontal bone on the contralateral (opposite) side (Fig. 3.5). Strabismus from ipsilateral superior oblique paresis and compensatory contralateral head tilt is present in 50–65% of cases of unilateral coronal synostosis [18,42]. It is recommended that the patient see an ophthalmologist familiar with craniofacial disorders for preoperative evaluation. Strabismus surgery is usually needed, as it rarely improves after craniofacial reconstruction [55]. However, strabismus surgery

corrects or improves the head tilt [18]. An anteroposterior skull film shows a harlequin appearance to the ipsilateral orbit as the superior orbital rim is elongated (Fig. 3.6).

### Metopic Synostosis

Metopic synostosis is characterized by a trigonocephalic or triangular shape to the head when viewed from above. There are various degrees of bitemporal narrowing, parietal bossing, hypotelorism (close-set

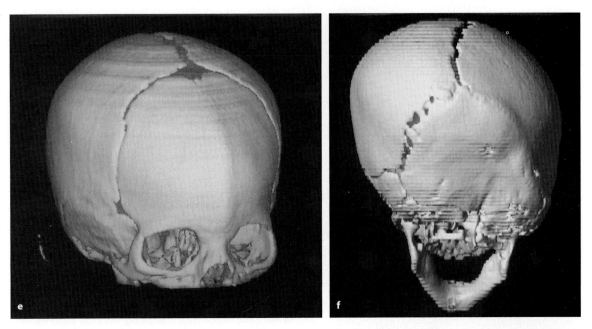

**Fig. 3.2 a–f.** Three-dimensional computed tomography reconstructions clearly show the stenosed sutures and skull shapes. **a** In sagittal synostosis the open sutures compensate for brain growth. **b** Top of the skull shows sagittal synostosis with a closed sagittal suture, open anterior fontanel, and open coronal and lambdoid sutures. **c** Left coronal synostosis showing closed left coronal suture, nasional deviation and elongation of the left superior orbital rim. **d** Metopic synostosis with trigonocephalic shape to the skull. **e** Closed metopic suture causes a vertical ridge or keel. **f** Right lambdoid synostosis

eyes), and ridging of the metopic suture that can resemble a keel (Fig. 3.7). A common variation is characterized by a normal shape to the skull, absence of hypotelorism, and just a slight ridging of the metopic suture. Although surgery is not considered in this instance unless the baby exhibits signs of increased intracranial pressure (vomiting, lethargy, extreme fussiness), the ridge can be "burred down" at a later date if it is still prominent.

### Lambdoid Synostosis

Lambdoid synostosis, or occipital plagiocephaly, is characterized by a trapezoid shape to the head when viewed from above, a tilted skull base (ipsilateral side displaced inferiorly), and ipsilateral ear displaced inferiorly and posteriorly. The fused lambdoid suture has a palpable ridge and there is an ipsilateral occipitomastoid bulge. When viewed from behind, the skull base appears tilted (Fig. 3.8). Care must be taken not to confuse true lambdoid synostosis with positional plagiocephaly (Table 3.2). Radiographically, a Towne's view skull film or CT scan will show a closed lambdoid suture.

### Positional Plagiocephaly

Deformational forces, such as the prenatal head on the mother's pelvic bone or the birth process itself, can shape the skull. The infant brain grows rapidly during the first several months after birth and it is this growth that expands the skull into its normocephalic shape. Infant head circumference increases 9 cm during the first 6 months and grows approximately 12 cm during the 1st year. In comparison, the head circumference increases by only 2.25 cm during the 2nd year after birth and just 0.75 cm between the 2nd and 3rd year. Therefore, deformational forces encountered when an infant head lies on a mattress, against a car seat, swing or stroller, or on any firm surface for prolonged periods of time, can have a significant influence during the period of rapid skull growth.

Most babies are born with normocephaly, but their skulls may become progressively more misshapen during the first several weeks after birth because of deformities from unrelieved pressure on the occipital bone. By the time a baby reaches 2 months of age he may have spent approximately 700 h sleeping. If the baby lies supine with his head turned to one side, ei-

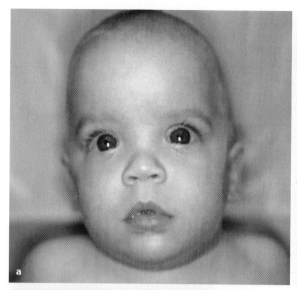

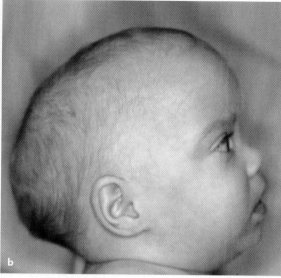

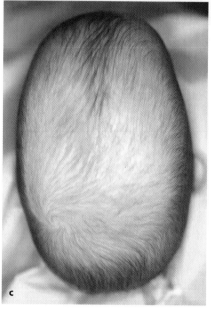

**Fig. 3.3 a–c.** Sagittal synostosis: note the long, narrow shape to the skull, bitemporal narrowing, occipital cupping, and frontal bossing

**Table 3.2.** Comparison of lambdoid synostosis and positional (deformational) plagiocephaly. *CT* Computed tomography

| Lambdoid synostosis | Positional plagiocephaly |
|---|---|
| Usually present at birth | Usually not present at birth |
| Trapezoid shape when viewed from above | Parallelogram shape when viewed from above |
| Ipsilateral ear displaced posteriorly and inferiorly | Ipsilateral ear displaced anteriorly |
| Bony ridge palpable over closed lambdoid suture | No bony ridge over lambdoid suture |
| Unilateral occipitoparietal flattening posteriorly | Usually unilateral occipitoparietal flattening, but can be bilateral |
| When viewed posteriorly there is an ipsilateral occipitomastoid bulge and the skull base appears tilted | When viewed posteriorly the skull base is horizontal and no occipitomastoid bulge |
| Radiographic evidence of closed suture (Towne's view, CT with bone windows, CT with three-dimensional reconstruction) | Radiographic evidence of open sutures |
|  | May have torticollis |

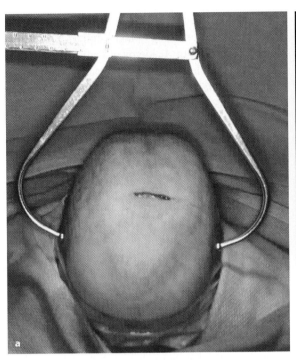

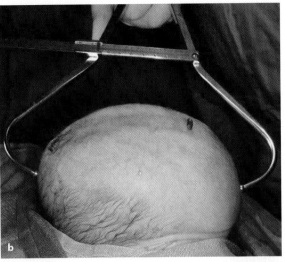

Fig. 3.4. Cranial calipers are used to measure the cephalic index. **a** Euryon to euryon. **b** Glabella to opistocranion

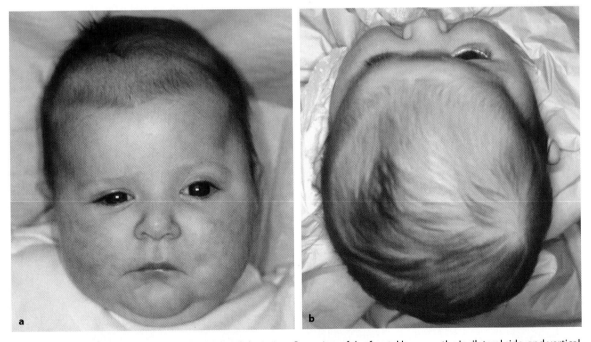

**Fig. 3.5 a, b.** Coronal synostosis: note the nasional deviation, flattening of the frontal bone on the ipsilateral side, and vertical dystopia

ther from preference or the head is not rotated to re-distribute the deformational forces of gravity, positional plagiocephaly can result. This condition can be further aggravated by torticollis (wry neck), which is a tightening of the sternocleidomastoid or cervical muscles that prevent the infant from turning his head 180° [46].

There has been a significant increase in "deformational" or "positional" plagiocephaly since 1992, when the American Academy of Pediatrics initiated the "back to sleep" campaign and recommended that infants sleep on their backs or sides to decrease the incidence of sudden infant death syndrome [30]. One referral center reported a tenfold increase in referrals for occipital plagiocephaly compared with 1991 [3]. It is important to differentiate positional plagiocephaly from craniosynostosis, as the treatment for craniosynostosis is surgery and the treatment for plagiocephaly is, with rare exception, non-surgical (Fig. 3.9).

A thorough history and physical examination will help differentiate between the two. Parents of infants with plagiocephaly frequently report that the head shape was normal at birth and that the occipital flattening was noticed later, often by the pediatrician at the 2-month well baby exam. They also recall their baby preferred to sleep in one position with the head turned to one side. Some babies may prefer to sleep with the back of the head on the mattress, not turning it to either side. These infants can have flattening of the entire occipital bone, which causes the face to appear very round when viewed from the front.

With positional plagiocephaly, there is no bony ridge palpated along the lambdoid suture and the base of the skull will be horizontal when viewed from be-

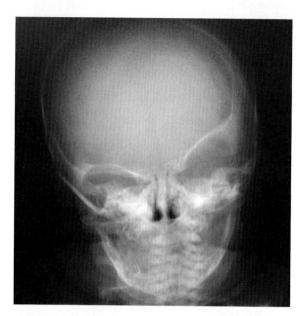

**Fig. 3.6.** Skull film shows "harlequin sign" as the superior orbital rim of the affected eye is elongated

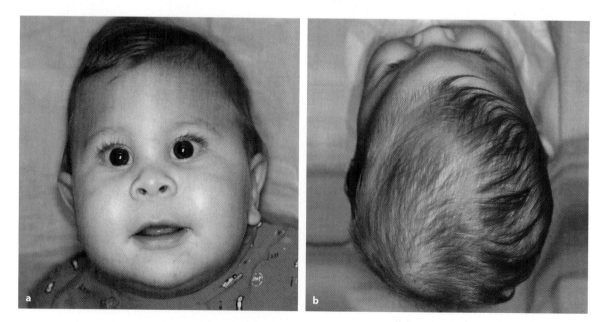

**Fig. 3.7 a, b.** Metopic synostosis: note the trigonocephalic shape of the skull, bitemporal narrowing, hypotelorism, and ridging of the metopic suture

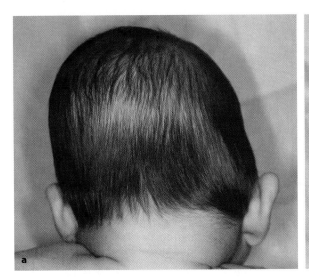

**Fig. 3.8 a, b.** Lambdoid synostosis: note the tilted skull base

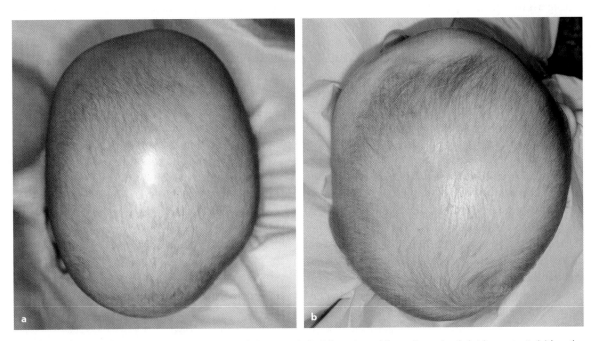

**Fig. 3.9 a, b.** Lambdoid synostosis versus positional plagiocephaly. When viewed from above, lambdoid synostosis (a) has the characteristic trapezoid shape to the skull while positional plagiocephaly (b) has the parallelogram shape to the skull

hind. When viewed from above, there is occipitoparietal flattening on the affected side with anterior displacement of the ear, forehead, and malar eminence on the ipsilateral side. This appears to resemble the shape of a parallelogram as one side of the skull is shifted forward (Fig. 3.10). A Towne's view x-ray or CT of the brain with bone windows will clarify the diagnosis by showing open lambdoid sutures.

### Treatment for Positional Plagiocephaly

Positional plagiocephaly can be prevented by teaching parents to reposition their infant's head from side to side when lying supine, starting from birth. Mild cases of flatness will resolve over weeks to months if the infant's head is repositioned on a flat surface. Toys or objects of interest can be placed on the nonpreferential side to encourage the infant to

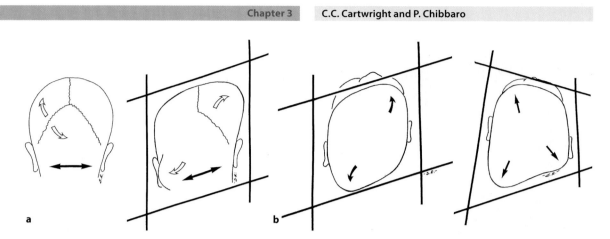

**Fig. 3.10.** These drawings illustrate the differences between positional plagiocephaly (*left*) and lambdoid synostosis (*right*). Used with permission [23]. **a** When the skull is viewed from behind, the *clear arrows* show the direction of skull growth and the *solid arrows* show the base of the skull. **b** When viewed from above, the skull with positional plagiocephaly (*left*) takes the shape of a parallelogram while the skull with lambdoid synostosis (*right*) takes the shape of a trapezoid

turn his head in the nonpreferential direction. Alternating arms to hold the baby when feeding will also encourage head turning to both sides. "Tummy time", or placing the baby prone while awake and observed, will decrease the gravitational forces on the skull.

A cranial orthotic device, such as a band or molding helmet, may be used to correct moderate to severe cases of positional molding, especially if parents have tried without success to reposition their baby. This is most effective between 4 and 12 months of age, during the time of rapid brain growth. Refer these patients to an orthotist experienced in cranial orthotic devices for positional plagiocephaly. In extremely rare cases of severe deformity, despite repositioning, correction of torticollis and use of a cranial molding device, surgery may be considered.

Torticollis (wry neck), or tightening of the sternocleidomastoid, can prevent an infant from turning his head to the nonpreferential side and cause further deformity to the face. Static stretching exercises can be done to gently stretch the affected sternocleidomastoid muscle. Confirm that there is no cervical spine defect before doing these exercises. Although physical therapy can be done by a therapist, parents can be taught to do these exercises at home 5–6 times a day. With the infant lying supine on a flat surface and the head in midline position, the parent can slowly turn the head 90° toward the nonpreferential side, holding the stretched position for 10 s, and then slowly turn the head back to midline. A second person may need to hold the shoulders so that they don't turn with the head. If a head tilt is present, the parent should slowly tilt the head to the contralateral side and hold that po-

sition for 10 s (Fig. 3.11). Parents should be informed that these exercises should be done slowly to prevent trauma to the muscle, and that the baby will cry the first few times. However, within a few days the muscle will relax and it will be easier to turn the head. The torticollis should resolve within a couple of weeks.

In sternocleidomastoid tumor of infancy, a tumor is palpable in the muscle and can restrict the infant's ability to turn the head. Stretching exercises may improve this condition, but surgery is usually necessary to remove the mass and lyse the muscle [30,46].

Although preventing positional plagiocephaly is ideal, treatment should be instituted as soon as the diagnosis is made. Early intervention during the period of rapid skull growth (first few months of age) will yield the best results.

## Syndromic Craniosynostosis

## Pathophysiology

Infants with craniosynostosis "syndromes" or "conditions" present with a characteristic group of clinical findings. They have multiple cranial suture synostoses, including the sutures of the cranial base, which result in complex skull and forehead deformities [2]. The cranial base abnormalities are manifested by hypoplasia of the midface and maxilla. These children often have hypertelorism, exorbitism, syndactyly, cleft palate, cardiac anomalies, and eye muscle abnormalities (e.g., strabismus). Depending on the degree of severity, there are frequently associated medical

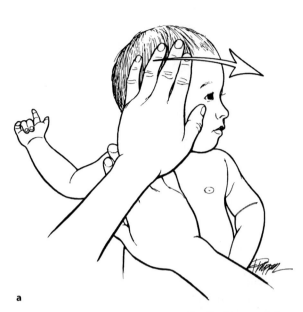

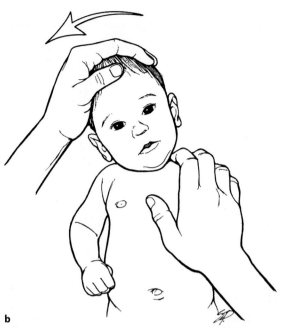

**Fig. 3.11.** Static stretching exercises. Used with permission [36]. **a** Slowly turn the head to the nonpreferential side, holding the stretch position for 10 s and then returning it to the midline. **b** Slowly tilt the head to the contralateral side and hold that position for 10 s

problems, including: hydrocephalus, papilledema, respiratory distress, and failure to thrive.

The most common of these conditions are Crouzon, Apert, and Pfeiffer syndromes. Although their etiology is not totally clear and the majority of the reported cases are sporadic, it is known that they have an autosomal dominant mode of inheritance. An affected individual always has a 50% chance of parenting a child who will be born with the same condition. Mutations in specific fibroblast growth factor receptor (FGFR) gene types for these syndromes have been identified [51,52].

### Crouzon Syndrome

First described by a French neurologist in 1912, this autosomal dominant condition has an approximate incidence of 1 in 25,000 births. It is caused by multiple mutations in the FGFR2. Common clinical findings in infants with Crouzon syndrome may include: bicoronal craniosynostosis, with a resulting short cranium, a broad/flat forehead, sometimes in combination with sagittal and/or lambdoid synostosis (often very severe, as in a child with a cloverleaf deformity), varying degrees of exorbitism, hypertelorism, and maxillary/midface hypoplasia – resulting in a "frog-like" face (Fig. 3.12). They are at very high risk for serious ocular abnormalities, including papilledema, optic atrophy, corneal exposure, and proptosis. In severe cases, the globe can actually herniate through the eyelids, often requiring emergency reduction or tarsorraphy (partial or complete suturing of the eyelids). They may also have a conductive hearing loss. In general, these children do not have anomalies of the hands or feet [2].

Depending on the severity of the midface hypoplasia (and whether there is choanal atresia), the child may have serious airway compromise and challenges with oral feeding, often requiring management by tracheostomy and/or gastrostomy placement. They are also at risk for development of hydrocephalus and/or a symptomatic Chiari malformation, possibly requiring early neurosurgical intervention [51].

### Apert Syndrome

Acrocephalosyndactyly type 1, more commonly known as Apert syndrome (after the French neurologist who described the syndrome in 1906) is the most complex of the craniosynostosis syndromes [40]. The incidence of this autosomal dominant condition is reported as 1/50,000 to 1/160,000 [2,18]. As with Crouzon syndrome, this condition results from a mutation of the FGFR2 gene. Infants with Apert syndrome also

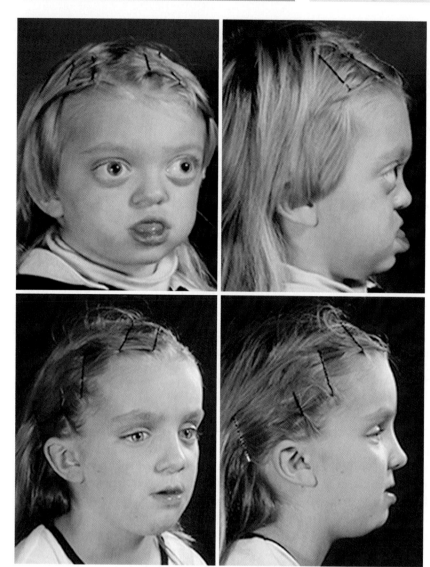

**Fig. 3.12.** Patient with Crouzon syndrome. Preoperative (*top*) – note the exorbitism and midface hypoplasia. Postoperative (*below*) – following cranial vault remodeling and midface advancement surgeries

characteristically have multiple-suture craniosynostosis. Their skulls are often very tall and turricephalic (tower-like). They usually present with an extremely flat and elongated forehead, bitemporal widening, and bilateral flattening of the occiput. The nose has a "beaked" appearance (Fig. 3.13). Hydrocephalus and agenesis of the corpus callosum are not uncommon in these children. They also have varying degrees of exorbitism, proptosis, midface/maxillary hypoplasia, and hypertelorism.

The classic distinguishing finding in infants with Apert syndrome is soft tissue and bony syndactyly (fusion) of the digits of the hands and feet. Many of these infants also have shortening of the upper extremities, dental abnormalities (e.g., anterior open bite), clefts of the secondary palate (they almost always have a very high arched palate), conductive hearing loss, cardiac anomalies, and chronic acne (first noted in infancy). Developmental delay and learning disabilities are higher in this group than in children with Crouzon syndrome, although many of these children develop normal intelligence [2].

## Pfeiffer Syndrome

This syndrome, also autosomal dominant, has an incidence of approximately 1 in 200,000. It is caused by mutations in FGFR1 or FGFR2 [41] and, like Apert syndrome, is characterized by multiple-suture craniosynostosis, varying degrees of developmental delay, midface hypoplasia, and upper airway anomalies

**Fig. 3.13 a, b.  a** Preoperative
patient with Apert syndrome.
Note the turribrachycephaly
and exorbitism. **b** Same patient
(bilateral syndactyly) pre- and
postoperative views
(handphotos courtesy of
Dr. Joseph Upton)

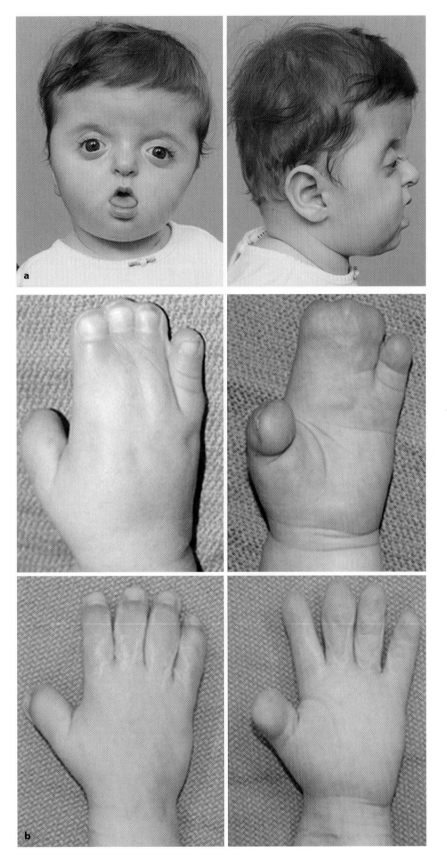

[51] (Fig. 3.14). These children commonly have very broad thumbs and great toes, and sometimes have syndactyly. They can be mistaken for a child with Apert syndrome, and require careful assessment and diagnosis by an experienced craniofacial team.

### Other Syndromes

There are several less commonly occurring craniosynostosis syndromes, including: craniofrontonasal dysplasia, Carpenter, Antley-Bixler, Saethre-Chotzen, and Jackson-Weiss Syndromes (Fig. 3.15). They also are characterized by craniosynostosis and midface deformities, and the affected infants can have associated neurosurgical, airway, and ophthalmologic problems, requiring assessment and management by a craniofacial team. In addition, there are almost 100 other "noncraniosynostosis" syndromes in which craniosynostosis may be a finding. Two common examples are Treacher Collins syndrome and craniofacial microsomia.

### Comprehensive Diagnosis/Assessment of the Infant with Syndromic Craniosynostosis

In order to comprehensively manage the syndromic child, there must be a team approach to diagnosis and assessment (Table 3.3). When a new patient is referred to a craniofacial center, the team assembles and obtains a full patient history, including the prenatal and birth course, and all medical/surgical information. A detailed feeding history is also obtained. The team psychologist and social worker interview the family

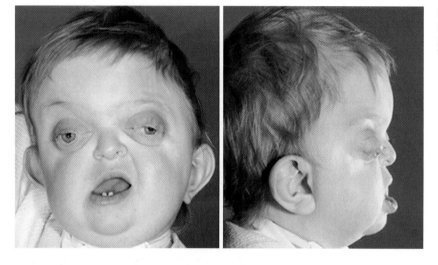

**Fig. 3.14.** Patient with Pfeiffer syndrome. Bilateral tarsorrhaphies were performed to prevent herniation of the globes

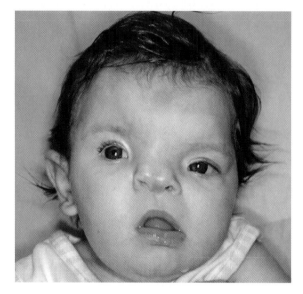

**Fig. 3.15.** Infant with frontonasal dysplasia and right coronal synostosis. Note the hypertelorism and bifid nose

**Table 3.3.** Craniofacial team

| | |
|---|---|
| Craniofacial surgeon | Nurse specialist |
| Neurosurgeon | Pediatrician |
| Orthodontist | Psychologist |
| Geneticist | Otolaryngologist |
| Speech pathologist | Ophthalmologist |
| Social worker | Prosthodontist |
| Audiologist | Pediatric dentist |

in private and complete a psychosocial profile. A complete physical examination is performed, including measurement of head circumference and intraoral evaluation. Any medical records brought to the consult by the family are reviewed, as well as skull films, CT, or magnetic resonance imaging (MRI) scans. All members of the team are given the opportunity to question the family and to examine the child.

The family is encouraged to express their concerns and to ask questions. The team then discusses the child and re-reviews all records without the family in the room, in order to allow for an open discussion and exchange of opinions. Treatment options will be prioritized, based on the patient's individual clinical findings. The team director meets with the family and presents a treatment plan. This may involve further medical workup, especially if there is a concern about airway, eye, or neurosurgical problems (e.g., if there is a suspicion of increased intracranial pressure, hydrocephalus, or a Chiari Malformation). Initial surgical intervention will depend on the age of the child at presentation to the team, as well as the presence of any medical problems. Often, prior to the initial cranial reconstruction, an infant might require placement of a tracheostomy, gastrostomy, ventriculoperitoneal shunt, or could need to undergo a posterior cranial decompression.

## ▪ Treatment for Craniosynostosis

The treatment for craniosynostosis is surgical. Unfortunately, some mistakenly believe that surgery is not necessary because the deformity is cosmetic, or that the surgery is cosmetic. The American Medical Association defines cosmetic surgery as "surgery performed to reshape normal structures of the body in order to improve the patient's appearance and self-esteem. Reconstructive surgery is performed on abnor-

mal structures of the body, caused by congenital defects, developmental abnormalities, trauma, infection, tumors or disease. It is generally performed to improve function, but may also be done to approximate a normal appearance" [1]. Craniosynostosis is a congenital defect and surgery to correct it is reconstructive. This may be an issue of importance for insurance companies or others with the authority to approve treatment.

Although surgery for craniosynostosis is reconstructive, it is also done for the cosmetic and psychological benefits, as well as to prevent neurological injury. Children with untreated craniosynostosis look "different" than their peers and are often teased and ostracized. Hats and protective helmets for sports such as biking, football, and baseball don't fit a misshapen head. Visual disturbances have been reported, especially the characteristic vertical dystopia seen in patients with coronal synostosis. Some children with craniosynostosis can have elevated intracranial pressure, which impairs mental development and can lower IQ [47–49]. Although a study of 22 infants with metopic synostosis failed to show a correlation between increased severity of deformity and decreased cognitive and motor development, those with isolated metopic craniosynostosis might show developmental delays in language acquisition [59]. Research on the incidence and extent of increased intracranial pressure is limited, due to the ethical considerations of placing intracranial monitors in healthy infants for research purposes. However, Cartwright and Jimenez studied 89 infants with untreated craniosynostosis and found a significant decrease in fussiness and irritability after suture release by endoscopic strip craniectomy as compared to preoperatively [4].

## ▪ Surgical Intervention

In 1888, LC Lane performed the first craniectomy to remove a stenosed suture on a 9-month-old infant with microcephaly [33]. Lannelongue, a French surgeon, performed bilateral strip craniectomies to treat sagittal synostosis in 1890 [34]. In 1894, Jacobi reported treatment of 33 microcephalic patients with poor results and high mortality rates [25]. This ended surgery for craniosynostosis for the next 30 years. Faber and Town proposed reviving the surgery in 1927 to prevent blindness and other complications [15]. In 1943, Faber and Town recommended operating at

1–3 months of age for optimal results, and this became generally accepted [16].

Currently, most craniofacial centers do not intervene surgically prior to age 3 months (except in the case of an infant with increased intracranial pressure that requires urgent decompression). The typical age range to operate is between 3–12 months, depending on the protocol of the center [2,29,44]. The types of techniques include: strip craniectomy (endoscopic or nonendoscopic approaches), fronto-orbital advancement with calvarial vault remodeling (for correction of metopic, unicoronal, bicoronal, and syndromic craniosynostoses), and the pi (extended strip craniectomy) and Hungspan procedures (specifically for correction of severe sagittal craniosynostosis) [38,39]. In syndromic infants with multiple suture synostoses, staged circumferential procedures may be required [2].

Infants with isolated craniosynostosis may be candidates for minimally invasive endoscopic wide vertex craniectomy with bilateral barrel stave osteotomies, or a more simple strip craniectomy in the case of sagittal synostosis, if diagnosed before the age of 6 months. Infants over age 6 months, as well as those with syndromic craniosynostosis, will require an intracranial fronto-orbital advancement with cranial vault remodeling. As stated previously, the age at which to intervene will depend upon both the child's age and clinical findings upon presentation, as well as the surgical protocol of the team (generally between ages 6 and 12 months). If the child is over age 18 months, bone grafting may be needed at the same time (rib or split cranium), as they are less likely to generate new bone to adequately cover the cranial defects that result from the fronto-orbital advancement. Children with Apert syndrome often require secondary cranial vault remodeling because of the severity of their abnormality (specifically the turricephaly of the skull).

In addition to cranial surgeries, syndromic children may require: shunt placement, correction of Chiari malformation, eye muscle surgery, choanal atresia repair, syndactyly reconstruction (several stages of surgery to separate the soft tissue and/or bony fusion of the hands), midface advancement, and definitive nasal reconstruction. They also will need many years of specialized orthodontic treatment [50].

Between ages 4 and 6 years (as early as age 3 years in tracheotomy-dependent children), the syndromic patient will often need to undergo correction of their midface hypoplasia, known as a midface advancement. This surgery accomplishes many things, including:

better eye coverage, improvement in breathing, correction of dental occlusion, and a more "acceptable" facial appearance. If the forehead requires further advancement, it can be addressed at the same time. The surgery can be performed by a "traditional" approach, using rib grafts to stabilize the advanced midface segments [40], or by a more gradual process, distraction osteogenesis, using either a rigid external halo-type fixation device, or an internal device [11]. Once the patient reaches skeletal maturity (age 16–21 years), definitive midface or maxillary advancement (as well as nasal reconstruction) may be indicated.

## Preoperative Preparation for Intracranial Surgery

Prior to intracranial surgery, all patients have a very specific and detailed preoperative workup, with some of the requirements being specific to the syndromic patient (Table 3.4). An MRI scan (brain and cervical spine) will document whether there is hydrocephalus or a Chiari malformation. If either is detected, the cranial reconstruction may need to be postponed until after a neurosurgical intervention (shunt placement or posterior cranial decompression). A CT scan can also detect hydrocephalus, but is most important in confirming the extent of the sutural synostosis, and the three-dimensional reconstructions will assist in surgical planning. A complete eye evaluation, including a dilated fundoscopic examination, is essential to identify the presence of papilledema. This finding will often result in performing an emergency strip craniectomy, or a cranial vault reconstruction prior to age 6 months. Other eye abnormalities, such as strabismus (a very common finding in patients with both syndromic and nonsyndromic craniosynostosis) should be identified preoperatively, as over 60% of children will require eye muscle repair after recovering from their cranial surgery [18].

A child with a tracheostomy or any breathing problems must have a thorough evaluation by a pediatric otolaryngologist, as well as a presurgical consult with a pediatric anesthesiologist. Preoperative medical photographs (all views) are essential for medical documentation. A complete genetics evaluation should be done prior to surgery, as the child's clinical examination will obviously be affected by the surgery. Presurgical screening (pediatric medical clearance, blood work, history/physical examination, obtaining surgical consent) and appointments with the craniofacial surgeon and the neurosurgeon are scheduled within 3–4 weeks of the procedure. The family is encouraged to donate blood for the patient. The entire family (including siblings and grandparents) is offered the opportunity to meet with the team psychologist and social worker in order to discuss any concerns, and to receive support in dealing with the surgical experience, which has an impact on everyone. Finally, the craniofacial nurse specialist meets with the parents for an extensive preoperative teaching session (Table 3.5). This includes written and verbal information/explanations about the hospitalization, the surgical procedure, postoperative course, and at-home management [6]. Pre- and postoperative photos of children who underwent the same procedure are shown, and networking to other families by phone or email is offered, as well as a tour of the preoperative waiting area and the pediatric units. The family is referred to craniofacial support groups and websites (Table 3.6).

## Surgical Experience

Whenever possible, any type of intracranial procedure should be scheduled as a first case, in order to minimize the physiologic and psychologic stress of waiting on the patient and family [6]. Many centers allow a parent to carry the infant into the operating room, in order to decrease separation anxiety. Once anesthesia is induced by mask, the parent is safely escorted back to the waiting area by the circulating nurse. After the child is induced with inhaled anesthetic and the parent leaves the room, he or she undergoes a "prep" period, which involves intubation, placement of cardiac and respiratory monitors, multiple intravenous lines (peripheral, central, and arterial), a Foley catheter, and corneal protectors. The hair is parted, but generally not shaved.

In order to minimize bleeding, the anesthesiologist will maintain the child in a hypotensive state, but one or two units of packed cells are often transfused during the procedure. Once the surgery is completed, one or two Jackson-Pratt drains are placed and the incision is closed with absorbable sutures. A gauze head dressing is applied, the corneal protectors are removed, the child is usually extubated and, once stable, is transferred either to the recovery room or the pediatric intensive care unit for initial observation. The total length of the procedure, including patient preparation, surgical intervention, extubation, and transfer to the postoperative unit, is approximately 4–6 h. This will obviously differ by the specific type of procedure, as well as by the center – the most important factor is that the family is prepared for what to expect.

**Table 3.4.** Preoperative workup for intracranial surgery.

| *ENT* **Ear, nose, and throat,** *MR* **magnetic resonance** |
| --- |
| MR scan (brain and cervical spine) |
| CT scan with three-dimensional reconstruction |
| Fundoscopic eye evaluation |
| Pediatric ENT evaluation |
| Anesthesia consult |
| Genetics evaluation |
| Medical photographs |
| Blood donation |
| Presurgical testing |
| Psychosocial consult |
| Preoperative nursing consult |
| Family networking |

**Table 3.5.** Preoperative nursing consult. *OR* Operating room, *ICU* intensive care unit, *IVs* intravenous lines

| Review of pre-/postoperative photographs | |
| --- | --- |
| Networking to families and support groups/craniofacial Websites | |
| Hospital information | Location of OR, waiting/recovery room, ICU, pediatric unit, visiting policies, rooming-In for parents |
| Procedure/postoperative | Length, description, possible complications, postoperative appearance (drains, IVs, dressings, swelling of eyes, overcorrection of forehead, Foley catheter), length of stay (ICU, hospital) |
| Home issues | Discharge instructions, signs/symptoms of infection/dehydration, prevention of swelling, activity, diet, postoperative appointments, return to childcare, parents return to work |

**Table 3.6.** Craniofacial resources/support groups

| Resource | Web site address |
|---|---|
| About Face | www.aboutfaceinternational.org / 800-665-FACE |
| | www.aboutfaceusa.org / 888-486-1209 |
| American Cleft Palate-Craniofacial Association | |
| Cleft Palate Foundation | www.acpa-cpf.org / 800-24-CLEFT |
| Children's Craniofacial Association | www.ccakids.com / 800-535-3643 |
| FACES – The National Craniofacial Association | www.faces-cranio.org / 800-332-2373 |
| Forward Face | www.forwardface.org / 800-393-FACE |
| Foundation for Faces of Children | www.facesofchildren.org / 617-355-8299 |
| Genetic Alliance | www.geneticalliance.org / 800-336-GENE |
| Let's Face It | www.faceit.org / 360-676-7325 |
| National Foundation for Facial Reconstruction | www.nffr.org / 212-263-6656 |
| National Organization for Rare Disorders | www.rarediseases.org / 800-999-6673 |

## Surgical Technique

### Fronto-orbital Advancement/Calvarial Vault Remodeling

The primary goal of this procedure is to expand the cranial vault (which increases the intracranial volume) by releasing the prematurely fused suture(s), thus maximizing brain growth and minimizing the possibility of increased intracranial pressure, hydrocephalus, and optic nerve damage. A second goal, which is especially important for the syndromic child, is to advance the retruded supraorbital bar, in order for the globe to receive more adequate coverage and protection. A third, very critical goal (sometimes the primary motivation to intervene surgically in the nonsyndromic infant) is to perform the above procedure in an attempt to normalize the appearance of the child [2,51].

Once the surgical preparation is completed, a coronal incision (across the top of the head, from ear to ear, often in a "zig-zag" pattern, to facilitate closure and help with scar camouflage) is made and the flap is "turned down" over the lower face [50]. The surgery is done as a team, by a pediatric neurosurgeon and a craniofacial surgeon. The neurosurgeon performs the frontal craniotomy. The frontal bone is removed and placed in sterile, saline-soaked gauze. The craniofacial surgeon creates a fronto-orbital bony segment (the "bandeau" or supraorbital bar). The brain is re-

tracted, and the bandeau and cranial bone plates (which are often split in two) are reshaped and advanced into an overcorrected position to allow for increased cranial vault growth [2]. The segments are then secured with sutures, wires, and/or absorbable miniplates/screws (Fig. 3.16).

### Hungspan Procedure

This procedure is frequently performed on children who require a secondary surgery for sagittal synostosis due to increased intracranial pressure. In some centers, it is the primary surgical intervention in very severely affected infants [38]. The extent of the cranial remodeling depends on the severity of the deformity. The child with a significant turricephaly will require a circumferential reshaping, involving advancement/remodeling of the frontal bone and supraorbital rim, as well as reduction of the vertical height of the skull. In the more mildly affected patient, only the frontal bone and supraorbital bar are remodeled and advanced into an overcorrected position (Fig. 3.17).

### Pi Procedure

The pi procedure is another type of cranial vault reconstruction designed to correct sagittal synostosis. It is so-named because the craniectomy is made in the shape of the Greek letter $\pi$. Barrel-stave osteotomies are made across the parietal bones and the skull is foreshortened to correct the scaphocephalic shape.

**Fig. 3.16.** Line drawing of intra-cranial fronto-orbital advance-ment/calvarial vault remodeling surgery. (used with permission; Mathes, S. Plastic Surgery, 2/E, © 2006 Elsevier Inc.)

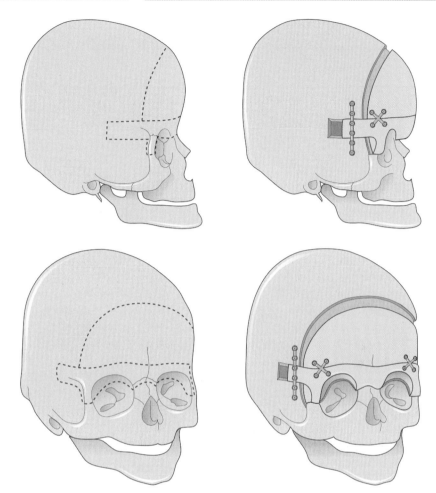

## Postoperative Nursing Management

Following an intracranial procedure, initial nursing care should focus on: assessment of neurologic status, postoperative hemostasis, fluid and electrolyte balance, pain management, and presence of infection. Frequent neurologic checks are needed to monitor the child's level of consciousness, observe for any signs of seizure activity and for a possible cerebrospinal fluid leak (bearing in mind that the craniotomy performed carries the potential risk of a dural tear). The drains and suture line need very close monitoring, as well as assessment of anemia (frequent hematocrit checks, evidence of hematuria, tachycardia, arrhythmia, and pale skin color). An additional blood transfusion may be needed on the operative day or on the first postoperative day. Intravenous antibiotics will continue until discharge; after this the child will remain on oral antibiotics for approximately 1 week.

The child is usually transferred to the general pediatric unit on the first or second postoperative day.

In almost all children, severe swelling of the forehead and eyelids will occur (the eyes will swell shut). Elevating the head of the bed may help make the child feel more comfortable; they often reject iced compresses and should not be forced to use them, as they will not prevent the edema. Parents are prepared for this preoperatively, but are often very anxious about it and need reassurance that the swelling will peak on the second postoperative day and will then resolve over a period of 1–2 weeks. The goal is to remove the Foley and most of the intravenous lines on postoperative day one, all remaining intravenous lines and the drains/head dressing by the second postoperative day, with hospital discharge by day three or four, depending on the child's ability to tolerate oral fluids [6,7]. Throughout the hospitalization, the nurse specialist is in contact with the family and serves as a resource to the nursing staff.

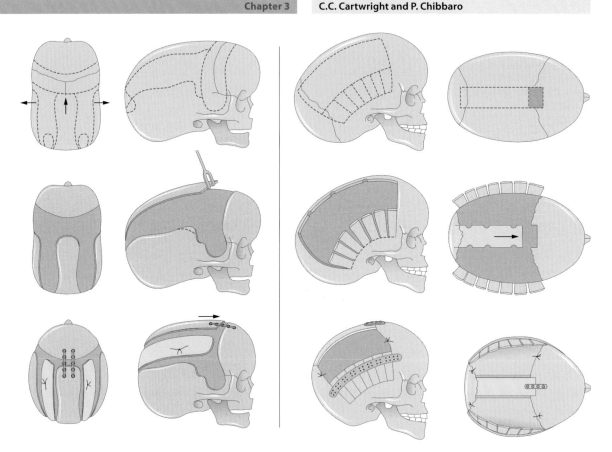

**Fig. 3.17.** Pi (*left*) and Hungspan (*right*) procedures for correction of sagittal craniosynostosis. (used with permission; Mathes, S. Plastic Surgery, 2/E, © 2006 Elsevier Inc.)

### Postdischarge Management

Prior to discharge, the nurse specialist will meet with the family and review with them the signs and symptoms of postoperative infection and dehydration. Suture line care is reviewed (this is also center-dependent, although most centers advocate showering upon discharge, with gentle shampooing to avoid formation of a hematoma). It is advised that the child should avoid contact with playmates or family members who may be ill for the first 2 weeks after surgery. They are reminded that the forehead and eye swelling will resolve, and that elevation of the head is helpful. Reassurance is given to parents that injury to the operative site is very unlikely (the bones are very well secured!) and that the child should be allowed to resume ambulation with their supervision. Parents are often very anxious about returning to work and bringing the child back to a caregiver, or to a daycare setting, and this will often require additional support and counseling. Postoperative visits are scheduled at 1–2 weeks and then as per the protocol of the craniofacial team.

### Strip Craniectomy

Although the extensive cranial vault remodeling for correction of craniosynostosis has shown good results, the lengthy operating times and blood transfusions to correct estimated blood loss from 25% to 500% have lead surgeons to use less invasive techniques [27]. The strip craniectomy, usually only done for sagittal synostosis, involves removing the stenosed sagittal suture. Blood loss is minimal and the hospital stay is 2–3 days. This is done in the young infant, before 6 months of age, to take advantage of the rapid brain growth during that time as well as the dura's ability to regrow bone. A custom-made molding helmet, worn postoperatively, helps to reshape the head during this period of rapid brain growth, as it overcomes the dural forces that caused the original deformity (Fig. 3.18).

The endoscopic wide vertex craniectomy with bilateral barrel stave osteotomies is a minimally invasive technique that uses endoscopes to visualize the intracranial area while a strip of bone containing the stenosed sagittal suture is removed [26]. Endoscopic

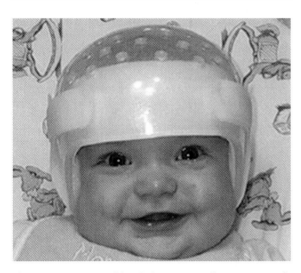

**Fig. 3.18.** Custom molding helmet is worn for approximately 1 year to overcome dural forces and reshape the skull

strip craniectomies have been done successfully on the sagittal, coronal, metopic and lambdoid sutures (and combinations thereof) with blood losses averaging less than 43 ml, and usually just an overnight stay in the hospital [5,27,28]. These strip craniectomies should be performed on infants less than 6 months of age and a custom-made molding helmet worn for approximately 1 year postoperatively for best outcomes. The cost of this procedure is substantially less than that of the traditional calvarial vault remodeling [5].

### Nursing Care

Although strip craniectomies are generally less of a surgical risk than cranial vault remodeling, they are not without risk. Preoperative preparation is similar to what is described for cranial vault remodeling, as these patients are also evaluated by members of the craniofacial team. Parents who prefer their infant not receive a blood transfusion for personal or religious reasons may choose the endoscopic strip craniectomy because of the minimal blood loss. Preoperative administration of erythropoietin may be considered to increase the baby's hematocrit. Preoperative photos and anthropometric measurements are taken.

Postoperatively, these infants also need frequent vital signs with neurological assessment to detect any early signs of blood loss, electrolyte imbalance, or neurologic deterioration. Any bleeding from the incision site should be immediately reported to the neurosurgeon. Although swelling of the head is expected, it usually peaks on postoperative day two or three and

has subsided by 1 week postoperatively. Preoperative diet and activity are usually resumed on the first postoperative day. Pain can be controlled with acetaminophen and ibuprofen, with nalbuphine for breakthrough pain. Discharge criteria include a stable hematocrit and vital signs, adequate oral intake, and pain controlled by oral medication. Parents should be instructed to call for increased fussiness not relieved by oral pain medication, decreased level of consciousness or lethargy, vomiting, or drainage from the incision site. The infants are measured for a custom-made molding helmet approximately 1 week after surgery. Because a strip of bone is missing, many parents become alarmed that their baby's brain may become injured during the time before they receive the helmet. Assure them that no extra precautions need to be taken, other than what they would usually do to protect a baby's head, as the dura, or covering to the brain, is very tough (dura mater means "tough mother").

The molding helmet is worn 23 h a day for about 1 year, with new helmets made as the head grows and changes shape. Usually three helmets are required over that year. Visits to a craniofacial clinic will be scheduled to check the head shape and fit of the helmet over the course of the year. Anthropometric measurements and pictures will be taken at each visit and compared to those taken preoperatively. Patients whose parents are not compliant with helmet use, or discontinue it too soon, will have less than optimum results. It is important that the helmet is worn as directed, to overcome the dural forces that continue to dictate skull growth and could recreate the deformity.

### Conclusion

The diagnosis of craniosynostosis can be a frightening one for the parents of a child with a skull deformity. It is important that craniosynostosis is differentiated from positional plagiocephaly early on, so the appropriate treatment can be instituted.

The patient with craniosynostosis requires comprehensive management by an experienced craniofacial team, with surgical intervention being the core component of their treatment. The nursing roles of provider of direct care, patient/family educator and liaison between the patient, their family and the rest of the team are key to a successful outcome.

## Pediatric Practice Pearls

■ Positional plagiocephaly can be prevented by rotating the infant's head when supine.

■ Early recognition and treatment of craniosynostosis versus positional plagiocephaly lead to improved outcomes.

■ Children with craniosynostosis should receive comprehensive care provided by a craniofacial team.

## References

1. American Medical Association Policy of House of Delegates (1989) Definitions of "cosmetic" and "reconstructive" surgery, H-435.992. Council of Medical Services Annual Meeting, June 1989, p A-89
2. Bartlett SP, Mackay GJ (1997) Craniosynostosis syndromes. In: Aston SJ, Beasley RW, Thorne CH (eds) Grabb and Smith's Plastic Surgery, 5th edn. Lippincott-Raven, Philadelphia, pp 295–304
3. Carson BS, James CS, VanderKolk CA, Guarnieri M (1997) Lambdoid synostosis and occipital plagiocephaly: clinical decision rules for surgical intervention. Neurosurg Focus 2:e5
4. Cartwright CC, Jimenez DF (2002) Fussiness and irritability in patients with craniosynostosis. Paper presented at the AANS/CNS Section on Pediatric Neurological Surgery Annual Meeting, December 2002, Phoenix, AZ
5. Cartwright CC, Jimenez DF, Barone CM, Baker L (2003) Endoscopic strip craniectomy: a minimally invasive treatment for early correction of craniosynostosis. J Neurosci Nurs 35:130–138
6. Chibbaro P (1994) Understanding and managing stressors facing the pediatric craniofacial patient and family. Plast Surg Nurs 14:86–91
7. Chibbaro P (1996) Nursing care of patients with craniofacial anomalies. In: Goodman T (ed) Core Curriculum for Plastic and Reconstructive Surgical Nursing. Anthony J. Jannetti, New Jersey, pp 267–283
8. Chumas PD, Cinalli G, Arnaud E, et al (1997) Classification of previously unclassified cases of craniosynostosis. J Neurosurg 86:177–181
9. Cohen MM (1986) Perspectives on craniosynostosis. In: Cohen MM (ed) Craniosynostosis. Diagnosis, Evaluation and Management. Raven, New York, pp 21–56
10. Cohen MM (1993) Sutural biology and the correlates of craniosynostosis. Am J Med Genet 47:581–616
11. Cohen SR, Holmes RE (2001) Internal Le Fort III distraction with biodegradable devices. J Craniofac Surg 12:264–272
12. Cohen MM, MacLean RE (2000) Craniosynostosis: Diagnosis, Evaluation and Management, 2nd edn. Oxford University Press, New York
13. Decker JD, Hall SH (1985) Light and electron microscopy of the new born sagittal suture. Anat Rec 212:81–89
14. Drake DB, Pershing JA, Berman DE, Ogle RC (1993) Calvarial deformity regeneration following subtotal calvariectomy for craniosynostosis: a case report and theoretical implications. J Craniofac Surg 4:85–89
15. Faber HK, Towne EB (1927) Early craniectomy as a preventive measure in oxycephaly and allied conditions. With special reference to the prevention of blindness. Am J Med Sci 173:701
16. Faber HK, Town EB (1943) Early operation in premature cranial synostosis for the prevention of blindness and other sequelae. Five case reports with follow up. J Paediatr 22:286
17. Frush DP, Donnelly LF, Rosen NS (2003) Computed tomography and radiation risks: what pediatric health care providers should know. Pediatrics 112:951–957
18. Gosain AK, Steele MA, McCarthy JF, Thorne CH (1996) A prospective study of the relationship between strabismus and head posture in patients with frontal plagiocephaly. Plast Reconstr Surg 97:881–891
19. Graham JM, Bardura RJ, Smith DW (1980) Coronal Synostosis: fetal head restraint as one possible cause. Pediatrics 65:995–999
20. Graham JM, deSaxe M, Smith DW (1979) Sagittal synostosis: fetal head restraint as one possible cause. J Pediatr 95:747–750
21. Higgenbottom MC, Jones KL, James HE (1980) Intrauterine constraint and craniosynostosis. Neurosurgery 6:39–49
22. Hoffman H, Raffel C (1989) Craniofacial surgery. In: McLaurin R, Venes JL, Schut L, et al (eds) Pediatric Neurosurgery: Surgery of the Developing Nervous System. WB Saunders, Philadelphia, pp 120–141
23. Huang MHS, Gruss JS, Clarren SK, Mouradian WE, Cunningham ML, Roberts RS, Loeser JD, Cornell C (1996) The differential diagnosis of posterior plagiocephaly: true lambdoid synostosis versus positional molding. Plast Reconstr Surg 98:765–774
24. Hunter AG, Rudd NL (1984) Craniosynostosis I. Sagittal synostosis: its genetics and associated clinical findings in 214 patients who lacked involvement of the coronal suture. Teratology 14:185–194
25. Jacobi A (1894) Non Nocere. Med Rec 45:609
26. Jimenez DF, Barone CM (1998) Endoscopic craniectomy for early surgical correction of sagittal craniosynostosis. J Neurosurg 88:77–81
27. Jimenez DF, Barone CM, Cartwright CC, Baker L (2002) Early management of craniosynostosis using endoscopic assisted strip craniectomies and cranial orthotic molding therapy. Pediatrics 110:97–104
28. Jimenez DF, Barone CM, McGee ME, Cartwright CC, Baker L (2004) Endoscopic-assisted wide-vertex craniectomy, barrel stave osteotomies, and postoperative helmet molding therapy in management of sagittal suture craniosynostosis. J Neurosurg (Pediatr) 100:407–417
29. Kabbani MD, Raghuveer TS (2004) Craniosynostosis. Am Fam Physician 69:2863–2870
30. Kane AA, Mitchell LE, Craven KP, Marsh JL (1996) Observations on a recent increase in plagiocephaly without synostosis. Pediatrics 97:877–885
31. Lajeunie E, Le Merrer M, Bonaiti-Pellie C, Marchac D, Renier D (1995) Genetic study of nonsyndromic coronal craniosynostosis. Am J Med Genet 55:500–504

32. Lajeunie E, Le Merrer M, Bonaiti-Pellie C, Marchac D, Renier D (1996) Genetic study of scaphocephaly. Am J Med Genet 62:282–285

33. Lane LC (1892) Pioneer craniectomy for relief of mental imbecility due to premature sutural closure and microcephalus. J Am Med Assoc 18:49–50

34. Lannelongue M (1890) De la craniectomie dans la microcephalie. C R Seances Acad Sci 110:1382–1385

35. Lemire LJ (1986) Embryology of the skull. In: Cohen MM (ed) Craniosynostosis. Diagnosis, Evaluation and Management. Raven, New York pp 105–130

36. Littlefield TR, Reiff JL, Rekate HL (2001) Diagnosis and management of deformational plagiocephaly. BNI Q 17:18–25

37. Mabutt LW, Kokick VG (1979) Calvarial and suture development following craniectomy in neonatal rabbit. Anatomy 129:413–422

38. McCarthy JG, Bradley JP, Stelnicki EJ, Stokes T, Weiner HL (2002) Hung span method of scaphocephaly reconstruction in patients with elevated intracranial pressure. *Plast Reconstr Surg* 109:2009–2018

39. McCarthy JG, Glasberg SB, Cutting CB, Epstein FJ, Grayson BH, Ruff G, Thorne CH, Wisoff Z, Zide BM (1995) Twenty year experience with early surgery for craniosynostosis. I. Isolated craniofacial synostosis – results and unsolved problems. Plast Reconstr Surg 96:272–284

40. McCarthy JG, LaTrenta GS, Breitbart AS (1990) The Lefort III advancement osteotomy in the child under 7 years of age. Plast Reconstr Surg 86:633

41. Mooney MP, Siegel MI (2002) Understanding Craniofacial Anomalies. Wiley-Liss, New York

42. O'Daniel TC, Milder BO, Marsh JL (1993) Ophthalmologic screening of infants with craniosynostosis. Scientific Program of the American Cleft Palate-Craniofacial Association, 50th Anniversary Meeting, April 12–24, Pittsburgh, PA, 1993

43. Ohman JC, Richtsmeier JT (1994) Perspectives on craniosynostosis facial growth. Clin Plast Surg 21:489–499

44. Panchal J, Uttchin V (2004) Management of craniosynostosis. Plast Reconstr Surg 111:2032–2048

45. Pritchard JJ, Scott JH, Girgis F (1956) The structure and development of cranial and facial sutures. J Anat 90:73–86

46. Rekate HL (1998) Occipital plagiocephaly: a critical review of the literature. J Neurosurg 89:24–30

47. Renier D (1989) Intracranial pressure in craniosynostosis: pre- and postoperative recordings: correlation with functional results. In: Persing JA, Edgerton MT (eds) Scientific Foundations and Surgical Treatment of Craniosynostosis. Williams Wilkins, Baltimore, pp 263

48. Renier D, Brunet L, Marchac D (1987) IQ and craniostenosis: evolution in treated and untreated cases. In: Marchac D (ed) Craniofacial Surgery. Springer-Verlag, Berlin, pp 114

49. Renier D, Sainte-Rose C, Marchac D, Hirsch JF (1982) Intracranial pressure in craniostenosis. J Neurosurg 57:370–377

50. Richard ME (1994) Common pediatric craniofacial reconstructions. Nurs Clin North Am 29:791–799

51. Ridgeway EB, Weiner HL (2004) Skull deformities. Pediatr Clin North Am 51:359–387

52. Rossi M, Jones RL, Norbury G, Bloch-Zupan A, Winter RM (2003) The appearance of the feet in Pfeiffer syndrome caused by FGFR1 P252R mutation. Clin Dysmorphol 12:269–274

53. Shillito J, Matson DD (1968) Craniosynostosis: a review of 519 surgical patients. Pediatrics 41:829–853

54. Sömmering ST (1800) Vom Baue des Menschlichen Körpers, 1st edn. Voss, Leipzig, Germany

55. Sun PP, Persing JA (1999) Craniosynostosis. In: Albright L, Pollack I, Adelson D (eds) Principles and Practice of Pediatric Neurosurgery. Thieme, New York, pp 219–242

56. Vander Kolk C, Carson B (1994) Lambdoid synostosis. Clin Plast Surg 21:575–584

57. Vermeij-Keers C (1990) Craniofacial embryology and morphogenesis: normal and abnormal. In: Strickler M, van der Meulen J, Rapheal B, et al (eds) Craniofacial Malformations. Churchill Livingstone, New York, pp 56–57

58. Virchow R (1851) Uber den cretinism, namentlich in franken und-ber pathologische schadelformen. Verh Phys Med Ges Wurzburg 2:230–244

59. Warschausky S, Angobaldo J, Kewman D, Buchman S, Muraszko K, Azengart A (2005) Early development of infants with untreated metopic craniosynostosis. Plast Reconstr Surg 15:1518–1523

# Neural Tube Defects

**4**

*Shona S. Lenss*

## Contents

## Introduction

Neural tube defects are a common birth defect, with an incidence rate in the United States of 1 in 1000 live births [1,9,11,29]. They are caused by abnormal embryological formation of the neural tube during the early weeks of pregnancy. Clinical outcomes are dependent on the characteristics of the defect; whether it is open or closed, the anatomic level and if there are associated brain abnormalities. The clinical deficit can range from a mild to severe disability or paralysis, and possibly death. There are several terms used to describe the open or closed forms of a neural tube defect (Table 4.1).

## Etiology

Both genetic and environmental factors play a role in the etiology of neural tube defects. The genetic role may involve mutations in genes that contribute to an abnormal or lack of closure of the neural tube. Clinical studies have shown that families with a known history of a neural tube defect are at a 2–5% higher risk for a recurrence, which is a 25–50 times higher

**Table 4.1.** What is in a name? The different terms applied to neural tube defects

| Open defect | Closed defect |
|---|---|
| Myelomeningocele | Occult spinal dysraphism |
| Spina bifida | Spina bifida occulta |
| Spina bifida aperta | Tethered cord syndrome |
| Spina bifida cystica | Spinal dysraphism[a] |
| Spinal dysraphism[a] | |

[a]Spinal dysraphism is a nonspecific term applied to both forms of neural tube defect

prevalence than in that of the general population [9,10]. Neural tube defects have also been linked to various genetic syndromes including Meckel syndrome, trisomies 13, 18, and 21, and other chromosomal abnormalities or deletion [9].

The environmental risk factors associated with neural tube defects are maternal health risk factors, medication use, and nutrition. There is a relationship between neural tube defects and disorders that affect metabolism of glucose, such as maternal diabetes and maternal obesity [9]. There is an increased incidence of spina bifida with prenatal use of antiepileptic medications (e.g., carbamazepine). Although rare, exposure to other teratogens, including thalidomide and Agent Orange may increase the risk for a neural tube defect [9].

Folic acid, a B vitamin, has shown the strongest link with the reduction of neural tube defects. Research has shown that prenatal folic acid use can decrease the prevalence of open neural tube defects by 50–70% [1,4,9]. Folate is the natural form of folic acid and is found in green leafy vegetables, beans, liver, and citrus fruits. It is not absorbed at a 100% ratio of the food that is ingested, therefore prenatal vitamin supplementation is recommended. Folic acid is a water-soluble synthetic compound that is used in vitamin supplements and fortified foods. The Centers for Disease Control and Prevention and the United States Public Health Service recommend that all women of childbearing age who are capable of becoming pregnant should take 400 µg of folic acid daily, whether or not they are planning a pregnancy. Women who have had a previous pregnancy or a family history of a neural tube defect should take 4000 µg of folic acid daily (Table 4.2) [1,4]. These recommendations are extremely important because the neural tube develops by gestational day 28, often before a woman discovers that she is pregnant. Further, approximately 50% of pregnancies in the United States are unplanned [1,12,24]. In January

1998, the United States Food and Drug Administration mandated food manufacturers to fortify certain grain products with folic acid [1,13]. Foods enriched with folic acid include breads, breakfast cereals, and pasta. Although the use of folic acid greatly reduces the risk of a neural tube defect, it does not eliminate the risk altogether. Nurses working with women who are capable of pregnancy can be highly effective in the education of folic acid supplementation.

## Epidemiology

Collectively, birth defects are the leading cause of death in infants under 1 year of age [9] and account for up to 21% of all infant deaths in the United States [22]. Neural tube defects are the second leading birth defect that can result in devastating outcomes in infants and children. In the United States, females are affected at a 2:1 higher ratio than males, Caucasians are diagnosed more often than other races and there is a higher incidence in the eastern states than in the western states [33]. Fortunately, the overall incidence of neural tube defects in the United States has steadily declined during the past few decades. This may be subsequent to an increased awareness of folic acid supplementation and prenatal diagnosis with elective termination of pregnancy. Prior to 1980, the incidence of neural tube defects in the United States was 1–2 per 1000 live births [18] and decreased further to 0.6 per 1000 live births in 1989 [33]. Many ongoing studies reporting incidence are specific to geographic location and cite ratios lower than 1 per 1000 [15,27,33], although most studies seem to cite the average ratio of 1 per 1000 live births.

## Pathophysiology

Neurulation is the embryologic formation of the neural plate, neural folds, and neural tube (Table 4.3). The neural tube is the cellular structure that later differentiates into the brain and spinal cord (Fig. 4.1). This process of human embryonic development occurs in 23 stages, each stage lasting 2–3 days. The development of the neural tube is complete by 28 days of gestation. The neural tube is formed by two different processes called primary and secondary neurulation. Primary neurulation begins immediately after fertilization, or day 1 of gestation, and consists of the formation of the neural tube from the rostral (head) to

**Table 4.2.** Folic acid for the prevention of neural tube defects [4]

**0.4 mg daily**
All women capable of becoming pregnant should take 0.4 mg (400 µg) of folic acid daily

**4.0 mg daily**
All women who have a family history of neural tube defect or have had a previous pregnancy affected by a neural tube defect should take 4.0 mg (4000 µg) of folic acid daily. *This is ten times the usual dose and must be prescribed by a qualified practitioner*

**Table 4.3.** Terminology

| |
|---|
| **Ectoderm** – the outer layer of cells in the developing embryo |
| **Neural crest** – a band of cells in the ectoderm at the margins of the neural tube that form into the cranial and spinal ganglia |
| **Neural fold** – one or two longitudinal elevations of the neural plate of an embryo that unite to form the neural tube |
| **Neural groove** – a narrow midline groove in the neural tube |
| **Neuropore** – an opening of the neural tube |
| **Neural plate** – a dorsal thickening of ectoderm in the developing embryo that develops into the nervous system |
| **Neural tube defect** – a defect in the embryologic development of the anterior or posterior neuropore during neural tube formation |

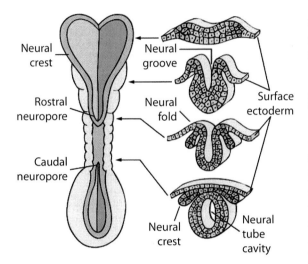

**Fig. 4.1.** Neural tube at the end of the 3rd week. Neural folds have begun to fold at the level of the future spinal cord. *Right* Cross sections of the neural tube at four different levels. The total length of the neural tube at this time is about 2.5 mm. Printed with permission from Padgett (2002) [23]

the caudal (bottom) neuropore, which forms into the brain and most of the spinal cord [24]. Secondary neurulation is the process by which the caudal end of the neural tube develops into the lower sacral and coccygeal segments (part of the conus medullaris or end of the spinal cord) [24]. The development of the neural tube begins at around 17–19 days of gestation with dorsal thickening of the ectoderm, forming into the neural plate. During days 19–21, the neural plate unfolds and forms a neural groove, and neural folds begin to develop laterally. During days 21–23, the neural folds continue to grow to the midline, which allows closure of the tube. The neural folds develop into a rostral neuropore and a caudal neuropore. Finally, the closure of the neural tube takes place over 4–6 days. Traditionally, researchers thought that the neural tube closed in the midline cervical area and then closure extended up and down. More recently,

evidence seems to indicate that the neural tube closes at several points simultaneously and then extends to the rostral and caudal ends to complete the closure.

## Myelomeningocele (Open Defect)

An open neural tube defect is a complex neurological defect of the central nervous system that results in permanent and sometimes severe disabilities. This defect is the result of a deficiency in primary neurulation. The spinal column does not fuse together, allowing outward growth of the spinal contents including cerebral spinal fluid (CSF), spinal cord, and nerves lined with meninges and sometimes skin (Fig. 4.2). An open defect in the spine is called a myelomeningocele (Fig. 4.3), and the disease process is spina bifida. The defect can occur anywhere in the spinal column, with 85% in the lumbosacral spine, 10% in the thoracic spine, and 5% in the cervical spine [5]. Finally, there is an open defect that involves the brain. Anencephaly is the most serious neural tube defect, where part or both cerebral hemispheres of the brain are absent, and are not covered by skull. The infant can have an intact brainstem, which can allow vital functions to continue for a short period, although these infants are often stillborn or die within days after birth.

The prognosis of a myelomeningocele is highly dependent on the size and location of the spinal defect and on the severity of its co-morbidities, which include hydrocephalus and Chiari II malformation. The most common clinical complications are paralysis, hydrocephalus, and bowel and bladder incontinence. The survival rate of spina bifida has increased with advanced and more aggressive surgical intervention. Historically, dating back to the 1960s, infants born with spina bifida were managed conservatively without surgery. Many infants who were not surgically treated died from perinatal problems, hydrocephalus

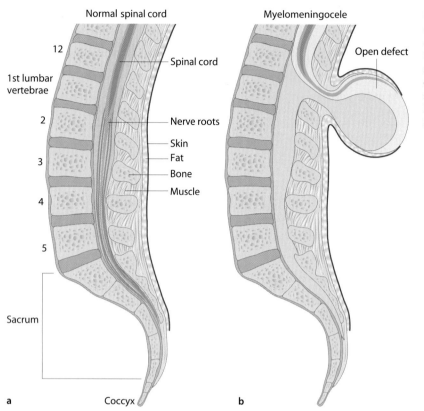

Fig. 4.2 a, b.  Normal spinal cord and myelomeningocele. **a** Anatomic diagram showing the normal anatomy of the spine and spinal cord. **b** A myelomeningocele defect. Printed with permission from University of Wisconsin Hospitals and clinics authority, Madison, WI, USA

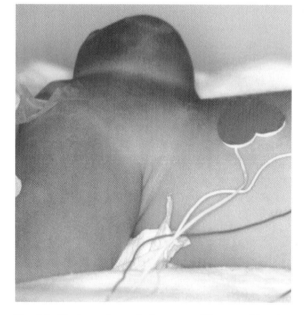

**Fig. 4.3.** Myelomeningocele (courtesy of Bermans Iskandar, Director of Pediatric Neurosurgery, University of Wisconsin, Madison, WI, USA)

or infection. A study by Laurence in South Wales evaluated children born between 1956 and 1962 that were not surgically treated and found that 11% of the children survived to 10–16 years old [19]. Although this is a high rate of mortality, demonstrating the natural progression of untreated myelomeningocele, the percentage of survival gave thought to more aggressive treatment. Throughout the 1960s, continued research showed a substantially higher rate of survival for infants who had immediate surgical repair of the myelomeningocele and surgical treatment of hydrocephalus [24]. Ames and Shut (1972) evaluated 171 patients with myelomeningocele who were treated surgically between 1963 and 1968. They found the survival rate continued to improve, climbing to 50–80% for children 3–8 years old [2]. Later, in the 1970s and 1980s, the trend for aggressive and immediate surgical intervention continued, and has become the current standard of care.

Today, we understand that although many of these infants are born with significant neurological deficits, many have normal intelligence and the capability to enjoy a productive and fulfilling life. Major factors that affect long-term clinical outcomes are intelligence quotient (IQ), ambulatory function, degree of bowel and bladder function, the presence of hydrocephalus, or the presence of a symptomatic Chiari II

Fig. 4.4 a–d. Mobility devices.
a Solid ankle foot orthosis.
b Lofstrand crutches. c Posterior
walker. d Fixed frame light-
weight manual wheelchair.
(Courtesy of Jim Miedaner,
University of Wisconsin Hospital
and Clinics, Rehabilitation Clinics, Madison, WI, USA)

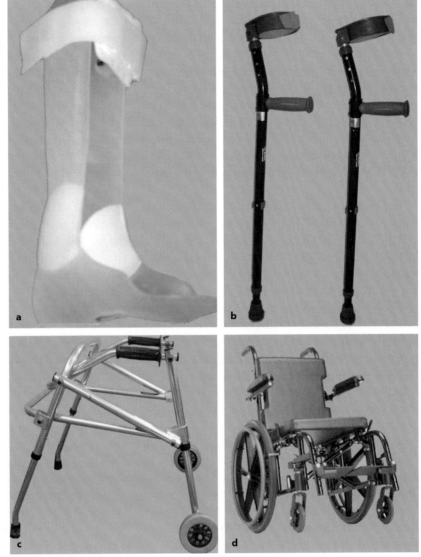

malformation. Intellectual ability is strongly influenced by the presence and severity of hydrocephalus,
level of the defect and associated handicap, and a history of having central nervous system infection (e.g.,
meningitis). It is known that with a lower level defect
there is less motor deficit (handicap) and higher intellectual capability. The ability to ambulate is directly
correlated to the anatomic level of the spinal defect
and subsequent neurological deficit. Children with a
lower spinal defect have a greater chance of ambulating. Approximately 95% of children with lower lumbar or sacral level defects can achieve walking, with
or without assistive devices [28]. The ability to ambulate ranges from independent walking, or requiring
assistive mobility devices (orthotic braces, crutches or

walker), to complete dependence on a wheelchair
(Fig. 4.4). Bowel and bladder dysfunction is a notable
determinant of social acceptance. Some patients may
be incontinent of bowel and bladder, while others can
achieve "social continence."

## Comorbidities of Myelomeningocele

## Hydrocephalus

Hydrocephalus is commonly known as "water on the
brain" and is the build up of CSF inside the ventricles
of the brain, causing increased intracranial pressure
(ICP). Hydrocephalus can be diagnosed prenatally
with an ultrasound or fetal magnetic resonance im-

age (MRI) to determine the presence and severity measured by the size of the ventricles in the fetus. Coniglio et al. (1997) have hypothesized that moderate to severe ventriculomegaly determined by a prenatal high-resolution ultrasound shows a correlation to an overall lower cognitive development quotient [7]. The researchers, however, recognized the need for further research of this hypothesis [7]. Clinically, it is noted that a higher incidence of hydrocephalus occurs with a high-level myelomeningocele lesion, such as those in the thoracic spine, as opposed to those in the sacral spine.

Approximately 90% of infants with spina bifida will require surgical treatment for hydrocephalus, and the majority of infants are shunted within days of birth [21]. Around 25% of infants with a myelomeningocele have obvious signs of hydrocephalus at birth, but the most common time of presentation is at 2–6 weeks after birth [26]. In cases with obvious signs of hydrocephalus at birth, the surgeon may place a shunt at the same time of surgical repair of the myelomeningocele, or within 24–48 h to reduce the risk of a CSF leak or wound breakdown after surgery [21]. In infants who are not shunted, many become symptomatic for hydrocephalus after a myelomeningocele repair due to a build up CSF.

More recent research by Warf (2005) has shown encouraging findings that support the treatment of hydrocephalus from a myelomeningocele with an endoscopic third ventriculostomy (ETV) and choroid plexus cauterization (CPC) [31]. An ETV is a procedure that creates an opening in the floor of the third ventricle to create free-flowing communication between the ventricle system and basal subarachnoid spaces [25]. A CPC is a procedure that destroys the choroid plexus, where CSF is made within the ventricles. The treatment of hydrocephalus from certain pathology with an ETV is not a new concept in neurosurgery and researchers are continuing studies to determine the long-term outcome of it used alone and in combination with CPC for treatment of infants with hydrocephalus related to a myelomeningocele.

### Chiari II Malformation

A Chiari II malformation is a herniation of the posterior fossa structures (cerebellum and medulla) into the spinal canal and is present in nearly all infants with myelomeningoceles. This may be the most serious comorbidity as it increases the mortality risk significantly due to potential depression of respiratory drive, episodic apnea, and bradycardia. It can also cause nystagmus and a lower cranial nerve palsy. Approximately 5–10% of infants become symptomatic from brainstem compression and will present with symptoms of stridor, drooling, increased tone in the arms and legs, or a posturing of the head [26]. Surgical decompression of a Chiari malformation can resolve these symptoms, except when they present immediately after birth, which may indicate irreversible problems from brainstem compromise. The surgery involves removal of part of the upper cervical vertebrae and expansion of the dura overlying the malformation in order to decompress, or make room for the herniating brain. Another complication that can occur with the presence of a Chiari malformation is syringomyelia, which is a fluid filled cyst (syrinx) that expands within the spinal cord causing neurological symptoms.

### Bowel and Bladder Dysfunction

The majority of patients with spina bifida have some degree of bowel and bladder dysfunction. The level of the defect is not always predictive of the degree of dysfunction. More than 90% of infants with a myelomeningocele have a neurogenic bladder [5]. Thus, it is important for the infant to be evaluated by a urologist. The urologist will evaluate the kidneys and the bladder integrity (elasticity and filling capacity). Common urological tests to evaluate these concerns are a renal ultrasound, voiding cystourethrogram and urodynamic bladder studies. Often, early management of the bowel and bladder dysfunction begins with baseline diagnostic testing, and concurrent testing throughout the lifetime to prevent deterioration of the urinary tract, preserve the current level of function and to ultimately decrease the risk of renal damage. Another goal of management for a neurogenic bladder is to provide socially acceptable continence, or "social continence" in the future (Table 4.4). Clean intermittent catheterization several times a day has improved regulation of bladder function and resulted in greater social continence.

### Prenatal Screening for Myelomeningocele

Prenatal screening is helpful in the detection of an open neural tube defect, and is extremely important in planning a timely and safe delivery. Screening and a consequent diagnosis can be determined with a

**Table 4.4.** A parent perspective: bowel and bladder continence

Our son was born with a sacral level myelomeningocele. When others see him, they don't see a child with a disability because he does not have any outward signs of spina bifida. He walks normally and has a shunt, but his biggest struggle is with bowel and bladder continence.

We have tried many things over the past 7 years to achieve bowel and bladder continence. We started catheterizing our son when he was 3½ years old. We were taught how catheterize him during a clinic visit and were sent home with supplies and our memory of what we had learned. After a few difficult weeks, we were on our way to a lifelong routine of catheterizing every 3–4 h. The bowel issues have been extremely difficult. We have tried several types of bowel programs; enemas and drinks that made him gag from the taste or texture. We were diligent and as patient as we could be with each program, but our emotions went up and down as each new promising method failed. After repeated failure to gain control of the bowel continence, we were told about a surgical procedure called the Malone antegrade continence enema (MACE) to help with bowel flushing.

He had the surgery when he was 8 years old. Since the surgery, things have improved, but he still has daily struggles. Every day after our son comes home from school, he has just enough time to do his homework and to eat supper before we begin our daily bowel program. We go to the "cinematography room" (what we call our bathroom), which is equipped with a TV/DVD player that is kept in the bathtub behind the shower curtain. He spends the next hour or more on the toilet while we do the "cleanout" procedure.

Our life revolves around the "cleanouts." He has little time to spend with friends or extracurricular activities, and overnights are almost impossible. We have to plan everything in advance. The stress of his situation is shared by the entire family. It has changed our family routine: Mom quit her job to stay home and tend to medical needs, Dad is the sole financial provider for the family, and his little sister feels left out at times.

We hope this helps medical professionals understand what goes on behind the scenes of a family dealing with ongoing medical needs. When doctors tell us "it's time to try something new," we brace ourselves for the implications this will have on our family life for the weeks to come.

maternal serum alpha-fetoprotein (MSAFP) test, ultrasound, or amniocentesis [7]. The MSAFP is done between 14 and 21 weeks, and is optimal between 16 and 18 weeks of gestation. If this number is higher than the normal value range, it may be an indicator of a possible neural tube defect. This is a screening test, and a normal MSAFP does not completely exclude the possibility of a myelomeningocele. An ultrasound is done between 15 weeks and up to the end of pregnancy for the assessment of the fetal age and general anatomy of the brain and spine [8]. If a neural tube defect is found, the patient is referred to a perinatologist for a high-resolution ultrasound and possible amniocentesis. Some medical facilities have the capability to do an MRI of the mother's abdomen to view the fetus (fetal MRI), which shows greater detail of anatomy and severity of hydrocephalus (Fig. 4.5). Fetal blood sampling and chorionic villus sampling are not useful in the determination of an open neural tube defects.

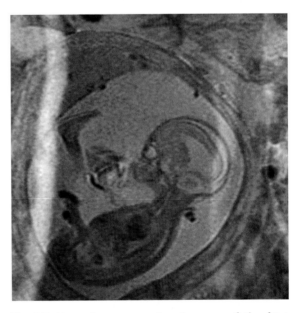

**Fig. 4.5.** Magnetic resonance imaging scan of the fetus showing ventriculomegaly (courtesy of Bermans Iskandar, Director of Pediatric Neurosurgery, University of Wisconsin, Madison, WI, USA)

## Management

### Medical Management

In many cases, an infant with a myelomeningocele is delivered by a planned cesarean section to minimize trauma to the defect during delivery. The infant is immediately assessed by neonatologists, neurosurgeons, and nurses. It is important to measure the head circumference (plot on growth chart) and palpate the fontanel (is it soft or tense) to detect immediate signs of hydrocephalus. A cranial ultrasound can be helpful to determine a baseline assessment of ventricle size, although a computed tomography (CT) or MRI scan will offer a more detailed assessment of the severity of hydrocephalus. A thorough neurological exam is done, the defect is carefully examined, and the spine is assessed for abnormal curvature. The myelomeningocele may appear as an obvious bubble that sits midline somewhere on the spine, filled with CSF, spinal cord, and nerves, with a membranous covering. It can also appear with a ruptured membrane or as an open defect with no membrane covering. Motor function is assessed by observing upper and lower extremities for spontaneous active movements, symmetry, and muscle bulk and tone. The sensory level is evaluated in the trunk and lower extremities. A thorough preoperative examination and appropriate diagnostic testing of medical abnormalities is important to ensure the best possible circumstance prior to surgery.

### Surgical Management

For a period of time, there was hope that fetal surgery would be beneficial for early treatment of myelomeningocele to decrease the devastation of the disease process (Table 4.5). In the past, doctors had observed the affected fetus by ultrasound and thought the leg and feet motion decreased throughout the pregnancy, lending to the idea of ongoing damage to the exposed spinal cord. As a result, prenatal surgery was developed. In 1994, doctors began doing myelomeningocele closure on the fetus while still in the mother's womb. Despite improvements in the surgical technique and positive outcomes, over time, surgeons were concerned about the benefits of surgery versus serious risk factors to the mother and fetus. It was observed, however, that prenatal repair was associated with a decreased incidence of hydrocephalus and Chiari II malformations. Later, in 2003, the National Institute of Child Health and Human Development and the National Institutes of Health began a 5-year study to determine whether prenatal surgery is more effective in comparison to the traditional surgery at birth [30]. The study is called the Management of Myelomeningocele Study. Pregnant mothers who have a fetus with a known myelomeningocele may elect to be a part of the study. The study is randomized. One-half of participants will be selected to have the prenatal surgery, and are required to stay near one of the designated medical centers from the time of prenatal surgery until delivery of the baby. The other half will stay at home during the remainder of the pregnancy and then return to one of the designated medical centers for delivery. Both groups will undergo a planned cesarean section delivery at 37 weeks gestation. The prenatal and postnatal surgeries are done by a team of neurosurgeons at one of three designated medical centers: the University of California at San Francisco in San Francisco, California, the Children's Hospital of Philadelphia in Philadelphia, Pennsylvania, and Vanderbilt University Medical Center in Nashville, Tennessee. The study is approximately half-completed; no preliminary data are available.

For now, postnatal surgery is the standard of care. Closure of the myelomeningocele is optimally done by a pediatric neurosurgeon, within the first postnatal day and at the latest by 72 h of life. Delay in surgical treatment can increase both morbidity and mortality because of the increased risk of meningitis. The goals of surgery are to close the defect, prevent infection, eliminate a CSF leak, and preserve neurological function. For a surgical repair of a myelomeningocele, the infant is placed in the prone position. The surgeon will open the sac, close the neural structures, and then close the dura, fascia, subcutaneous tissues, and finally, the skin.

### Nursing Considerations

The birth of a child with a chronic and debilitating disease is a time of high anxiety, and nurses can play a vital role in making this a more positive experience for the parents and extended family members. The family is at the start of an event that will bring a pattern of change to their role as parents and in the dynamics within their family. Nurses have a dual responsibility in caring for a patient with special medical needs: the first is to provide quality nursing care to the patient, and the second is to care for the emotional needs of the family (Table 4.6). It is important

**Table 4.5.** A parent perspective: an unexpected journey

After settling my three small boys for the night, I was beyond my typical nervous laughter when I told my husband that we were expecting our fourth child. I was definitely surprised and cautiously guarded as I wondered how I was going to manage four children under the age of 5 years. Nothing seemed out of the ordinary, until the day of my scheduled ultrasound. We learned that our baby had spina bifida. We were told of our options: to continue or to terminate the pregnancy. After sharing our strong desire to continue the pregnancy, we were told about maternal-fetal surgery. Initially, we were not interested because of the risks involved, but after learning more about some of the promising medical outcomes and the reduced need for a shunt to treat hydrocephalus, we decided to learn more about how the risks outweighed the benefits. We traveled over 1,000 miles away to a center where it was done.

After an agonizing 3-day consultation and medical tests, we decided to undergo the surgery, at 24 weeks gestation. We hoped that we made a good decision to improve the quality of life for our unborn child. Four days after the surgery as I was flying back home, my thoughts turned to my other children as I looked down at the Terbutaline pump flowing medicine into my body to keep me from going into premature labor. Our commitment to surgery required many volunteers, friends, and family to keep things going at home. It seemed to be going alright, but what came later tested my strength and endurance.

My unborn son was doing fairly well until around the 28th week of gestation when I started losing amniotic fluid internally from a tear in my uterus at the surgical site. I was hospitalized until my son's delivery at 34 weeks gestation. When he was born his lungs were underdeveloped and he was immediately placed on a ventilator. He was hospitalized for 3 weeks and sent home on oxygen and oral tube feedings. Ironically, I had met another family during my pregnancy and they too were expecting a son with spina bifida. He was born a day later than my son, by a planned C-section with surgery scheduled immediately after birth. It was hard not to compare our babies. I thought about how fetal surgery had impacted our situation. While their baby had the typicalclosure at birth and was discharged from the hospital a few days later, my son was still in the neonatal ICU on a ventilator and very sick from prematurity.

Both my son and I had multiple complications as a result of the fetal surgery and it was one of the most challenging experiences I have gone through. I am glad we had the option of surgery, but my husband and I still wonder if this was the best decision, especially since he ended up requiring a shunt for hydrocephalus. It was difficult to come to terms with having a child with spina bifida. And it was more difficult with the added stressors of having gone through a prenatal surgery, a complicated recovery, premature delivery, and our son's ongoing medical issues.

Our son is 4 years old now and he is doing great and making progress by leaps and bounds. When I look at him, it is hard to believe that he had so many challenges early on in his life.

to assess the family's ability to cope with their stress and emotions; naturally they may feel overwhelmed or in a state of shock. Finally, nurses should listen empathetically as they offer support and reassurance throughout the process of educating the family.

### Preoperative Care

As nurses care for families who have a newborn with a myelomeningocele, it is important to assess the parents' current level of understanding of the disease and their ability or willingness to learn. Although many parents have had time to prepare for the birth if the diagnosis was made through prenatal testing, others may have learned about the diagnosis for the first time after delivery. Obviously, in both instances this is a stressful and overwhelming time for the family. It is important to educate the family about what to expect during the first hours of their baby's life. Initially,

the infant will be examined by many professionals to determine the presence of other associated abnormalities such as genetic disorders, and cardiac, urologic, or orthopedic problems. Routine medical care of the infant prior to surgery may include the following: (1) cover the myelomeningocele defect with a sterile-saline-soaked dressing to avoid drying out, (2) place the infant in a prone or lateral recumbent position until surgery, (3) withhold oral feedings to maintain an "aseptic bowel" thereby decreasing the risk of infection to the open defect, (4) administer intravenous antibiotics if ordered by the surgeon, and (5) administer intravenous fluids in lieu of no oral intake until after surgery. Nurses can help a new mother understand that impending surgery should not be a deterrent to breastfeeding. If the mother is interested in breast feeding, nurses or a lactation consultant can help to initiate pumping and storing of milk until the

**Table 4.6.** A parent perspective: a myelo-what?

My second pregnancy seemed to be going along without complications. The triplescreen was negative and I had three ultrasounds, ordered by my physician; the first to confirm a due date, the second for routine screening at 20 weeks gestation, and a third late in pregnancy to evaluate amniotic fluid: they were all "normal"! The day my daughter was born was the day we learned that she had spina bifida.

After a short, but difficult delivery, the medical staff whisked away a somewhat "purple" – looking newborn to the next room with my husband following behind. After several moments of silent panic, I sighed in relief as I heard her cry for the first time. "Thank You, God" I remember mumbling as the doctor worked to repair the trauma my body had endured. Several more minutes passed before a very calm and reassuring female neonatologist approached my bedside to inform me that my daughter had a lesion on her backed called a myelomeningocele. "A myelo-what?", I thought to myself. She explained that my daughter would need surgery to repair the lesion as soon as possible. They gave me a quick peek at my daughter and then they took her to neonatal intensive care to prepare her for surgery.

My husband and I sat together in a quiet hospital room. He tried to explain what the surgeon had told him about the surgery and complications of hydrocephalus and the possibility of needing a shunt. The staff gave us a book and some other literature to read as we waited for her to get out of surgery. I hadn't even held my daughter and here I was, looking at lifeless diagrams and words that would affect the rest of our lives. Although we knew this was important information, nobody wants their child defined by a book or pamphlet. We didn't need to know that this happens 1 in every 1000 births. When it comes to any newborn, it is more important for medical professionals to remember that the "human connection" needs to come first. What we needed, right then, was to know that our daughter was going to be OK. We didn't need a book to tell us who our daughter was. We knew that she would show us who she is and that each detail would emerge in its own order, not like a book divided neatly into chapters.

From our experience, we believe that medical professionals should pass on information with great compassion. Preface the information with the fact that all cases are based on the individual and the unique characteristics of the type of myelomeningocele they have. Shortly after birth, we told our pediatrician that "She is going to write her own book, the story of her life, and spina bifida will only be part of it." Now 5 years old, each day we learn that our daughter has defied many of the "statistics" that we first read about.

---

baby can be put to breast. Finally, educate parents about the surgery, anesthesia care, and what to expect for the immediate recovery.

Patients with spina bifida are at high risk for developing a latex sensitivity or allergy. The natural history of a latex allergy is not well understood. It is believed that an allergy or sensitivity to latex develops from repeated exposure in the hospital environment and from multiple surgeries, particularly when latex comes into contact with mucous membranes (e.g., the urinary catheter). Latex is a form of rubber derived from a plant source, the *Hevea brasiliensis* tree. Latex is found in many medical and home supplies (Table 4.7). Latex reactions vary from mild contact dermatitis to anaphylactic shock or death [20]. Children with a known sensitivity can be treated preoperatively with antihistamines and epinephrine.

### Postoperative Care

It is important to have a well organized discharge plan in mind as you care for the infant and family for the remainder of the hospitalization. Nursing education is best achieved by the use of a variety of teaching modalities; written materials, verbal instruction, and demonstration as you prepare a family for discharge. Routine postoperative care of the infant after surgery may include the following: (1) place the infant in a prone or side lying position for up to 3 days (or per the surgeon's preference) to minimize the risk of CSF leaking or wound compromise, (2) cover the incision with a dressing to protect the wound from soiling of urine and feces (Fig. 4.6), (3) administer intravenous antibiotics (per surgeon preference) to minimize risk of infection, and (4) administer intravenous fluids for the first 24 h or until the infant is breastfeeding or taking oral feedings well.

Beyond the initial postoperative period, it is important to educate the family about care of the infant at home so they feel more confident transitioning out of the hospital. The family is instructed to monitor for signs of progressive hydrocephalus and for signs and symptoms of infection including fever or wound changes of drainage, swelling or redness. Signs or symptoms of hydrocephalus include fullness of the

**Table 4.7.** Latex products

| Patient care items and mechanical equipment | Home and community items | Anesthesia equipment |
|---|---|---|
| Adhesive tape | Baby bottle nipples | Ambu bags |
| Bandages | Elastic on diapers and clothes | Airway mask |
| Blood pressure cuffs, tubing, and bladders | Pacifiers | Nasal airway |
| Catheters (gastric, urinary) | Many toys and balloons | Anesthesia bags and tubing |
| Catheter leg bag straps | | |
| Dental equipment (dental dams, bite blocks) | Avoid bananas, avocados, kiwi fruit, raw potatoes, tomatoes, chestnuts (latex-sensitive individuals can have a cross-sensitivity to foods that contain the polypeptides found in latex) | |
| Electrocardiogram pads | | |
| Medication vial ports, intravenous injection ports, syringe plunger tips | | |
| Stethoscopes | Condoms | |
| Rubber gloves | | |

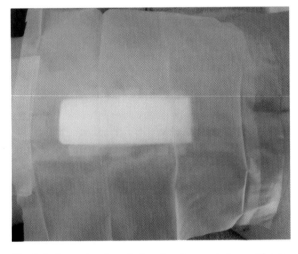

**Fig. 4.6.** Example of occlusive dressing and drape. The incision is covered by a 4×4 gauze and occlusive dressing. A plastic drape is secured to the top of the buttocks and draped over the back and torso to avoid soiling from the diaper (courtesy of Bermans Iskandar, Director of Pediatric Neurosurgery, University of Wisconsin, Madison, WI, USA)

fontanel, irritability, decreased interest in feedings, lethargy, or projectile vomiting. Daily measurement of head circumference is useful to detect rapid head growth. It is equally important to observe the infant for symptoms indicative of a problem from the Chiari malformation including abnormal breathing, such as stridor or apnea. It is important that families are informed to contact the medical team immediately with

concerns of progressive hydrocephalus or breathing difficulties.

Finally, a multidisciplinary care approach is vital for the long-term management of the complex medical needs of a child with spina bifida. The medical team often consists of a neurosurgeon, orthopedic surgeon, rehabilitation specialist, urologist, nurses or nurse practitioners, physical/occupational therapist, and a psychologist. Sometimes, collaborative care with neurology and endocrine specialists is required. This approach to healthcare is essential to offer each child the greatest potential to lead a healthy and productive life.

## ■ Spina Bifida Occulta (Closed Defect)

A closed neural tube defect is a less devastating neurological defect of the central nervous system, but can result in progressive and possibly permanent neurological deficits. This defect is the result of a deficiency in primary and secondary neurulation. It occurs later in embryologic development, causing abnormal formation of the spine from failure of the vertebral lamina to fuse together properly. The abnormal development of the neural tube and abnormal fusion of the bony vertebrae allows ingrowth of tissues, such as fat or skin, which creates abnormal attachment or tethering of the spinal cord (Fig. 4.7). The closed defect is called spina bifida occulta or occult spinal dysra-

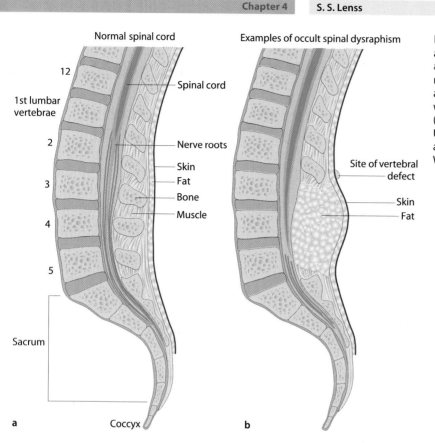

Normal spinal cord

12
1st lumbar vertebrae
2
3
4
5

Sacrum

a    Coccyx

Spinal cord
Nerve roots
Skin
Fat
Bone
Muscle

Examples of occult spinal dysraphism

b

Site of vertebral defect
Skin
Fat

**Fig. 4.7 a, b.** Normal spinal cord and occult spinal dysraphism. **a** Anatomic diagram showing normal anatomy of the spine and spinal cord. **b** Spinal cord with closed neural tube defect (printed with permission from the University of Wisconsin Hospitals and clinics authority, Madison, WI, USA)

phism (OSD), which occurs predominantly in the lumbosacral spine [32]. There are a spectrum of clinical abnormalities of OSD, and each have a different clinical presentation.

These abnormalities include a lipoma or lipomyelomeningocele, dermal sinus tract, split cord malformation (diastematomyelia or diplomyelia), dermoid cysts and tumors, meningocele manque, or a tight filum terminale. All forms of OSD result in a tethered spinal cord. A tethered spinal cord is characterized by a spinal cord that is positioned abnormally low in the spinal canal because it is attached or anchored to the surrounding structures. The prognosis of a tethered cord is good when it is diagnosed and surgically treated before neurological deficits occur.

■ **Clinical Presentation**

Unlike the open defect, the clinical presentation of OSD is variable. In the majority of patients signs are obvious on examination, but in some cases there are no signs until symptoms occur. Normally, the end of the spinal cord (conus medullaris) floats freely in the

spinal column. At birth, the conus is located at vertebral level L3 and ascends to its normal position of vertebral level L1 by 3 months of age. In a child with OSD, the spinal cord is tethered caudally and natural linear growth causes progressive tension and stretching of the spinal cord. This causes decreased local blood flow, or ischemia to the nerve cells, thereby causing overt symptoms. The common presentation of signs and symptoms are a skin lesion, pain or weakness of the legs, back pain, change in bowel or bladder control, or orthopedic problems such as scoliosis. The majority of patients diagnosed with a tethered cord will present with one or more of the six characteristic skin lesions of OSD (Table 4.8). These are a hemangi-

**Table 4.8.** Cutaneous stigmata of spina bifida occulta

| |
|---|
| Hemangioma |
| Hypertrichosis (tuft of hair) |
| Atretic meningocele (cigarette burn) |
| Dermal sinus tract |
| Lipoma |
| Caudal appendage |

oma, hypertrichosis, atretic meningocele, dermal sinus opening, subcutaneous lipoma, or a caudal appendage. Other medical problems that have an association with tethered spinal cord are imperforate anus, cloacal exstrophy, and history of previous spinal surgery. Previous spinal surgery, such as myelomeningocele repair, causes scar tissue and subsequent risk of retethering of the spinal cord. The incidence for a patient with a myelomeningocele to retether at some point in their lifetime is 15–20% [11].

## Cutaneous Anomalies of OSD

One or more of the six characteristic cutaneous lesions occur in up to 70% of patients diagnosed with a tethered spinal cord [6]. All midline lesions on the spine are clinically significant for a possible tethered cord, making it important to distinguish between abnormal and benign skin markings. All the skin lesions described in the section to follow are clinically significant for OSD when observed on the back and located in the midline lumbosacral spine.

A hemangioma is a flat or raised, pink or red skin lesion that consists of capillary vessels (Fig. 4.8). The examiner needs to distinguish differences between common skin finding and a true hemangioma. For example, infants commonly have a nevus at the base of the skull called a "stork bite", which is benign. A Mongolian spot (a pigmented black or blue spot) or a nevus (pigmented circumscribed area on skin) may be found in the lumbosacral region and have no clinical significance for OSD.

Hypertrichosis is a localized patch or tuft of hair (Fig. 4.9). Hair that is localized and sometimes diffuse is "baby" hair that dissipates over the first months of life and is not indicative of OSD. Hypertrichosis is highly correlated to the malformation called diastematomyelia, which is a split or double spinal cord [6].

An atretic meningocele is a skin lesion that looks like a scar and is sometimes called a "cigarette burn" (Fig. 4.10). The skin over this lesion may be sensitive to touch. An atretic meningocele presumably indicates that a meningocele (malformation of the meninges) was once present during fetal life and had partially repaired itself. The lesion can be connected to the spinal cord by a tract of fixed fibrous band that extends from the skin to the spinal cord.

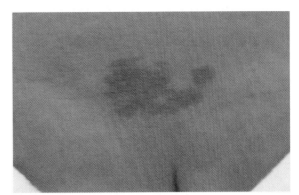

**Fig. 4.8.** Lumbar hemangioma (courtesy of Bermans Iskandar, Director of Pediatric Neurosurgery, University of Wisconsin, Madison, WI, USA)

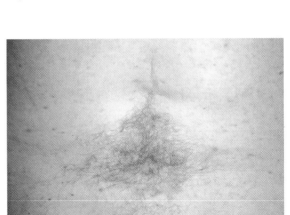

**Fig. 4.9.** Hypertrichosis (courtesy of Bermans Iskandar, Director of Pediatric Neurosurgery, University of Wisconsin, Madison, WI, USA)

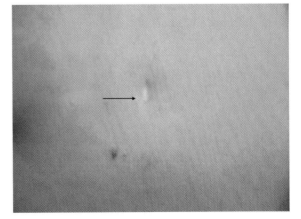

**Fig. 4.10.** Atretic meningocele (courtesy of Bermans Iskandar, Director of Pediatric Neurosurgery, University of Wisconsin, Madison, WI, USA)

A dermal sinus is a small hole or opening in the skin that appears as a dimple in the skin (Fig. 4.11). It is often connected to underlying structures by a subcutaneous tract lined with epithelium, bone, dura, or the spinal cord. A dimple found at the level of the coccyx is not suspicious, and is termed a benign sacrococcygeal dimple (Fig. 4.11).

A lipoma or lipomyelomeningocele is a soft tissue mass that is completely covered with skin (Fig. 4.12). It can grow larger over time as fat grows in proportion to the patient's body weight. A lipoma or lipomyelomeningocele may be an extension of an intramedullary mass within the spinal cord.

A caudal appendage appears as a tail or "pseudotail," which presents as a skin-covered round structure that is attached to the skin of the back (Fig. 4.13). It can be discolored or covered with hair, and sometimes it contains cartilage, fat, or other organ-specific tissues. In contrast, a "true" human tail is the remains of an embryonic structure that may contain vertebrae, spinal cord, notochord, sacral artery and vein, muscle, fat, or connective tissue.

## Orthopedic Findings of OSD

The orthopedic signs of OSD vary and may not be easily identified at birth. In fact, clinical signs or symptoms may not be evident until a child has a growth spurt or is walking. Scoliosis or kyphosis, asymmetry of the legs and feet, or deformities of the feet are signs of OSD. For example, one calf may be thinner and the foot on the same side may be smaller, or have a higher arch or hammering of the toes. Another orthopedic finding is asymmetry of the buttocks, identified by lateral curve of the upper part of the gluteal crease. On examination, evaluate the spine for abnormal curve, and assess soles of the feet for asymmetry, difference in size or arch, unilateral or bilateral club feet, or for the presence of valgus or varus positioning. If the child is walking, evaluate for inversion or forefoot adduction. It is important to identify the underlying cause of orthopedic anomalies and refer to a specialist for further evaluation if appropriate. Finally, vertebral deformities are commonly present with OSD and include anomalies of the laminae, vertebral bodies, disc space, pedicles, or sacrum (sacral agenesis/dysgenesis).

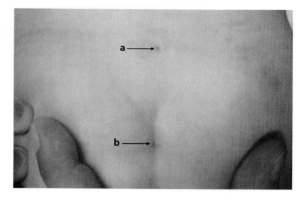

**Fig. 4.11.** Dermal sinus and sacral dimple. **a** Dermal sinus with flat hemangioma. **b** Sacrococcygeal dimple. (courtesy of Bermans Iskandar, Director of Pediatric Neurosurgery, University of Wisconsin, Madison, WI, USA)

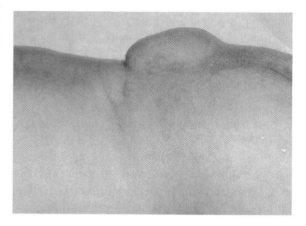

**Fig. 4.12.** Lipomyelomeningocele (courtesy of Bermans Iskandar, Director of Pediatric Neurosurgery, University of Wisconsin, Madison, WI, USA)

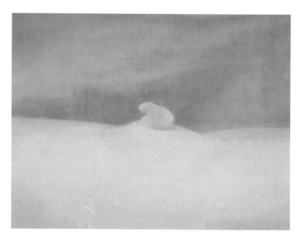

**Fig. 4.13.** Caudal appendage (courtesy of Bermans Iskandar, Director of Pediatric Neurosurgery, University of Wisconsin, Madison, WI, USA)

## Urologic Dysfunction of OSD

Urinary dysfunction may be the first sign of OSD if it has not already been diagnosed from other presenting signs or symptoms. Bladder dysfunction occurs from neurologic injury or defective development of the spinal cord. The overall incidence of urinary problems associated with OSD is not clear. Urinary symptoms may not be evident until a child learns to toilet train. In the presence of OSD, bladder dysfunction can present at anytime throughout life as urgency, urinary retention, or enuresis [28]. Another presenting sign of OSD can be recurrent urinary tract infections.

## Management

### Surgical Management

Surgery is the treatment of choice for OSD to prevent future neurological deterioration or complications from a tethered spinal cord. There is little data in the literature that compares the natural progression of OSD to cases that are treated surgically, due to ethical considerations of conducting such studies. It is known, however, that management without surgery can be associated with neurological deterioration, and that surgical intervention can halt this progression and sometimes improve function. Early surgical treatment is important to prevent permanent neurological deficits, and surgery can be done any time after birth. The surgical procedure is called a tethered cord release, and it releases the spinal cord so that it can hang freely in the spinal column. Often, intraoperative monitoring, called somatosensory evoked potentials, electromyography, and bladder cystometry is done to monitor the bladder, anal sphincter, and nerve conduction to the lower extremities. Overall, the outcome of surgery is positive. There are many research studies that demonstrate a low risk of developing neurological deterioration from the surgery [3,6,16].

### Medical Management

After surgery, the patient is followed by a neurosurgeon and urologist. The urologist monitors bowel and bladder function through the use of diagnostic testing if necessary. The neurosurgeon monitors neurological status through examination and sometimes will order a postoperative MRI of the lumbar sacral spine. Further radiographic imaging is done if there is a return of symptoms suggestive of retethering of the spinal cord. Finally, although rare, if there are chronic problems with lower extremity weakness or difficulties with ambulation, a rehabilitation physician or physiatrist will provide continued medical care.

## Nursing Considerations

The diagnosis of a medical condition is stressful for the patient and family. Nurses can guide families through this process while promoting a positive experience. It is important to provide age-appropriate education to the patient and family about the tethered cord, diagnostic testing, and about referrals, if any, to other specialists. Many parents are concerned about surgery and the possibility of a permanent bowel and bladder deficit or weakness in the lower extremities.

The preoperative nursing care of a patient with OSD is limited. After the diagnosis is made, appropriate referrals and outpatient diagnostic studies are done. A tethered cord is not an emergency and the patient will stay home until surgery is scheduled. Prior to surgery, the patient should avoid repetitive flexion and extension of the spine, or sudden forceful movements of the body. Back or leg pain is managed with oral medications. Many surgeons will withhold nonsteroidal anti-inflammatory drugs for up to 1 week prior to surgery to minimize intraoperative bleeding.

The postoperative care of a patient with a tethered cord is similar to that of a patient with a myelomeningocele (Table 4.9). As with any hospitalized patient, it is important to have a discharge plan in mind as you prepare the patient and family for transition to home. The family is instructed to monitor their child for signs and symptoms of infection including fever or wound changes of drainage, swelling or redness, and to notify medical staff immediately with concerns. After a surgery for tethered cord release, when applicable, the child is to avoid all contact sports for a minimum of 4–6 weeks.

**Table 4.9.** Postoperative care guidelines for tethered cord release. *CSF* Cerebrospinal fluid, *I & O* input and output, *IV* intravenous, *PO* per os

| |
|---|
| Observe for adverse effects from anesthesia (irritability, nausea, vomiting) |
| Assess pain and medicate as needed |
| Obtain frequent vital signs and neurologic checks |
| Keep the head of bed flat for up to 5 days to minimize the risk of CSF leak |
| Log roll every 2 h |
| Apply protective barrier to incision to avoid exposure to stool or urine |
| Observe dressing frequently for discharge; if present observe amount, color and notify surgeon |
| Administer IV hydration until taking PO fluids well |
| Record I & O |
| Foley catheter care if needed |
| Latex precautions (if applicable) |

## Diagnostic Studies for Neural Tube Defects

An ultrasound is a low cost and often readily available tool. It can be used for screening of OSD in newborns before 5–6 months of age; before the posterior elements of the spine are ossified, which obstructs visualization of the spinal cord [14,17]. An ultrasound, however, does not show the detail for complex anatomy of the spine and possibly the complicated spinal cord abnormalities associated with tethered cord. Postnatal ultrasound is not a common diagnostic test for a myelomeningocele.

## Radiographic Imaging

Evaluation with plain radiograph anteroposterior and lateral views of the affected part of the spine can be helpful in determining vertebral anomalies. This is beneficial as an initial screening for OSD, but is not diagnostic for either the open or closed defect.

An MRI is a noninvasive and radiation-free test that is used commonly for screening of spinal anomalies. It shows complete and clear anatomical detail of the spine, spinal cord, filum terminale, fat, tumors, or dermoids. A disadvantage to traditional MRI imaging is that it takes a long time and necessitates sedation of the infant.

A CT scan is an excellent screening tool for detail of bony anatomy. It is used commonly for the diagnosis of hydrocephalus in a patient with a myelomeningocele. A CT scan is quick and does not require sedation; however, there is a small risk of exposure to radiation with each scan.

## Conclusion

Neural tube defects affect thousands of children in the United States each year. Over the past four decades, there have been progressive changes in medical practices and we have observed greater longevity and overall improved quality of life in these patients. A major breakthrough in research has proved that prenatal folic acid use can prevent the incidence of neural tube defects in up to 70% of children. Ongoing research about fetal surgery may not only determine the most promising surgical option for treatment of children with a myelomeningocele, but may also show a positive impact on the severity of comorbidities. Advances in our knowledge of timely treatment and appropriate diagnostic tests for occult spina bifida can decrease the occurrence of long-term neurological deficits. In conclusion, spina bifida and spina bifida occulta can be devastating to the lives of many children. Through the continued research and implementation of evidence-based practice, we can continue to make great strides in the treatment of this potentially devastating neurological disorder.

## Pediatric Practice Pearls

- Become familiar with the multidisciplinary care needs of a patient with spina bifida to better address their educational and emotional needs while providing holistic nursing care.
- Cover the surgical incision with an occlusive dressing and rectangular drape secured to the buttocks under the top of the diaper and drape upwards over the back to avoid soiling from feces and urine.
- Provide timely nursing education through a variety of teaching modes at a time that is right for the family. An overwhelmed parent is less ready to learn. Observe nonverbal cues in order to pace your "teachable moments".

## References

1. AAP Policy Statement Committee on Genetics (1999) American Academy of Pediatrics: folic acid for the prevention of neural tube defects. Pediatrics 104:325–327
2. Ames MD, Shut L (1972) Results of treatment of 171 consecutive myelomeningoceles, 1963 to 1968. Pediatrics 50:466–470
3. Anderson FM (1975) Occult spinal dysraphism. a series of 73 cases. Pediatrics 55:826–835
4. Centers for Disease Control and Prevention (2004) Spina bifida and anencephaly before and after folic acid mandate – United States, 1995–1996 and 1999–2000. MMWR Morb Mort Wkly Rep 53:362–365
5. Cohen AR, Robinson S (2001) Early management of myelomeningocele. In: McLone DG (ed) Pediatric Neurosurgery; Surgery of the Developing Nervous System. WB Saunders, Philadelphia, pp 241–259
6. Coniglio SJ, Anderson SM, Ferguson JE (1997) Developmental outcomes of children with myelomeningocele: prenatal predictors. Am J Obstet Gynecol 177:319–324
7. d'Ercole C, Shojai R, Desbriere R, Chau C, Bretelle F, Piechon L, et al (2003) Prenatal screening: invasive diagnostic approaches. Childs Nerv Syst 19:444–447
8. Detrait ER, George TM, Etchevers HC, Gilbert JR, Vekemans M, Speer MC (2005) Human neural tube defects: developmental biology, epidemiology, and genetics. Neurotoxicol Teratol 27:515–524
9. Elwood JM, Little J, Elwood JH (1992) Epidemiology and Control of Neural Tube Defects. Oxford University Press, Oxford, UK
10. Gaskill SJ (2004) Primary closure of open myelomeningocele. Neurosurg Focus 16:1–4
11. Henshaw SK (1998) Unintended pregnancy in the United States. Fam Plann Perspect 30:24–29, 46
12. Honein MA, Paulozzi LJ, Mathews TJ, Erickson JD, Wong LY (2001) Impact of folic acid fortification of the US food supply on the occurrence of neural tube defects. JAMA 285:2981–2986
13. Hughes JA, De Bruyn R, Patel K, Thompson D (2003) Evaluation of spinal ultrasound in spinal dysraphism. Clin Radiol 58:227–233
14. James CCM & Lassman LP (1981). Spina bifida occulta: orthopaedic, radiological and neurosurgical aspects. London New York, Academic Press: Grune & Stratton
15. Jorde LB, Fineman RM, Martin RA (1984) Epidemiology of neural tube defects in Utah, 1940–1979. Am J Epidemiol 119:487–495
16. Keating MA, Rink RC, Bauer SB (1988) Neurourological implications of the changing approach in management of occult spinal lesions. J Urol 140:1299–1301
17. Korsvik HE, Keller MS (1992) Sonography of occult dysraphism in neonates and infants with MR imaging correlation. Radiographics 12:297–306
18. Lary JM, Edmonds LD (1996) Prevalence of spina bifida at birth – United States, 1983–1990: a comparison of two surveillance systems. MMWR CDC Surveill Summ 45:15–26
19. Laurence KM (1974) Effect for early surgery for spina bifida cystica on survival and quality of life. Lancet 1:301–304
20. Mazagri R, Ventureyra EC (1999) Latex allergy in neurosurgical practice. Childs Nerv Syst 15:404–407
21. McLone DG (1998) Care of the neonate with a myelomeningocele. In: Neurosurgery of the neonate. Neurosurg Clin N Am 9:111–120
22. National Center for Health Statistics (1993) Annual summary of births, marriages, divorces, and deaths: United States, 1992. Mon Vital Stat Rep 41:1–36
23. Padgett K (2002) Alterations of neurologic function in children. In: McCance KM, Huether SE (eds) Pathophysiology: The Biologic Basis for Disease in Adults and Children, 4th edn. Mosby, St. Louis, MO, p 567
24. Park TS (1999) Myelomeningocele. In: Albright AL, Pollack IL, Adelson PD (eds) Principles and Practice of Pediatric Neurosurgery. Thieme, New York, pp 125–139
25. Petronio J, Walker ML (2001) Ventriculoscopy. In: McLone DG (ed) Pediatric Neurosurgery; Surgery of the Developing Nervous System. WB Saunders, Philadelphia, pp 559–562
26. Rekate HL (1999) Treatment of hydrocephalus. In: Albright AL, Pollack IL, Adelson PD (eds) Principles and Practice of Pediatric Neurosurgery. Thieme, New York, pp 125–139
27. Roberts HE, Moore CA, Cragan JD, Fernhoff PM, Khoury MJ (1995) Impact of prenatal diagnosis on the birth prevalence of neural tube defects, Atlanta, 1990–1991. Pediatrics 96:880–883
28. Sakakibara R, Hattori T, Uchiyama T, Kamura K, Yamanishi T (2003) Uroneurological assessment of spina bifida cystica and occulta. Neurol Urodyn 22:328–334
29. Sebold CD, Melvin EC, Siegel D, Mehltretter L, Enterline DS, Nye JS, et al (2005) Recurrence risks for neural tube defects in siblings of patients with lipomyelomeningocele. Genet Med 7:64–67

30. United States Department of Health and Human Services (2003) NICHD study to test surgical technique to repair spinal defect before birth. Retrieved March 19, 2006, from http://www.nih.gov/news/pr/apr2003/nichd-25.htm

31. Warf BC (2005) Comparison of endoscopic third ventriculostomy alone and combined with choroid plexus cauterization in infants younger than 1 year of age: a prospective study in 550 African children. Journal of Neurosurgery: Pediatrics 103:475–481

32. Yamada S, Won DJ, Yamada SM (2004) Pathophysiology of tethered cord syndrome: correlation with symptomatology. Neurosurg Focus 16:1–5

33. Yen IH, Khoury MJ, Erickson JD, James LM, Waters GD, Berry RJ (1992) The changing epidemiology of neural tube defects: United States, 1968–1989. Am J Dis Child 146:857–861

# Chiari Malformation and Syringomyelia

**5**

*Susan McGee and Diane Baudendistel*

## Contents

## ■ Introduction

Chiari malformations are a group of abnormalities of the hindbrain that were originally described in 1891 by Hans Chiari, a German professor. His work, based on autopsy results, created the classic definitions of hindbrain herniation now described as Chiari type I (CIM), Chiari type II (CIIM), and Chiari type III (CIIIM) malformations. CIM consists of displacement of the cerebellar tonsils below the foramen magnum (FM). CIIM, usually associated with myelomeningo-cele (MM), includes caudal displacement of the inferior cerebellar vermis, the fourth ventricle, and the medulla into the cervical canal. CIIIM, a rare and severe form, includes a low occipital or high cervical encephalocele in combination with downward displacement of most of the cerebellum, the fourth ventricle, and possibly portions of the brainstem [3, 10, 19].

## ■ Chiari Type I

Historically, Chiari malformations were described as developmental anomalies. However, currently there is evidence to indicate that some CIMs are acquired [10].

### ■ Developmental Anomaly

CIM is anatomically the simplest of the three (Fig. 5.1). Typically there is descent of the cerebellar tonsils 5 mm or more below the FM and rarely found below the second cervical (C2) level. Cerebellar tonsils that enter the cervical canal, but descend less than 5 mm, are described as cerebellar ectopia. Hydrocephalus is uncommon in patients with CIM. Fibrous adhesions or scarring may develop between the dura, the arachnoid, and the cerebellar tonsils. This in turn may cause obstruction of the flow of cerebrospinal fluid (CSF)

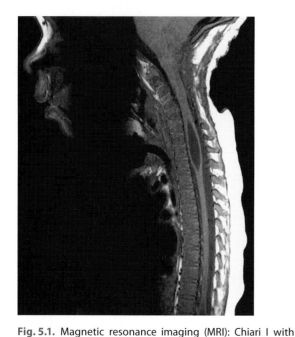

**Fig. 5.1.** Magnetic resonance imaging (MRI): Chiari I with syrinx

**Table 5.1.** Etiology of Chiari malformations [9,10]

| Theory | Mechanism |
|---|---|
| Hydrodynamic | Hydrocephalus the primary cause |
| Mechanical | a. Spinal cord tethering causing abnormal development or<br>b. Abnormal bony structures not providing enough space in the posterior fossa (cephalocranial disproportion) |
| Variation in pressure gradient | Pressure gradient between the intracranial and spinal compartments forcing the cerebellar tonsils to migrate caudally (craniospinal pressure gradient) |
| Traumatic birth | Birth trauma causing tonsillar edema and arachnoid scarring |

from the fourth ventricle. Skull-based deformities, such as a small posterior fossa and steep incline of the tentorium, may be present. Basilar impression or invagination, concavity of the clivus, and atlantoaxial assimilation have been associated with CIM [19]. Although this has historically been considered a condition of adulthood, CIMs have been identified in all age groups, including the neonatal population [5, 6, 9, 21].

## Acquired Anomaly

CIMs may develop in patients treated for hydrocephalus or pseudotumor with a lumboperitoneal shunt or ventriculoperitoneal shunt [11, 19]. Over time, overshunting from the lumbar subarachnoid space to the peritoneal cavity may cause the cerebellar tonsils to move caudally below the FM. This descent of the cerebellar tonsils may be reversed by removal of the shunt. In patients with ventriculoperitoneal shunts, it has been reported that the overdrainage of the ventricles caused increase CSF in the subarachnoid space, theoretically changing the pressure gradient and contributing to the downward movement of the cerebellar tonsils. Other authors report that with specific patients and techniques to prevent overshunting, this phenomenon can be avoided (Table 5.1) [12].

## Chiari Type II

CIIM is present in nearly all children with MM [2]. CIIM is probably a primary dysgenesis of the brainstem associated with the neural tube defect and multiple other developmental anomalies present in these MM patients [3]. However, there is evidence that patients undergoing intrauterine repair of MM may not have the typical low-lying tonsils of the CIIM [16–18], placing into question the theory that this is a primary dysgenesis, and giving support to the hydrodynamic theories of Chiari malformations. Up to 90% of MM patients also develop symptomatic hydrocephalus, with 50% of infants showing evidence of hydrocephalus at birth [1]. For these patients, the Chiari malformation is more than hindbrain herniation, but also includes anatomic changes in the supratentorial structures and the skull. The posterior fossa abnormalities include caudal descent of the pons, medulla, cerebellar vermis, and fourth ventricle, "kinking" of the brainstem, "beaking" of the tectum, and aqueductal stenosis (Fig. 5.2). Some associated anomalies of the cerebral hemispheres include polymicrogyria (multiple small convolutions of brain with thickened cortex), cortical heterotopias, dysgenesis of the corpus callosum, and a large massa intermedia. Skull deformities include "Luckenschadel" (copper-beaten appearance), shortening of Blumenbach's clivus, and enlargement of the FM [3]. Hindbrain dysfunction is the leading cause of death in children with myelodysplasia [10].

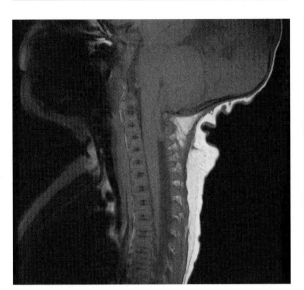

**Fig. 5.2.** MRI: Chiari II

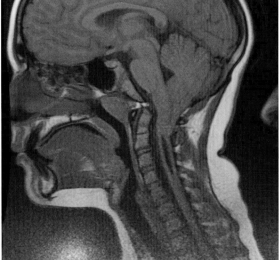

**Fig. 5.3.** MRI: cervical syrinx

## Chiari Type III

CIIIM involves descent of most of the cerebellum and brainstem below the FM and may be associated with a cervical or occipital encephalocele. The encephalocele may contain cerebellum, occipital lobes, and brainstem. Herniation of the fourth and lateral ventricles may occur. Hydrocephalus is often present. Even with treatment, the prognosis for the CIIIM is much poorer than for either CIM or CIIM [10, 19].

## Etiology

Despite being identified in the 1800s, a debate still continues about the spectrum of Chiari malformations. Although these three malformations have abnormalities of the cerebellum and the craniocervical junction in common, they are thought to be distinct conditions with differing etiologic factors [3, 15]. Many theories about their etiology have been proposed. Ongoing research brings hope for information that will help in determining best treatment options for this challenging spectrum of disorders.

## Syringomyelia

Syringomyelia (or syrinx) refers to a cavitation or cyst within the substance of the spinal cord extending over many segments. Hydromyelia is a term that describes a distended central canal, which is therefore lined by ependymal tissue. The technical difference between these two terms has little clinical significance because the hydrodynamics of both types of cavitations are identical, as evaluated by current imaging techniques. Therefore, the medical literature currently uses the term syringomyelia to describe all intramedullary cysts with CSF-like content [10]. Although syringomyelia most often occurs in association with posterior fossa abnormality, a syrinx can also be associated with tumors, injury or inflammatory processes, or may be idiopathic.

Syringomyelia is often associated with CIMs and CIIMs. Syringomyelia is present in 30–85% of patients with CIM [13]. The medical literature has posed a variety of mechanisms for the development of the syrinx in patients with Chiari malformations. In general, there is agreement that the abnormal CSF dynamic associated with Chiari malformations forces CSF into the central canal to form cysts within the spinal cord, creating the syrinx (Figs. 5.3 and 5.4). The presence of syringomyelia will have an impact on symptom presentation, treatment options, and long-term outcomes [2, 10, 19]. A new finding of syringomyelia may be associated with a shunt malfunction in CIIM patients.

## Presentation

## Chiari Type I

Occipital and upper cervical headache is the most common presenting symptom in CIM, present in 63–

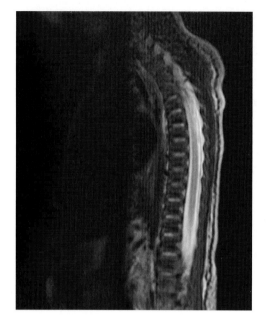

**Fig. 5.4.** MRI: thoracic syrinx

spasticity, and ataxia [10, 19]. The literature indicates, however, that 10% of all patients with CIM present with headache only and have a normal neurological examination. In addition, this percentage may be higher in the pediatric population. In a recent study reporting findings about 130 children with CIM, 21% of patients presented with headache only and a normal neurological examination [20]. Diagnoses of CIM in children and adolescents are often based on history, symptoms, and radiographic studies, in the absence of focal neurological findings (Table 5.2).

### Chiari Type II

CIIMs are present at birth in patients with an open neural tube defect. The literature reports that 18–33% of these patients will demonstrate symptoms related to the CIIM [2, 19]. Those patients who demonstrate a symptomatic CIIM in infancy have a more rapid and severe onset of symptoms than those who become symptomatic later in childhood. Symptom presentation early in life is related to higher morbidity and mortality.

Most patients are asymptomatic at birth, but a small group of neonates have respiratory distress. These patients demonstrate a poor respiratory drive, probably related to brainstem dysfunction. In infancy, respiratory distress, including cyanotic spells, central or obstructive apnea, inspiratory stridor, and hoarse or high-pitched cries, are the most common presenting signs. New or worsening stridor, accompanied by oxygen desaturation, in an infant with CIIM is considered a medical emergency.

Swallowing dysfunction is the second most common sign of a symptomatic CIIM [2]. Patients demonstrate poor suck-and-swallow coordination, nasal regurgitation, projectile emesis, choking, drooling, or

69% of patients [2, 4]. The headache may be triggered or exacerbated by the Valsalva maneuver or extreme neck movement. Weakness or numbness of one or both arms may be present. Some patients report gait unsteadiness, sensory changes, and dysphagia. The nonverbal child may present with persistent crying and irritability as well as arching of the neck. Respiratory irregularities and recurrent aspirations may be noted in the patient's history. CIM may also present as developmental delay, although this has not yet been methodically evaluated.

On physical exam, nystagmus, facial hyperesthesia, dysarthria, palatal weakness, or tongue atrophy may be present. Vocal cord paralysis may be present in rare cases. Other possible findings include hyperactive upper extremity reflexes, positive Babinski, weakness of upper and lower extremities, scoliosis,

**Table 5.2.** Categories of patients with Chiari type I based on predominant clinical symptoms [19]

| General | Spinal | Brainstem | Cerebellar | Combination |
|---|---|---|---|---|
| Headache | Extremity paresthesias | Apnea | Ataxia | Multiple symptoms from different categories |
| Nausea/vomiting | Weakness | Bradycardia | Clumsiness | |
| Irritability | Scoliosis | Dysphagia | | |
| | | Hypotonia | | |
| | | Spasticity | | |

pooling of food in the posterior pharynx. As a result, these patients may suffer from failure to thrive, repeated episodes of aspiration pneumonia, and chronic gastroesophageal reflux. Nystagmus and vocal cord paralysis may also be present. This combination of symptoms reflects brainstem and lower cranial nerve dysfunction [2, 19]. Infants may also present with decreased upper extremity tone.

The clinical presentation of symptomatic CIIM in the older child is usually more gradual, with milder symptoms that are often responsive to surgical intervention. Symptoms in this age group include upper extremity weakness, spasticity, decreased function of the lower extremities, headache, neck pain, nystagmus, ataxia, and scoliosis. This group of symptoms is related to dysfunction of the cerebellum and spinal cord. Because these symptoms may progress very slowly, a complete history to identify subtle and gradual changes is vital. Presentation in adulthood is rare, but would mimic the progression of symptoms of the older child (Table 5.3).

### Chiari Type III

CIIIMs are present at birth and are identified by the occipital or high cervical encephalocele. Multiple anomalies of the cerebellum and brainstem accompany the encephalocele, which contains varying amounts of brain tissue. The severity of the anomaly usually makes it incompatible with life. Even with treatment, patients have a short life expectancy.

### Syringomyelia

The neurologic examination should include a thorough sensory evaluation and testing of the reflexes, in addition to strength testing. Syringomyelia should be suspected in patients that present with scoliosis, leg or foot asymmetries, or abnormal sensory examination. Dysesthetic pain of the trunk or extremities may be present. New or progressive spasticity is another symptom of concern for syrinx. Clumsiness, weakness, and atrophy of the upper extremities also may occur. In MM patients, a worsening of urodynamics should be noted. In patients with CIM, urinary incontinence may be a late sign of syringomyelia [2, 10, 19].

### Diagnostic Tests

Cervical radiographs are needed if there is any concern about bony instability of the neck. Ultrasonography provides identification of Chiari malformations and syringomyelia in the neonate and infant, but decisions about surgical intervention are based on mag-

**Table 5.3.** Comparison of Chiari I and II malformations [6,19]. *FM* Foramen magnum

| | Chiari I Malformation | Chiari II Malformation |
|---|---|---|
| Brain | Caudal herniation of cerebellar tonsils > 5–7 mm below the FM<br>Peg like or pointed<br>Often asymmetric | Caudal herniation of cerebellar vermis, brainstem and fourth ventricle below the FM |
| **Common associated findings** | | |
| Skull | Underdeveloped occiput<br>Small posterior fossa<br>+/- enlarged FM<br>Basilar impression | Craniolacunia<br>Lemon sign<br>Small posterior fossa<br>Enlarged FM<br>+/– Basilar impression |
| Spine | Assimilation of the atlas<br>Scoliosis<br>Klippel-Feil deformity | +/– Assimilation of the atlas<br>Enlarged cervical canal<br>Klippel-Feil deformity |
| Ventricles and cisterns | Hydrocephalus rare (3–10%) | Hydrocephalus (90%)<br>Intrinsic malformation of ventricles including asymmetry, pointed frontal horns and colpocephaly |
| Spinal cord | Syrinx (30–85%) | Syrinx (20–95%) |

netic resonance imaging (MRI) findings. Intraoperative ultrasound is used to identify whether bony decompression establishes adequate CSF flow. If CSF flow remains impaired with bony decompression, the surgery proceeds to include duraplasty [14].

MRI of the brain, craniocervical junction and spine is the best tool to diagnose Chiari malformations and syringomyelia. MRI provided a breakthrough in the diagnosis of Chiari malformations, which often present with vague and nonspecific signs and symptoms. Identifying compression of the hindbrain and cervical spine as the possible cause of discomfort in these patients aided clinicians in providing useful treatment options. Recognition of CIM in the very young child provided them with an opportunity to benefit from advances made in the surgical approach to this condition. Cine MRI may be used to assess CSF flow around the cerebellar tonsils. The location and extent of syringomyelia is best defined by spinal MRI [14].

Computed tomography is of limited value in diagnosing Chiari malformations, but provides information about the presence of hydrocephalus. Sleep and swallow studies help identify signs of brainstem or cranial nerve compression. Consultation for evaluation of vocal cord motility may be indicated.

## Treatment Options for CIM

### Medical

A child diagnosed with CIM presents a variety of challenges related to developmental considerations and the nonspecific symptoms often associated with this condition. Because the CIM may present with only headache, care must be taken to confirm that the malformation itself is causing the headaches. Children, as well as adults, are subject to a variety of types of headaches. Taking a thorough history of the type, pattern, and location of the headache, and evaluating the effect of conservative treatment is a key component of the medical management of these patients. If the headaches can be managed medically, the child may avoid a major surgical procedure.

Children with known CIM should be followed annually for evaluation of symptom development or progression. MRI imaging with cine of the craniocervical junction to assess CSF flow may be indicated.

The parents and child should be advised that the child should avoid contact sports and lumbar punctures.

### Surgical

Early surgery is recommended for symptomatic patients [4]. Patients who have CIM identified on MRI, and have occipital headaches unrelieved by medical management, and/or other signs/symptoms associated with CIM, are candidates for surgery. MRI evidence of a syrinx is an additional reason for surgical intervention. Common goals are improvement of presenting symptoms, radiographic reduction of syringomyelia, and arrest or remission of associated scoliosis [3]. If the patient also has hydrocephalus, treatment with a CSF diversionary shunt should precede surgery to treat the CIM.

The surgical procedure is planned to decompress the posterior fossa sufficiently to allow room for CSF to circulate around the cerebellum and the cervical spinal cord. A vertical occipital incision is made to allow for bony decompression of the FM. Initial decompression may also include partial laminectomy to the level of cerebellar descent [3]. If the removal of bone allows for adequate CSF flow, as determined by intraoperative ultrasound, the procedure may be completed at this stage [14]. If there is continued evidence of impingement on the brainstem and cerebellum, the surgeon may perform a variety of procedures to further decompress the space. This may include intradural exploration, partial dural removal or scoring, duraplasty with graft material or pericranium, plugging of the obex, shunting of the fourth ventricle, and coagulation of the cerebellar tonsils [2, 8, 14].

### Nursing Care

The main concerns for nurses taking care of these patients postoperatively are pain management and respiratory compromise. In addition, if the dura was opened, the patient is at risk for CSF leak and infection. Surgical treatment without disrupting the dura is limited to the pediatric population and has decreased the incidence of postoperative complications [14]. The patient is monitored overnight in the intensive care unit (ICU) for prevention and early detection of potential complications.

Pain and stiffness of the neck is due to the incision through the semispinalis capitis and splenius capitis muscles, as well as from opening the dura. Pain management in the early postoperative period includes use of narcotics, preferably by patient- (or parent-) controlled analgesia. Twenty-four hours after surgery, adding ibuprofen scheduled around the clock can improve pain scores and decrease the need for narcotics for breakthrough pain. Antispasmodics for neck spasm may also be indicated.

Monitoring patients for respiratory compromise is vital. The combination of potential irritation to the brainstem and the need for narcotics can make these patients susceptible to decreased respiratory drive. ICU monitoring until most of anesthesia effects are eliminated limits this complication.

Pseudomeningocele is the most common surgical complication when the dura has been disrupted. This occurs when CSF leaks into the subcutaneous space, causing a fullness of the surgical site [14]. To minimize the risk of CSF leak in patients with dural compromise, the operative site should be closely monitored and the patient's head should be kept in midline position for 48 h. A short course of dexamethasone may minimize symptoms from postoperative edema. Another possible complication is chemical meningitis (or aseptic meningitis). The symptoms include nuchal rigidity, low-grade fever, and headache. If bacterial meningitis has been ruled out, a short course of dexamethasone is the treatment of choice.

The usual hospital length of stay is 3–5 days. Discharge criteria include normothermia, adequate oral fluid intake, and pain controlled with oral medications. In addition, it is particularly important for patients who have undergone duraplasty to have a bowel regime that keeps their movements soft and regular to prevent disruption of the surgical site by straining.

## Treatment Options for CIIM

### Medical

Imaging for CIIM is indicated only when new symptoms occur or when baseline status deteriorates. Symptoms of concern may include swallowing difficulties, weakness or increased weakness of the upper extremities, new spasticity, or occipital headaches. If the child has shunted hydrocephalus, the shunt should be evaluated first and revised if it is malfunctioning.

In the presence of a functioning CSF shunt, evaluation of the CIIM by an MRI of the brain and craniocervical junction is the next step. If the symptoms persist and the MRI shows brainstem compression or obstruction of CSF flow, surgical treatment is indicated.

### Surgical

The surgical intervention for CIIM parallels that for CIM. A suboccipital incision is made to allow for removal of the posterior arch of C1 and excision of any extra dural constrictive band. A laminectomy is performed to the level of descent of the cerebellar tonsils, which may require a 1-, 2-, or 3-level laminectomy. MM patients, unlike CIM patients, have an elongated FM and, thus, do not require further expansion. The dura should be opened to create CSF flow around the CIIM.

### Nursing Care

As with CIM, these patients are monitored after surgery in the ICU or the neonatal ICU. Postoperatively, patients with CIIM are at increased risk for respiratory complications, including late extubation and feeding problems after surgery, especially when respiratory distress was a presenting feature. The risk for CSF leak and infection exists when dura has been opened. Neck movement limitation and steroids may be indicated to minimize symptoms related to dural opening and postoperative edema. Neck pain and stiffness occur in these patients and must be managed carefully in light of the presence of respiratory compromise preoperatively, especially in very young patients.

Like CIM patients, discharge criteria include normothermia, adequate oral fluid intake, and pain controlled with oral medications. A bowel regime is needed to keep stool soft and regular to prevent disruption of the surgical site by straining.

## Treatment Options for Syringomyelia

When syringomyelia is associated with a Chiari malformation, treatment by posterior fossa decompression of the hindbrain malformation often results in resolution of the syrinx. Primarily in CIIM, symptomatic syringomyelia may persist despite decompressive surgery. In the absence of Chiari malformation, asymptomatic syringomyelia may be observed clinically with yearly examinations and intermittent MRI.

Direct shunting of the syrinx may improve symptoms in those patients who have persistent symptoms after successful posterior fossa decompression or in those patients who have a symptomatic syrinx without a Chiari malformation. Options include syringoperitoneal, syringopleural, and syringosubarachnoid shunts. The shunt acts to decompress the fluid build-up within the spinal cord, diverting the fluid to another space for reabsorption [7].

### Nursing Care

Postoperative care includes incision care, pain management, and evaluation of shunt function. With syringoperitoneal shunting, there will be an incision over the spine at the level of the syrinx and an incision over the abdomen for insertion of the distal catheter. Abdominal pain and bowel function are key areas for nursing assessment.

The syringopleural shunt will have a similar back incision but with the distal catheter incision in the lateral chest. Observation of respiratory status is important with this treatment option. Decreased breath sound and oxygen desaturation may indicate a symptomatic pleural effusion. Serial chest radiographs may be used to evaluate the patient's ability to accommodate the pleural fluid being diverted by the shunt.

The syringosubarachnoid shunt requires only one incision to accommodate both the proximal and distal catheters and may be effective in symptom relief.

The use of a shunt to treat syringomyelia requires ongoing follow up to observe for signs of shunt failure.

### Patient and Family Education

1. Informed consent: major risks of surgery include excessive bleeding, CSF leak, infection, persistence of symptoms, neurological deficit, and anesthesia complications.
2. Preoperative history and physical examination.
3. Preoperative diagnostic tests, which may include swallow evaluation, sleep study, MRI, and developmental assessment.
4. Educational handouts about Chiari malformations, Web site information recommendations.
5. Incision care after removal of the dressing.
6. Sutures either dissolvable or removed in about 2 weeks.
7. Activity restrictions: no driving while on narcotics or while neck is stiff; return to school or work in 4–6 weeks.
8. Follow-up imaging; MRI in 4–6 weeks, then annually for 5 years (more frequently if syrinx present).
9. Signs and symptoms of shunt failure, for patients requiring shunting of the syrinx.
10. Discharge instructions: incision care with observation for infection or pseudomeningocele; call surgeon's office for headache not responsive to medication and fever greater than 101ºF.

### Outcomes: Short and Long Term

### Chiari I Malformation

Successful decompression can provide rapid relief of headache. Symptoms due to cranial nerve or brainstem dysfunction will show improvement over several weeks to months. Follow-up swallow studies are useful to evaluate the effects of treatment when done 6 or more weeks postoperatively. Ataxia or weakness may also gradually improve. Patients with symptoms other than isolated headaches on presentation benefit from appropriate therapies postoperatively, such as occupational, physical, and/or speech therapy.

MRI should demonstrate improvement in CSF flow around the craniocervical junction approximately 6 weeks after surgery. A syrinx should radiographically resolve or decrease in size within 3–6 months of posterior fossa decompression. Symptoms may persist in spite of the radiographic improvement [2].

### Chiari II Malformation

Better outcomes occur with older children who present with cerebellar dysfunction, spasticity, and weakness. Results in the neonatal and infant population have been varied, but in general, their outcomes are poorer. CIIM may cause death as a result of respiratory failure [2]. The rapidity of neurologic decline and immediate preoperative neurologic status are the most important factors affecting prognosis.

## Conclusions

The spectrum of Chiari malformations and syringomyelia present a continuum of challenges to the pediatric patient. The range of effect on quality of life varies from mild, with effective treatments available, to very severe, with minimal or no benefit from medical intervention. Advances in radiographic imaging and surgical techniques have provided opportunities to improve the health status of many of these patients. Advances in nursing research provides the opportunity for nurses and the allied health professionals to further enhance the functional level and optimal development of children with this varied spectrum of disorders. Incorporating the best practice for the pediatric neurosurgical patient in the areas of wound healing, pain management, prevention of postoperative complications, and effects of hospitalization on child development and psychosocial wellness will further enhance the quality of life of this young population.

---

### Pediatric Practice Pearls

- For pain management after posterior fossa decompression, use patient/parent-controlled analgesia; start ibuprofen 24 h after surgery and when the patient is taking fluids orally. Gradually decrease narcotics while continuing the ibuprofen.
- Straining with constipation can disrupt the surgical site and is particularly a risk when the dura has been disrupted. Start a bowel regime when the patient is taking fluids orally to avoid constipation.
- Relaxation techniques and gentle massage can be helpful during recovery from posterior fossa decompression. Muscle spasms often complicate the pain cycle.
- In patients who have had the dura disrupted, keeping the head midline for 24–48 h postoperatively may minimize the risk of a CSF leak.

---

## References

1. Detwiler PW, Porter RW, Rekate HL (1999) Hydrocephalus – clinical features and management. In: Choux M, Di Rocco C, Hockley AD, Walker ML (eds) Pediatric Neurosurgery. Churchill Livingstone, London, pp 253–271
2. Dias MS (1999) Myelomeningocele. In: Choux M, Di Rocco C, Hockley AD, Walker ML (eds) Pediatric Neurosurgery. Churchill Livingstone, London, pp 33–59
3. Greenberg MS (2001) Handbook of Neurosurgery. Thieme Medical Publishers, New York
4. Hida K, Iwasaki Y, Koyanagi I, Sawamura Y, Abe H (1995) Surgical indication and results of foremen magnum decompression versus syringosubarachnoid shunting for syringomyelia associated with Chiari I malformation. Neurosurgery 37:637–639
5. Lazareff JA, Galarza M, Gravori T, Spinks TJ (2002) Tonsillectomy without craniectomy for the management of infantile Chiari I malformation. J Neurosurg 97:1018–1022
6. Menezes AH (1995) Primary craniovertebral anomalies and the hindbrain syndrome (Chiari I): data base analysis. Pediatr Neurosurg 23:260–269
7. Menezes AH (1999) Craniovertebral anomalies and syringomyelia. In: Choux M, Di Rocco C, Hockley AD, Walker ML (eds) Pediatric Neurosurgery. Churchill Livingstone, London, pp 151–184
8. Narvaro R, Olavarria G, Seshadri R, Gonzales-Portillo G, McLone DG, Tomita T (2004) Surgical results of posterior fossa decompression for patients with Chiari I malformation. Childs Nerv Syst 20:349–356
9. Nohria V, Oakes WJ (1991) Chiari I malformation: a review of 43 patients. Pediatr Neurosurg 16:222–227
10. Oakes, WJ, Tubbe RS (2004) Chiari malformations. In: Winn HR (ed) Youmans Neurological Surgery, 5th edn. Saunders, Philadelphia, pp 3347–3361
11. Payner TD, Prenger E, Berger TB, Crone KR (1994) Acquired Chiari malformations: incidence, diagnosis, and management. Neurosurgery 34:429–434
12. Rekate HL, Wallace D (2003) Lumboperitoneal shunts in children. Pediatr Neurosurg 38:41–46
13. Schijman E (2004) History, anatomic forms, pathogenesis of Chiari I malformation. Childs Nerv Syst 20:323–328
14. Sherman J, Larson JJ, Crone KR (1999) Posterior fossa decompression without dural opening for the treatment of Chiari I malformation. In: Rengachary SS, Wilkins RH (eds) Neurosurgical Operative Atlas, vol 8. American Association of Neurological Surgeons, Park Ridge, IL, pp 179–183
15. Strayer A (2001) Chiari I malformation: clinical presentation and management. J Neurosci Nurs 33:90–104
16. Sutton LN, Adzick NS, Bilaniuk LT, Johnson MP, Crombleholme TM, Flake AW (1999) Improvement in hindbrain herniation demonstrated by serial fetal magnetic resonance imaging following fetal surgery for myelomeningocele. JAMA 282:1826–1831
17. Tulipan N, Hernanz-Schulman M, Bruner JP (1998) Reduced hindbrain herniation after intrauterine myelomeningocele repair: a report of four cases. Pediatr Neurosurg 29:274–278
18. Tulipan N, Hernanz-Schulman M, Lowe LH, Bruner JP (1999) Intrauterine myelomeningocele repair reverses preexisting hindbrain herniation. Pediatr Neurosurg 31:137–142

19. Weprin BE, Oakes WJ (2001) The Chiari Malformations and associated syringohydromelia. In: McClone DG (ed) Pediatric Neurosurgery. WB Saunders, Philadelphia, pp 214–235

20. Yeh DD, Koch B, Crone KR (2006) Intraoperative ultrasonography used to determine the extent of surgery necessary during posterior fossa decompression in children with Chiari malformation type I. J Neurosurg 105:26–32

21. Yundt KD, Park TS, Tantuwaya VS, Kaufman BA (1996) Posterior fossa decompression without duraplasty in infants and young children for treatment of Chiari malformation and achondroplasia. Pediatr Neurosurg 25:221–226

# Tumors of the Central Nervous System

*Tania Shiminski-Maher*

**6**

## Contents

## Introduction

Brain tumors are the most common solid tumor in childhood. For example, there are approximately 2000 brain tumors diagnosed in children each year in the United States. The incidence of brain tumors is higher among males than females, and higher among white children than any other group. While the incidence of reported pediatric brain tumors has been increasing over the past few decades, this is probably because of improvements in diagnostic capabilities and reporting. Recent advances in diagnostic capabilities, aggressive surgical techniques, and multimodal therapy, including radiation and/or chemotherapy, have lead to longer survival and even cure of some classifications of pediatric brain tumors [17].

Because there are many different kinds of brain tumors, the number of children diagnosed with each particular type is small. Advances in successfully treating each subset of tumor have been a direct result of children being enrolled in clinical trials. The majority of those trials are part of the Children's Oncology Group (COG). Such trials accurately evaluate treatments and recommend standard best treatments for each tumor type. In addition to clinical treatments, COG also conducts biological research focused on identifying possible causes of central nervous system (CNS) tumors [27].

## Etiology

Despite the research to date, the cause of pediatric CNS tumors remains unknown. Pediatric CNS tumors have been associated with phakomatoses in children. Children with tuberous sclerosis may have tubers within their ventricular system or astrocytomas elsewhere in the CNS. Hemangioblastomas are common in children who have Von Hippel-Lindau syndrome. Radiation exposure has been linked to children with pediatric brain tumors. Children who received cranial irradiation either in low or moderate doses have had a higher incidence of brain tumors [30].

Recent advances in molecular biology and cytogenetics have begun to identify possible sites of oncogenesis. Alterations in chromosome 17 have been associated with medulloblastoma and astrocytoma, and loss of chromosome 10 has been associated with glioblastoma. There have been reports of correlation of breast cancer in mothers of children who have medulloblastoma [30]. Clinical research in pediatric CNS tumors on the cooperative group level is focusing on biology, not only to identify causes, but as a step to develop new treatment strategies [5, 21].

## Nervous System Anatomy

It is essential to have an understanding of normal anatomy to understand the diagnosis and treatment of CNS tumors. The brain sits inside a solid calvarium, the bony structure that is a fixed volume once the sutures are fused. The spinal cord sits inside the hollow vertebrae of the spine. It is the brain and spinal cord that make up the CNS. The brain and spinal cord communicate with the arms, legs, and other organs through the peripheral nervous system. Control of blood pressure, breathing, and hormonal function is carried out primarily in the brainstem by the autonomic nervous system [10].

The largest region in the brain is called the cerebrum (also called the supratentorial region). It is made up of two cerebral hemispheres (left and right). The two hemispheres are separated by a large groove, called the cerebral fissure. Deep within the cerebral fissure are a bundle of nerve fibers called the corpus callosum, which transmits information between the two sides. The cerebrum interprets sensory input from all parts of the body and controls body movements. It is the part of the brain responsible for thinking, emotions, memory, reasoning, learning, and movement. Symptoms of CNS tumors in this area can be generalized (as a result of changes in intracranial pressure regulation) or focal (as a result of tissue destruction or compressions from the tumor). Focal symptoms include seizures, memory difficulties,

headaches, weakness or paralysis of arms and legs, speech abnormalities, personality changes, and visual loss or changes. Generalized symptoms include irritability, lethargy, early morning vomiting, headache, loss of appetite, and behavior changes [27].

The cerebrum is divided into four areas (called lobes) on each side of the brain: the frontal, temporal, parietal, and occipital lobes. The corpus callosum connects the two parts of each lobe. In general, motor function for one side of the body is controlled by the opposite cerebral hemisphere. For example, movement of the arms and legs on the right side of the body is controlled by the left cerebral hemisphere. By early school age, around 5 years, a hand preference is usually identified. A person's speech center is located in the hemisphere opposite hand dominance. This is important when planning treatment for a tumor that is within or adjacent to the speech or motor cortex. In this situation, special preoperative testing may be needed, along with intraoperative monitoring to minimize damage to that area. Younger children have the ability to switch dominance after an injury to the dominant side has occurred, or have mixed dominance in terms of speech or motor functioning [27].

The frontal lobes process and store information that helps you think ahead, use strategy, and respond to events based on past experiences and other knowledge. A small part of the frontal lobe is involved in articulating speech. Another small strip of the frontal lobe helps to control movement. Malfunctions in the frontal lobe may lead to poor planning, impulsiveness, and certain types of speech problems. Symptoms are most pronounced if the tumor crosses the corpus callosum and affects both frontal lobes. Symptoms of tumors of the frontal lobe include seizures, changes in ability to concentrate, poor school performance, or changes in social behaviors and personality. The posterior section of the frontal lobe is the motor area, which controls movement of the head and body parts on the opposite side of the body [27].

The temporal lobes, located at the sides of the brain, are responsible for speech, language, hearing, and memory. They are also believed to be the center where information taken in from the various senses is integrated, permitting complex thoughts, movements, and sensations to be formulated and acted upon. Within the temporal lobe is the amygdala, which controls social behavior, aggression, and excitement. The hippocampus is involved in storing memory of recent events. Depth perception and sense of time are also controlled by the temporal lobes [10].

Tumors in the temporal lobes can cause atypical seizures, such as staring spells, and memory problems associated with poor school performance. When a tumor grows in the temporal lobes, the brain has a hard time filtering out extra information. Sensory information and memories may start to blend together in unfamiliar ways, resulting in feelings of deja vu in some cases [27].

Directly behind the frontal lobes and above the temporal lobes are the parietal lobes. The parietal lobes process sensory information coming in from the body, including data about temperature, pain, and taste. The parietal lobes also control language and the ability to do arithmetic. When the parietal lobes are not functioning properly, sensory information is not processed correctly, and an individual may have a hard time making sense of the environment. The posterior aspect of the parietal lobe, next to the temporal lobe, is important in processing the auditory and visual information needed for language. Abnormal movements or weakness in the arms and legs, memory problems, and seizures are associated with tumors in the parietal areas. During a seizure affecting the parietal lobe, strange physical sensations may be felt, such as a crushing pressure or a tingle in part of the body [27].

The occipital lobes serve as the visual centers of the brain. They are responsible for making sense of the information that comes to the brain from the eyes through the optic nerves. The left occipital lobe deals with input from the right eye, and the right lobe deals with input from the left eye. Tumors in the occipital lobe are associated with visual field cut (loss of peripheral vision) on one side or the other [27].

The posterior fossa or infratentorium contains the cerebellum, the brainstem, and the fourth ventricle. The cerebellum controls balance, coordination, and the ability to judge distances. The brainstem, which contains the cranial nerves, is the relay center for transmitting and coordinating messages between the brain and other parts of the body. It consists of the midbrain, including the thalamus, pons, and medulla. The midbrain contains cranial nerve nuclei that processes vision and hearing; it also coordinates the sleep and wake cycles. Eye and facial movement are controlled by cranial nerve nuclei located in the pons, which also serves as a link between the cerebellum and cerebrum. The medulla contains the cranial

nerves that control breathing, swallowing, heart rate, and blood pressure. The fourth ventricle is a fluid-filled space that connects the upper fluid chambers to the spinal cord and subarachnoid space surrounding the brain [27].

Sixty percent of all childhood brain tumors originate in the posterior fossa. Symptoms of tumors in this area of the brain include signs of increased intracranial pressure, weakness of cranial nerves (cranial nerve palsies), and ataxia. If the tumor grows toward or puts pressure on the fourth ventricle, normal flow of cerebrospinal fluid (CSF) is blocked, causing hydrocephalus [24]. Please refer to Chap. 2 (Hydrocephalus) for an overview of this physiology.

The spinal cord contains the 31 pairs of spinal nerves that exit at various levels in the cervical, thoracic, lumbar, and sacral regions. The spinal cord sits inside the vertebral column, a series of bones that sit upon one another. Nerve impulses travel from the brain down the spinal cord and exit at various levels. They provide sensory and motor stimulation, which result in contraction of muscles in organs in the body, as well as movement of the extremities [10]. Figure 6.1 illustrates normal brain anatomy.

## ■ Diagnosis

The diagnosis of a CNS tumor in a child is often difficult to establish. The presenting symptoms of a CNS tumor may be vague, or similar to the symptoms of many common childhood illnesses. As there are only approximately 2000 children diagnosed with CNS tumors annually in the United States, the likelihood of a pediatrician seeing a CNS tumor in the practice in his/her career is thus remote. It is not unusual to get a history from the family of many trips to a healthcare provider before the actual diagnosis is made [27].

Signs and symptoms vary depending upon the rate of growth and location of the tumor. Table 6.1 summarizes symptoms based upon tumor location and tissue type. Tumors with a short history (less than 1 month) and/or an acute onset of symptoms tend to be more rapid growing, and may be described as aggressive, high grade, or histologically malignant. Those with a long history of vague symptoms or those picked up incidentally tend to be slower growing, low grade, or histologically benign [29].

On physical examination, the child with a CNS tumor may have specific neurological deficits that are

# Normal Brain Anatomy

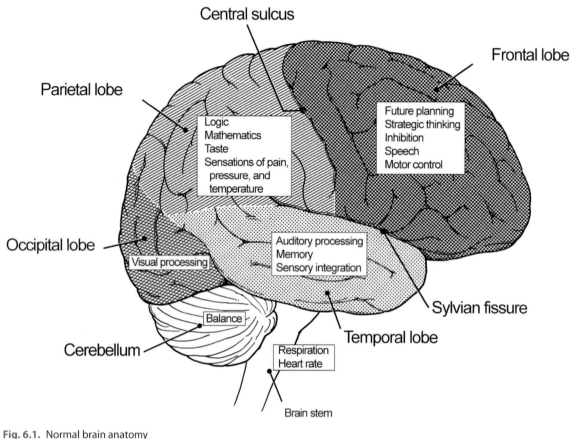

**Fig. 6.1.** Normal brain anatomy

correlated with the tumor location. It is possible for a child to have a normal examination, for example, in a situation where the tumor is diagnosed incidentally because of a diagnostic test being performed for another reason [27].

Posterior fossa tumor symptoms are most commonly associated with increased intracranial pressure. Symptoms of increased intracranial pressure include double vision, papilledema, headache, nausea, vomiting, ataxia, and lethargy. This may be due to the pressure exerted by the mass itself, or by obstruction of the normal flow of CSF by the tumor. Signs of increased intracranial pressure will be discussed in de-

tail in the next section. Other signs associated with posterior fossa tumors include ataxia, nystagmus, and cranial nerve problems. Cranial nerve deficits are indicative of brainstem involvement [30].

Symptoms of supratentorial tumors include hemiparesis, hemisensory loss, seizures, visual field changes, and intellectual problems. Midline tumors, such as those in the hypothalamic or pituitary region, are associated with increased intracranial pressure, visual changes, and/or endocrine issues such as diabetes insipidus (DI) or precocious puberty [30].

Spinal cord tumors usually present with scoliosis, back or leg pain (which often awakes the child from

**Table 6.1.** Brain tumors: diagnosis based on location and symptoms. Adapted from Shiminski-Maher et al. (2002) [27]. *CNS* Central nervous system, *DNET* dysembryoplastic neuroepithelial tumors, *PNET* primitive neuroectodermal tumors

| Part of the CNS | Symptoms of tumor | Types of tumor |
|---|---|---|
| Frontal lobes (cerebral hemispheres) | Problems with learning and concentration, changes in behavior, personality changes, seizures, weakness of an arm or leg on opposite side of tumor | Astrocytoma Glioma Rarely PNET or Ependymoma |
| Parietal lobes (cerebral hemispheres) | Seizures, difficulty processing information, language difficulties | Astrocytoma Glioma DNET |
| Temporal lobes (cerebral hemispheres) | Atypical/partial complex seizures, behavior problems (aggressiveness, impulsiveness) | Astrocytoma Glioma DNET |
| Occipital lobes (cerebral hemispheres) | Loss of peripheral vision | Astrocytoma Glioma |
| Cerebellum (posterior fossa) including the fourth ventricle | Problems with balance, uncoordinated gait, increased intracranial pressure, nausea and vomiting | Astrocytoma Glioma Medulloblastoma Ependymoma |
| Brainstem (posterior fossa) including the fourth ventricle | Increased intracranial pressure, headache, nausea and vomiting, Cranial nerve problems including eye movement disruption, decreased hearing, facial asymmetry, breathing or swallowing difficulties and problems with balance and strength | Astrocytoma Glioma Ependymoma Medulloblastoma (rare) |
| Midbrain/thalamus | Altered level of consciousness, memory problems, weakness of arms or legs | Astrocytoma Glioma |
| Diencephalon (hypothalamus, sella, pituitary) Optic Pathway | Hormonal secretion disruption (decreased growth, diabetes insipidus, thyroid deficiency, puberty problems) memory and academic problems Visual changes: acuity or field cut | Astrocytoma Gliomas Craniopharyngioma Germ Cell |
| Ventricular system | Increased intracranial pressure, hydrocephalus, memor or academic problems, hormonal changes | Ependymoma Choroid Plexus Astrocytoma Glioma Medulloblastoma |
| Spinal cord | Back pain, scoliosis, weakness in arms or legs, bowel and bladder problems | Astrocytoma Ependymoma |

sleep), weakness or sensory changes in the arms or the legs, and/or bowel and bladder dysfunction. Occasionally, a brain tumor will metastasize to the spinal cord and produce similar symptoms to those just described [27].

### Increased Intracranial Pressure and Hydrocephalus

Increased intracranial pressure occurs from the mass of the tumor occupying space within the brain. It can also occur when the tumor causes an obstruction in the flow of CSF, resulting in hydrocephalus. Symptoms of increased intracranial pressure include: head-

ache (that awakens from sleep), nausea, vomiting (which often temporarily relieves the nausea and headache), lethargy, double vision or other visual changes, gait instability, memory problems, and decline in academic functioning. Nausea is especially problematic, as the nausea centers are located near the medulla, which may be compressed or infiltrated by a tumor. Infants whose sutures are open can increase their head circumference to compensate for the pressure. Infants and children have the ability to compensate for increased intracranial pressure, especially if the tumor is slower growing and pressure increases are subtle. In addition, these symptoms are typical of many childhood illnesses and, therefore, may go un-noticed. Late signs of increased pressure are papill-edema, vital sign changes, and severe altered level of consciousness [18,25].

## Diagnostic Tests

The diagnosis of a CNS tumor is confirmed with a radiographic study, which is usually ordered by the primary care provider in a child with symptoms sug-gestive of intracranial or intraspinal pathology. Sev-eral other diagnostic tests may also be performed prior to treatment. Obviously, the extent of testing will depend upon the clinical condition of the patient. In general, the more information available to the treating team, the better to plan for maximal surgical removal of the tumor followed by appropriate adjunc-tive therapy [6].

Until the last decade, the computed tomography (CT) scan was the most frequently ordered imaging test. This has been essentially replaced by the mag-netic resonance imaging (MRI) scan. Nurses are gen-erally familiar with this diagnostic test, but not neces-sarily with how it works. A patient having an MRI scan is placed in a machine that contains a strong magnetic field. This magnetic field causes protons in the water molecules in the body to align parallel or antiparallel within the field, and this generates a pic-ture of the neuroaxis [6].

MRI is a much more sensitive diagnostic test than the previously utilized CT scans. Its sensitivity allows for the detection of smaller tumors that may be missed with a CT scan. In addition, an MRI provides greater anatomic detail in multiple planes. The administra-tion of a contrast agent (gadolinium diethylenetri-aminepentaacetic acid) allows for better visualization of some tumors. Moreover, newer imaging sequences are continually being developed to assist in determin-ing whether a tumor's pathology is malignant or be-nign, or to differentiate between recurrent tumor and treatment changes [6].

Magnetic resonance angiography utilizes the mag-netic field to display blood vessels within the brain. It is helpful in visualizing the blood supply to a tumor, or in identifying vessels that may be compromised be-cause of the tumor. It is a noninvasive way of looking at the blood supply within the CNS and has replaced conventional angiography in many situations. Angi-ography is used in a small group of CNS lesions whose differential diagnosis includes tumor versus aneu-rysm/cavernoma, or where hemorrhage into the tu-mor cavity is suspected [6,30].

Because the quality of the MRI images is depen-dent upon the patient lying motionless throughout the study, younger children, and some older ones, will require conscious sedation or anesthesia to perform the test. Sedation protocols vary with the institution, and larger pediatric centers may have blocks of time set aside with anesthesiologists present to efficiently utilize scanner time. If the child shows clinical signs of increased intracranial pressure or has hydrocepha-lus, it may be the physician's preference to insert a drain prior to the MRI scan, especially if the child is intubated [30].

A CT scan may be the first diagnostic test per-formed. Some tumors, especially small ones, may not be seen on a CT scan, and most tumors will not be visualized on a CT scan unless contrast is given. CT scans are most often used during the treatment pro-cesses as a screening tool for children who have expe-rienced a change in their neurological status. It can be performed in less than 5 min and is not as sensitive to the child moving as an MRI. The CT scan does ex-pose the child to radiation during the test, and there is a growing awareness of the potential harmfulness of cumulative radiation after many CT scans during the course of the illness [4].

Other radiodiagnostic tests include positron emis-sion tomography and single-photon-emission com-puted tomography. Both of these tests have been evolving over the past decade, but still remain un-common because of the high cost and limited avail-ability of equipment. Larger academic centers have the ability to perform these tests, which focus on a tumor's metabolism, thereby helping clinicians to de-termine the rate of cell growth and to differentiate between active tumor cells and treatment effects. These tests are usually utilized after a specific treat-ment, to evaluate its effectiveness [6].

An electroencephalogram (EEG) measures the electrical activity within the brain and may be per-formed on a patient whose clinical presentation in-cludes a seizure. Patients with tumors that are associ-ated with seizures that are difficult to control or gen-eralized seizures undergo continuous EEG monitoring with videotaping in a special epilepsy-monitoring unit. Subdural grids are inserted in some cases to lo-calize speech or motor centers prior to surgical re-moval of the tumor. A Wada test (intracarotid sodium amobarbitol test) may be performed to determine which side of the brain is responsible for speech and memory. This test is slowly being replaced with the functional MRI scan, which attempts to obtain the same information in a noninvasive manner [27].

Visual acuity and visual field studies performed by an ophthalmologist are utilized if a patient presents with visual abnormalities. Laboratory tests, including blood and CSF workups, which are necessary to look for tumor markers or endocrine abnormalities, may also be part of the initial workup. Serum electrolytes, thyroid levels, and growth hormone levels are necessary to check for hypothalamic/pituitary tumors. Serum and CSF tumor markers of human chorionic gonadotrophin (HCG) or alpha-fetoprotein are needed for suprasellar tumors that may be germ cell tumors [6].

## Treatment

Technical advances in medicine and surgery have dramatically changed the management of pediatric CNS tumors over the past two decades. Imaging allows us to diagnose tumors earlier, to plan and carry out treatment plans, and to monitor the effects of those treatments. Evolution in the surgical equipment, radiation therapy equipment, and use of chemotherapy for CNS tumors has improved long-term survival and the quality of that survival. Treatment consists of any combination of surgery, radiation therapy, chemotherapy, and observation. Treatment depends upon the location and type of CNS tumor. The tumor location determines the surgical approach. Tumors near eloquent areas may require special planning. The type of tumor refers to its cellular make-up and rate of growth [27].

### Surgery

Surgery is the primary and front-line treatment for virtually all CNS tumors. On radiology confirmation of a tumor, the child is seen by a neurosurgeon and evaluated for surgery. The goals of surgery are for maximal safe surgical removal and to provide a tissue diagnosis. It is optimal for a child diagnosed with a CNS tumor to be operated on by a pediatric neurosurgeon whose practice comprises at least 50% children. This is because pediatric neurosurgeons are more likely to extensively remove pediatric tumors than general neurosurgeons, and the extent of surgical resection is a significant prognostic indicator [2,8].

Ideally, surgery should be carried out as efficiently as possible under elective, controlled conditions. This is possible for the child who has minimal clinical symptoms or for whom medical management can temporize symptoms. Placing a child with subtle symptoms of increased intracranial pressure on steroids may temporarily relieve the symptoms as they decrease edema around the tumor. Diuretics such as mannitol may also be utilized to decrease intracranial pressure. The child should be monitored carefully for any change in status. In severe situations of increased intracranial pressure, intubation with mechanical ventilation is necessary to assure adequate oxygenation to the brain. Any child with significant symptoms or who is unstable should be operated upon immediately. If the child has hydrocephalus, the surgeon may place a ventricular drain to relieve the symptoms prior to the craniotomy for tumor removal. Simply removing the tumor, however, may open blocked CSF pathways and thus relieve the hydrocephalus [3].

Tumors of the hemispheres and posterior fossa are often readily accessible, allowing for gross total surgical resections. Surgical debulking of tumors in the areas of the third ventricle, hypothalamus, optic nerve, and pituitary regions has also become possible. Surgery is not indicated in children with diffuse intrinsic brainstem tumors (most of which are malignant in histology), because the surgical risks outweigh the benefits of a radical surgical procedure; the overall prognosis is thus not changed with surgery. The exception is the focal tumor that is isolated to one area within the brainstem (either only in the medulla or only in the pons, or those at the cervicomedullary junction). These tumors are benign in histology and it is possible to remove them surgically, thus delaying or avoiding adjunctive treatments [30].

Staged surgical procedures and second-look operations have become a frequently used modality to increase the extent of tumor resection and to decrease morbidity. Deep tumors can be approached from two different trajectories to maximize the resection. A surgeon will choose to perform a second operation when the postoperative imaging study shows residual tumor and the pathology is low grade. Second-look operations after a specific treatment modality has been given to allow for evaluation of the tumor response to the treatment, as well as the potential for rendering the patient free of disease [30].

Standard neurosurgical tools utilized by the surgeon in the operating room include the operating microscope, ultrasonic surgical aspirator, carbon dioxide laser, ultrasound, endoscopy, and intraoperative monitoring, such as electrocorticography and sensory and motor evoked potentials (Fig. 6.2). An MRI scan obtained prior to surgery can provide preoperative and intraoperative localization using a frameless navigational system, as shown in Fig. 6.3. In some situations, this allows the surgeon to use a smaller craniotomy to maximally remove the tumor. An ultrasound is used to localize the tumor and it is usually removed with the ultrasonic surgical aspirator. An endoscope may be used to remove or biopsy a tumor within the ventricular system. The laser is commonly used to remove spinal cord tumors. The endoscope can also be used to perform an anterior third ven-

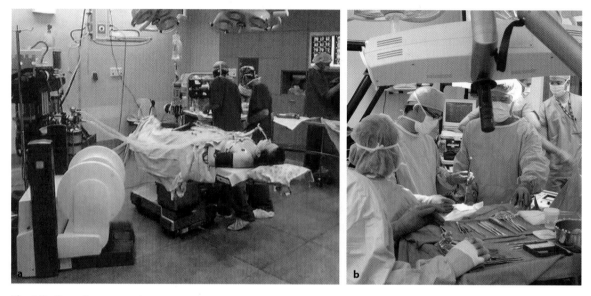

**Fig. 6.2.** Operating room setup

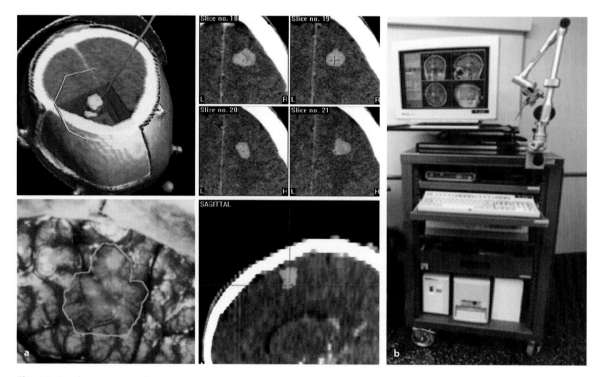

**Fig. 6.3.** Intraoperative guidance systems

triculostomy to treat obstructive hydrocephalus, thus avoiding insertion of a ventriculoperitoneal shunt [16].

Intraoperative monitoring (called evoked potentials) involves watching the nerve impulses travel from the brain to important functional areas, such as arms, legs, face, eyes, and bowels, and bladder (Fig. 6.4). By using this technology during the operation the sur-

geon can determine the location of the tumor in relation to important body function, thus maximizing resection while attempting to minimize injury. Electrocorticography, as shown in Fig. 6.5, allows the surgeon to place electrodes or grids into the cavity after a tumor resection to ensure that any abnormal tissue that can generate a seizure is also removed [2,30].

**Fig. 6.4.** Use of evoked potentials during tumor resection to monitor motor function. *CST* cervical sympathetic trunk

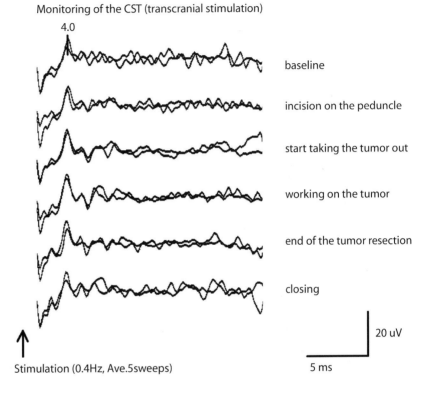

Monitoring of the CST (transcranial stimulation)

4.0

baseline

incision on the peduncle

start taking the tumor out

working on the tumor

end of the tumor resection

closing

20 uV

Stimulation (0.4Hz, Ave.5sweeps)

5 ms

**Fig. 6.5.** Grid placement for evaluation of seizure focus outside tumor cavity

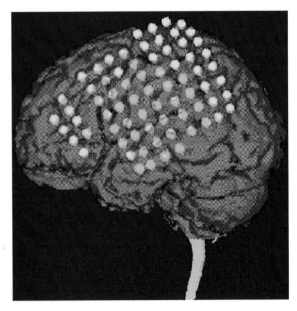

Localization of the tumor using intraoperative guidance systems has become common in the last decade. An MRI scan is obtained preoperatively, with surface markers placed on the scalp. The computerized scan is then sent to the navigational system in the operating room. In the operating room, the surgeon can touch the surface markers upon the scalp and the computer then generates a picture of the lesion in relation to that specific marker. This allows for surgical removal of a tumor through a much smaller craniotomy, reducing both the recovery time and the duration of hospitalization. It is an extremely efficient tool for localizing small lesions within the brain. These systems continue to be modified and improved upon with each generation of equipment [16].

Hydrocephalus that does not resolve with the removal of tumor, and for which an anterior third ventriculostomy is not possible, is treated with insertion of a ventriculoperitoneal shunt. The clinicians must also monitor for the development of hydrocephalus in the weeks or months following surgery secondary to scarring of the CSF pathways from surgery or adjunctive treatments [23,24]. See Chap. 2 (Hydrocephalus) for detailed information about the treatment of hydrocephalus.

### Observation

A postoperative MRI scan is performed, usually within the first few days after surgery. The purpose of the scan is to evaluate the amount of tumor removed. This scan, combined with the histology of the tumor, will determine the next treatment step. For tumors that are very slow growing, and for which a significant surgical removal has been possible, observation with frequent MRIs may be the only recommendation. The ability to detect subtle changes in tumor growth with the MRI has made clinicians more comfortable in observing these tumors. By such observation it has been found that many lesions lie dormant or even regress over time. It has also been noted that growth may not be at a steady rate, but in "pulses" at certain intervals. Observation may delay the use of more surgery or other treatments [27].

Observation may be the treatment of choice at the original diagnosis if the tumor is very small and/or was diagnosed incidentally. MRI is again utilized to monitor the lesion for any change in size over time. Observation is also required following any adjunctive treatment that may be used following surgery. Once a child or adolescent has completed additional treatments for their tumor, MRI scans and other pertinent diagnostic tests are performed on an interval basis [27].

### Radiation

Many CNS tumors are very sensitive to radiation treatments, also called radiotherapy. Prior to the technical advances in surgery, radiation was the primary treatment for CNS tumors in children. It became clear as children began to survive their CNS tumors, however, that radiation treatments also carry acute and long-term side effects that dramatically impacted the individual's ability to function. These side effects include cognitive, growth, hormonal, and hearing issues. The intensity of the side effects was directly related to the age of the child at the time radiation was given. In general, younger children were much more vulnerable to significant toxicity than were older children. Radiation treatments can only be administered once and, therefore, should be employed at the time of minimal disease based upon the tumor type and the age of the patient. Beginning in the late 1980s, clinicians chose to treat younger children requiring adjunctive treatment with chemotherapy first in an attempt to withhold radiation for as long as possible. This past quarter century has brought about technological advances that allow for MRI and CT computerized planning of radiation treatments. This enables focused treatments to the tumor while sparing as much normal brain tissue as possible. Currently, radiation treatments (especially more targeted treatment plans) are being considered for younger children if the tumor is not responsive to chemotherapy [19,31].

Radiotherapy directs high-energy x-rays called photons at targeted areas within the CNS to destroy tumor cells. Radiation can be given internally or externally, with the majority of pediatric CNS tumors treated with external radiation. A large machine called a linear accelerator delivers external radiation via x-rays (photons) to the precise portion of the CNS where the tumor is located. These photons enter the patient at a high dose and deposit that radiation to the tumor target and beyond. Treatment doses for the majority of CNS tumors are between 45 and 60 cGy. If the tumor has the potential of spreading, or has already spread beyond the primary site, the entire CNS will receive external radiation dosing between 18 and 24 cGy. Radiation treatments are normally given once a day at around the same time. Twice-a-day treatments (called hyperfractionation) are another way of delivering radiation treatments. The daily dose is split into two fractions and delivered approximately 12 h apart with the intent of hitting the tumor cells at different times of their cycles and therefore increasing cell death [9].

Conformal radiation therapy is a technique used to target radiation doses to the tumor, while limiting the dose to normal tissues. Conformal radiation therapy requires brain imaging with MRI and CT so that the tumor target and critical normal structures can be accurately defined. It is now the accepted standard for radiation treatments for pediatric CNS tumors. There are several specific types of conformal radiation therapy that utilize photons. Three-dimensional conformal radiation therapy uses radiation fields from several directions that overlap at the tumor. In this manner, the tumor receives the high-dose radiation while the normal tissue surrounding it receives a smaller dose. Intensity-modulated radiation therapy is a sophisticated type of three-dimensional conformal therapy that modifies the radiation beam based on the shape of the target to be treated. Another type of sophisticated three-dimensional technique is stereotactic radiosurgery/radiotherapy, which delivers radiation to a small, precisely defined target. Stereotactic radiosurgery is delivered as one single treatment, while stereotactic radiotherapy is multiple fractionated treatments [14].

Proton-beam radiation is another type of conformal treatment. Unlike the other therapies that utilize photons, this uses protons. Protons, unlike photons, enter the patient with a relatively low dose and deposit their energy within the tumor with no exit dose of radiation to the normal tissues beyond the tumor. At this time, however, there are only a handful of centers with a proton machine. Long-term studies documenting the effectiveness of protons on tumor control and toxicity are needed to justify the construction of more proton facilities [31].

Internal radiation, or brachytherapy, implant therapy or interstitial therapy, is used much less than external radiation to treat childhood CNS tumors. Brachytherapy uses radioactive seeds or implants that are surgically placed into the tumor cavity. Brachytherapy may be useful in treating CNS tumors because it delivers high-dose radiation directly to the tumor site while sparing surrounding healthy tissue. Unlike external radiation, it provides a continuous low dose of radiation to the tumor rather than intermittent bursts once or twice a day [27].

Children should receive radiation therapy at major medical centers with experience in treating children with CNS tumors. This will ensure that treatments conform to the standards set up by COG. Immobilization devices are necessary to ensure that the radiation beam is directed with precision. Sedation or anesthesia may be required on a daily basis for those who cannot tolerate the immobilization process [27].

### Chemotherapy

Until the 1980s chemotherapy was not used to treat pediatric CNS tumors. It was felt that the blood–brain barrier would prevent the penetration of chemotherapy into a tumor within the CNS. Chemotherapy, either alone or as part of a multimodality treatment, is used to treat all malignant CNS tumors and has been shown to be effective in the treatment of some benign tumors. Cooperative group studies within COG have allowed for testing of specific chemotherapeutic protocols, and have been responsible for increasing the progression-free survival in children with CNS tumors. In the past decade the use of higher doses of chemotherapy followed by stem cell rescue have been used in treating tumors in infants (while delaying radiation treatments) or resistant tumors [12,30].

The goal of chemotherapy includes destruction or interruption of the growth of tumor cells. The destruction occurs when the chemotherapeutic agent enters the cell and disrupts its proliferative process. In addition to destroying the abnormally growing tumor cells, the chemotherapy also affects normal-growing cells such as hair, skin, and blood cells, with common adverse effects, including immunosuppression, hair loss, and nausea and vomiting. For more information, see Table 6.2. [24].

Chemotherapy is given either as a single agent alone, or in combination with other drugs. Most treatment plans have a schedule or road map that outlines the drugs given over the treatment plan. Chemotherapy is sometimes given simultaneously with radiation therapy in an attempt to increase radiation's effectiveness. In this case the chemotherapy is referred to as a radiosensitizer. When these drugs are given in high doses or at frequent intervals over a long period of time, bone marrow suppression can be a major side effect. Autologous stem cell reinfusion can

**Table 6.2.** Common chemotherapy drugs and their side effects. Adapted from Shiminski-Maher et al. (2002) [27]

| Chemotherapy group | Specific drugs in group | Side effects of group |
|---|---|---|
| **Alkylating agents:** poison cancer cells by interacting with DNA to prevent cell reproduction | Busulfan<br>Carmustine (BCNU)<br>Carboplatin<br>Cisplatin<br>Cyclophosphamide (Cytoxan)<br>Dacarbazine (DTIC)<br>Ifosfamide<br>Lomustine (CCNU)<br>Procarbazine<br>Temozolamide (Temodar)<br>Thiotepa | Common side effects:<br>Myelosuppression<br>Nausea and vomiting<br>Anorexia and weight loss<br>Stomtitis<br>Alopecia<br>Less common but potential side effects:<br>Hearing loss (cisplatin, carboplatin)<br>Kidney damage (cisplatin, carboplatin)<br>Hemorrhagic cystitis (cytoxan, ifosfamide) |
| **Antimetabolites:** starve cancer cells by replacing essential cell nutrients necessary during synthesis phase of the cell cycle | Hydroxyurea<br>Methotrexate | Myelosuppression<br>Skin rashes<br>Photosensitivity<br>Mouth sores |
| **Antibiotics:** prevent cell growth by blocking reproduction, weakening the membrane of the cell, or interfering with certain cell enzymes | Bleomycin | Alopecia<br>Mouth sores<br>Nausea and vomiting<br>Anorexia and weight loss<br>Lung toxicity |
| **Alkaloids:** derived from plant, interrupt cell division by interfering with DNA synthesis, specific enzyme activities, cell division or disrupting the membrane of the cell to cause cell damage or death | Ironotecan (CPT-11)<br>Topotecan<br>Vinblastine<br>Vincristine | Anorexia<br>Myelosuppression<br>Nausea and vomiting<br>Alopecia<br>Peripheral neuropathy<br>Constipation |
| **Hormones/steroids:** create a hostile environment that slows cell growth | Dexamethasone<br>Methylprednisolone<br>Prednisone | Increased appetite<br>Mood changes<br>Weight gain<br>Sleep loss |
| **Antiangiogenesis:** disrupt the blood supply to a tumor, depriving it of nutrients necessary to grow | Thalidomide | Peripheral neuropathy<br>Drowsiness<br>Constipation<br>Myelosuppression |

regenerate the bone marrow, thus allowing for dose-intensive treatments [27].

## Rehabilitation

Rehabilitation services are a necessary treatment for the majority of children with CNS tumors. The tumor itself, or effects of treatments may impair the use of or coordination in an extremity. Problems with speech, language, memory, and processing may also occur. Physical, occupational, and speech therapy as indicated should be initiated immediately, and often will continue for months or years depending upon individual needs. Therapies are incorporated into school educational plans, with exercise supplements built into daily activities [27].

## Types of Tumors

Tumors of the CNS are classified based on the cell from which they originate and by their rate of growth. CNS tumors develop from astrocytes or neuroglial cells. Other tumors develop from neuronal or premature cell lines. After a sample of the tumor is obtained during surgery, a neuropathologist looks at the tumor under a microscope. He determines the type of tumor, depending upon the cell from which it develops, and the rate of cell growth. Unfortunately, there is no uniform classification of brain tumors. Different pathologists may look at the same tumor and give it a different name. This can be very frustrating and confusing for families. Names for different types of CNS tumors include: astrocytomas, gliomas, glioblastoma multiforme, ependymomas, oligodendrogliomas, gangliocytoma, ganglioglioma, medulloblastoma, primitive neuroectodermal tumors (PNETs), pineal cell tumors, choroid plexus tumors, germ cell tumors, craniopharyngiomas, hemangioblastomas, and dermoid and epidermoid tumors [21, 27].

The terms malignant and benign are confusing when applied to many CNS tumors. In order to identify if a tumor is malignant or benign, it must be looked at in terms of rate of growth and location. Unlike adult brain tumors, which are primarily histologically malignant or fast-growing, childhood brain tumors have a greater likelihood of being histologically benign or slow growing. Slow-growing tumors are technically classified as benign. These tumors, if they are totally removed with surgery, rarely regrow. Many slow-growing tumors, however, are found deep within the brain or brainstem, where aggressive surgery is not possible because of significant risk of damaging adjacent structures. In these cases other treatments (e.g., chemotherapy and/or radiation) are used in an attempt to shrink or halt further tumor growth. Thus, even if a tumor deep in the brain is slow growing, it may require the same treatments as malignant brain tumors – and these treatments can cause the same long-term side effects. Some healthcare providers call this "malignant by location." Figure 6.6 shows the microscopic histology of a slow-growing tumor [27].

All fast-growing tumors are considered malignant and cancerous. Figure 6.7 shows the microscopic histology of a malignant CNS tumor. Even if totally removed with surgery, these tumors will usually grow back without further treatment (radiation and/or chemotherapy). Malignant CNS tumors rarely spread to other parts of the body like breast or liver cancer, but most healthcare professionals still consider them to be a type of cancer [30].

### Treatment Based upon Histology

Once the tissue diagnosis has been made with a surgical procedure, the next step is to formulate a treatment plan. Postoperative imaging is obtained to determine the extent of tumor removal that has been obtained. This information, along with any other preoperative testing, is summarized, and the next step of care is recommended. Many large centers utilize a tumor board to make treatment decisions. This is a multidisciplinary group including surgeons, oncologists, neuro-oncologists, radiation therapy physicians, radiologists, and other appropriate specialists. A case may be presented to the Tumor Board at various times during the course of the illness when treatment decisions need to be made. A summary of treat-

**Fig. 6.6.** Histology of slow-growing tumor

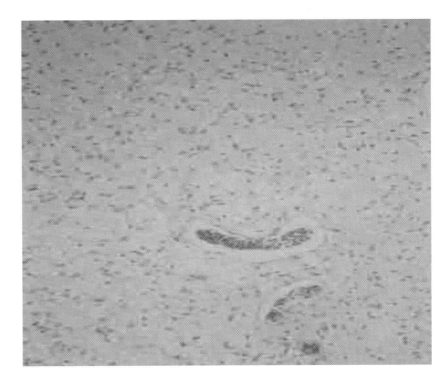

**Fig. 6.7.** Histology of fast-growing tumor

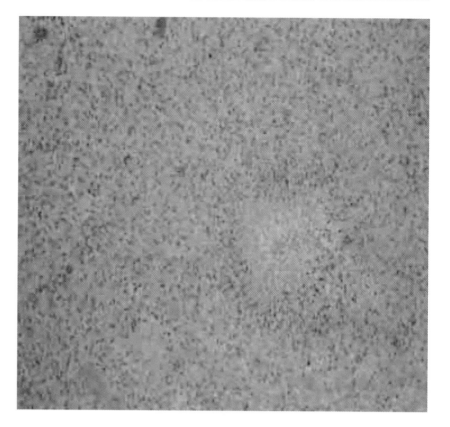

ments based upon tumor histology is found in Table 6.3. A discussion of treatment plans based on specific pathologic diagnosis follows [27].

### Low-Grade Astrocytomas

Astrocytomas (also called gliomas) make up about one-third of CNS tumor in children, and are the most common type thereof. They may be slow growing or very fast growing and can arise anywhere in the brain and spinal cord. About 80% of astrocytomas are slow growing in the pediatric population. This includes juvenile pilocytic astrocytoma, low-grade astrocytoma, and optic pathway or hypothalamic gliomas. Slow-growing astrocytomas in the brain arise in the cerebral hemispheres, the cerebellum, or the spinal cord. Surgery is the primary treatment for slow-growing astrocytomas. This is possible in many areas of the cerebrum and always possible in the cerebellum. The most potentially curable form is the cerebellar pilocytic astrocytoma (Fig. 6.8). If there is question of residual tumor after surgery, the surgeon can either reoperate, or follow closely with frequent MRI scans and reserve surgery if there is an increase in tumor size. Cerebellar or hemispheric low-grade astrocyto-

mas rarely spread throughout the neuroaxis; spine imaging is therefore not necessary [17].

Slow-growing astrocytomas account for 75% of all spinal cord tumors in children (Fig. 6.9). Surgery is the primary treatment, and multiple surgical procedures are usually needed to maintain tumor control. The use of intraoperative monitoring has dramatically improved the safety of radical tumor removal. Radiation therapy is used for tumors that grow despite multiple surgical procedures. Chemotherapy historically has not been given to children with low-grade spinal cord tumors, so its effectiveness is unknown [20].

Low-grade astrocytomas also occur in the diencephalons, specifically in the hypothalamus and optic chiasm (Fig. 6.10). They can be sporadic or associated with neurofibromatosis syndromes. In children, the histological diagnosis is made with the presence of Rosenthal fibers and they are generally very low in cellularity. The clinical course varies, with many lesions remaining dormant for extended periods of time. Treatment is indicated if there are either worsening clinical symptoms or radiographic evidence of tumor growth. Observation with careful clinical examina-

**Table 6.3.** Brain tumors: treatment based upon type and location of tumor. Adapted from Shiminski-Maher et al. (2002) [27]. *MRI* magnetic resonance imaging

| Part of the CNS | Type of tumor | Treatment |
|---|---|---|
| Frontal lobes<br>Parietal lobes<br>Temporal lobes<br>Occipital lobes | Astrocytoma<br>Glioma<br>DNET<br>Rarely PNET or Ependymoma | Maximal surgical removal using intraoperative guidance, monitoring, electrocorticography, and MRI. Observation between surgical treatments for tumors that are slow growing.<br>Chemotherapy and or radiation may be considered for disease progression in low grade lesion r for adjunctive treatment for high grade astrocytomas or gliomas, PNET or ependymoma. |
| Cerebellum | Astrocytoma<br>Glioma<br>Medulloblastoma<br>Ependymoma | Maximal surgical removal. Observation following surgery for slow growing tumors with reoperation at progression. Chemotherapy and/or radiation for medulloblastoma and ependymoma. |
| Brainstem/fourth ventricle | Astrocytoma<br>Glioma<br>Ependymoma<br>Medulloblastoma | Radiation +/− chemotherapy is standard treatment for diffuse brainstem tumors.<br>Surgery is possible for focal lesions followed by observation, chemotherapy or radiation. |
| Midbrain/thalamus<br>Diencephalon<br>Optic pathway<br>Ventricular system | Astrocytoma<br>Glioma<br>Craniopharyngioma<br>Germ Cell<br>Choroid Plexus | Conservative surgery or observation for low grade tumors. Observation +/− chemo for low grade. Chemotherapy and radiation for germ cell or other high grade tumors. |
| Spinal cord | Astrocytoma<br>Ependymoma | Maximal surgery then observation.<br>Radiation for high grade tumors or tumor progression. |

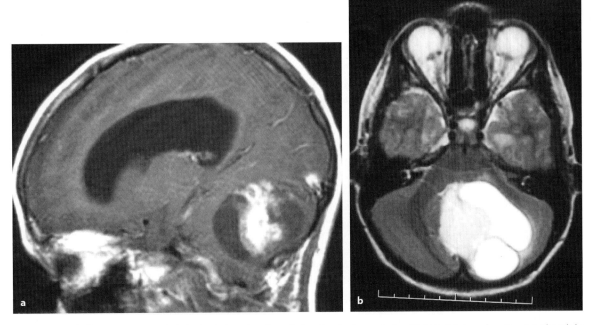

**Fig. 6.8.** Cerebellar astrocytoma. *Left* Sagittal view showing obstructive hydrocephalus. *Right* Axial view showing mural nodule

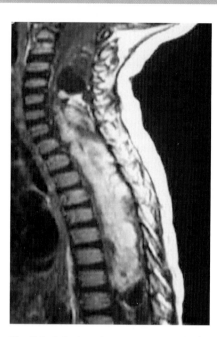

**Fig. 6.9.** Spinal cord astrocytoma: sagittal view of a solid enhancing tumor with a cyst above and below

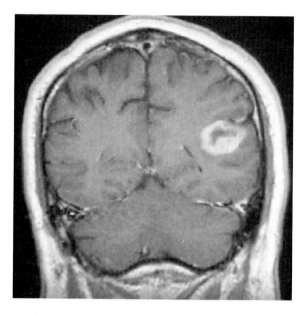

**Fig. 6.11.** Anaplastic astrocytoma: enhancing tumor adjacent to motor strip

tion and serial MRI scans is the treatments of choice. Surgery is indicated only for tissue diagnosis, or for partial reduction in the size of the tumor. Surgical management of hydrocephalus may be required if the tumor is obstructing normal CSF pathways [6, 30].

Additional treatment is given if the MRI shows tumor growth or if the child develops symptoms (usually visual or hormonal). The type of treatment depends upon the age of the child and the growth pattern of the tumor. Treatment may include surgery, but usually chemotherapy (especially in children less than

10 years old). Radiation therapy is the third treatment option, recommended for the patient with progressive tumor who has failed initial chemotherapy or for the child or adult over age 10 years. Most neuro-oncologists try to delay radiation therapy for these tumors for as long as possible, because of the increased risk of damage to the developing nervous system [27].

**Malignant Astrocytomas**

A small number of astrocytoma tumors in the pediatric population grow rapidly; these are known as malignant astrocytomas. They usually grow in the cerebrum or brainstem, and are rarely found in the spinal cord. Types of rapid-growing astrocytomas include high-grade anaplastic astrocytoma, glioblastoma multiforme, and gliomatosis cerebri [27].

High-grade astrocytomas are difficult to cure even with the most aggressive treatments (Fig. 6.11). Maximal surgical resection appears to be the only significant variable in extending time to progression for this resistant tumor. Radiation therapy remains the standard adjunctive treatment for children with malignant astrocytomas and, when given after aggressive surgery and with chemotherapy, will prolong time to progression. Chemotherapy windows have included single and multiple agents along with high-dose chemotherapy with autologous marrow or stem cell rescue. To date, despite multiple cooperative group clini-

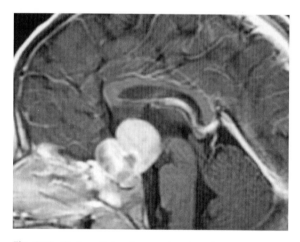

**Fig. 6.10.** Optic pathway low-grade astrocytoma

**Fig. 6.12.** Brainstem glioma. **a** Sagittal view of a ring enhancing tumor. **b** Axial image of diffuse appearance on T2-weighted image

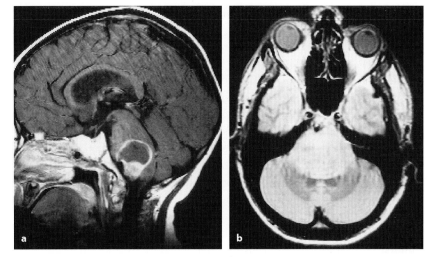

cal trials where chemotherapy was given before, during, and following radiation therapy, there has been no significant improvement in event-free survival [17].

### Brainstem gliomas

Astrocytomas that grow in the brainstem are called brainstem gliomas. They make up 10–15% of all pediatric brain tumors. Brainstem tumors can be either low-grade or high-grade astrocytomas. Ninety percent of these tumors are fast growing and cause rapidly developing symptoms. They involve multiple levels of the brainstem and have a diffuse appearance on the MRI scan (Fig. 6.12). Surgery is not an option because aggressive surgery in the brainstem would result in severe neurological impairment. The majority of children diagnosed with a brainstem glioma do not survive more than 2 years beyond diagnosis [1].

Radiation therapy is the primary treatment, and usually results in an initial decrease in tumor size and improvement in clinical symptoms. Chemotherapy has been added to radiation with no improvement in survival. Unfortunately, usually within 1 year, the tumor begins to grow again, and adjunctive treatments may provide palliation but are ineffective in curing the tumor [27].

About 10% of brainstem tumors are slow-growing brainstem gliomas. They are usually focal tumors located in the medulla, pons, or midbrain, and symptoms develop over a long period of time. Unlike the diffuse high-grade lesions, these tumors usually remain confined to one component of the brainstem. Surgical debulking may render the tumor dormant

for an extended period of time. Adjunctive treatment alternatives include observation, radiation, and/or chemotherapy [1].

### Spinal Cord Malignant Astrocytomas

Anaplastic astrocytoma, or glioblastoma multiforme, is a rare entity in children, but a handful are diagnosed each year. Like the high-grade astrocytomas of the brain, the extent of surgical resection may impact time to progression, and radiation treatments may temporarily reduce the size of the tumor. Tumor progression usually occurs within the 1st year to 18 months, with event-free survival at five-years being rare [20].

### Subependymal Giant Cell Astrocytomas

Subependymal giant cell astrocytomas are tumors that are always associated with tuberous sclerosis, which is an autosomal dominant inherited phakomatosis. Clinical symptoms include adenoma sebaceum, seizures, and mental retardation. These tumors only occur in 6–15% of children with tuberous sclerosis. Most subependymal giant cell astrocytomas arise in the lateral ventricle near the foramen of Monroe and cause obstructive hydrocephalus. Because death can occur from undiagnosed tumor and hydrocephalus, all children with tuberous sclerosis should be screened radiographically every 2 years for the presence of a lesion. A gross total removal of the tumor is usually possible, with surgery being the only known effective treatment [17].

### Oligodendrogliomas/Gangliogliomas/ Gangliocytomas

This group of slow-growing glial tumors is rare in children and as a total may comprise less than 5% of all pediatric CNS tumors. They are so slow growing that a diagnosis is obtained because of headache complaints or a seizure, which results in radiological imaging. They can also be diagnosed incidentally. If surgically accessible, a gross total removal is curative. Observation, with further surgery or radiation therapy if the tumor begins to grow, is recommended [6].

### Ependymoma

Ependymomas make up 8–10% of childhood brain tumors. They arise from the cells that line the ventricular system. About 70% of ependymomas occur in the posterior fossa, usually in the fourth ventricle (Fig. 6.13). Ependymomas also occasionally grow in the cerebral hemispheres and in the spinal cord. Because of the risk of spread of tumor to other areas of the neuroaxis, preoperative imaging of the entire CNS is recommended [17].

Surgery is the first treatment for ependymomas. Surgical management of hydrocephalus is also required because of the tumor obstructing flow through the fourth ventricle. It is difficult, however, to totally remove an ependymoma from the fourth ventricle because it is close to the brainstem. As with other tumor types, the extent of surgical removal is correlated with increased progression-free survival, thus children with fourth-ventricular ependymomas tend to have a worse prognosis. Treatment of ependymomas after surgery is controversial. Radiation has been shown to be beneficial in a small group of patients. Chemotherapy has shown some efficacy and continues to be considered along with radiation for tumors that cannot be surgically removed. Although various subtypes of histology have been identified, there appears to be no significant difference in the length of time to either survival or recurrence. Ependymomas tend to recur locally and most recurrences occur within 5 years of diagnosis [17].

### Medulloblastoma

Medulloblastomas are the most common malignant tumor and account for about 20% of all CNS tumors in children. These are, by definition, posterior fossa lesions originating in the cerebellum with potential extension into the fourth ventricle and/or brainstem. Because these lesions can interfere with the normal flow of CSF, hydrocephalus is often present at diagnosis. Medulloblastoma can also grow in the cerebral hemispheres (Fig. 6.14). Unlike most other CNS tumors, medulloblastoma cells can spread throughout the brain and the spinal cord. Medulloblastoma tumors spread far from the primary tumor in 25–40% of cases. For this reason, children should have an MRI scan of the entire brain and spine at diagnosis to determine if the tumor has spread. An analysis of CSF (for the presence of tumor cells) by lumbar puncture is also done. Rarely, bone metastases occur, usually in less than 5% of children [29].

Treatment plans vary depending upon the child's age at diagnosis, the amount of tumor removed, and the extent of tumor spread. Surgery (in one or several

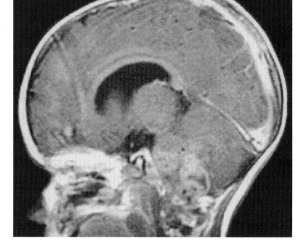

**Fig. 6.13.** Ependymoma: sagittal image of enhancing tumor filling the fourth ventricle causing obstructive hydrocephalus

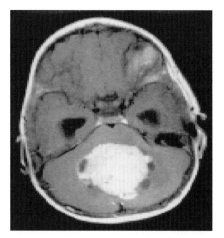

**Fig. 6.14.** Medulloblastoma

operations) is the first treatment for medulloblastoma. Total removal is the goal. This is sometimes difficult if the tumor has spread to the brainstem or the floor of the fourth ventricle. About 30–50% of all children will require treatment for hydrocephalus with either a shunt or an anterior third ventriculostomy. If not done preoperatively, a neuroaxis MRI scan for drop metastases and a spinal tap for cytology to determine CSF spread must be done immediately postoperatively. Medulloblastoma is very responsive to radiation therapy and to many chemotherapy drugs [27].

Medulloblastoma tumors are grouped into two broad categories: standard risk and high risk. A tumor that has been completely removed by surgery and has not spread to other areas of the CNS is called standard risk. Children with standard-risk medulloblastoma receive craniospinal radiation and chemotherapy during induction, with a chemotherapy backbone for maintenance. Progression-free survival for this group of children is approximately 75–90% at 5 years. Those children who are younger than age 3 years at diagnosis, who have spread of their disease within the neuroaxis, or who have greater than 5 cm$^3$ of tumor after surgery are considered high risk. Treatment for these children varies with age. For those younger than age 3 years, intensive chemotherapy with a tandem stem-cell rescue is indicated to achieve a remission, until the child is older than 3 years of age, at which point radiotherapy can be used. Older children receive radiation with or without a radiosensitizing chemotherapy, followed by intensive chemotherapy with autologous stem-cell rescue, if necessary [27].

### Primitive Neuroectodermal Tumors/ Pineoblastoma

PNETs and medulloblastoma were once considered the same type of tumor that arose in different locations in the brain. For many years, the two names were used interchangeably regardless of where the tumor grew. Historically, medulloblastoma was the name given to this tumor when it grew in the posterior fossa and PNET when it grew outside of the posterior fossa in the cerebral hemispheres. A PNET of the pineal gland is referred to as a pineoblastoma. Even though a gross total surgical removal is possible for PNETs depending upon location, their prognosis is generally worse than for children with posterior fossa medulloblastoma; however, they are usually treated with the treatment protocols for high-risk medulloblastoma [27].

### Dysembryoplastic Neuroepithelial Tumors

Dysembryoplastic neuroepithelial tumors (DNETs) are very rare, low-grade neuroepithelial tumors that are most common in the first two decades of life. They arise in the supratentorial cerebral cortex, often in the temporal lobes. Clinical presentation is almost always partial complex seizures. Surgery is the primary treatment and employed not only to remove the tumor, but to treat the seizure disorder as well. If the entire tumor is not removed, the patient is observed with serial scans [17].

### Craniopharyngiomas

Craniopharyngiomas are the most common suprasellar brain tumor in children, accounting for 6–8% of all CNS tumors (Fig. 6.15). They occur most frequently in children and are rarely seen in the adult population. Despite clinically benign features, their location in the sella is in close proximity to the hypothalamus, pituitary gland, and optic chiasm, resulting in significant morbidity and mortality. They precipitate multisystem abnormalities, including endocrinopathies, and visual, cognitive, and social problems either at the time of tumor presentation or in conjunction with treatment. Treatment is controversial because aggressive surgery often cures the child, but can cause lifelong memory, visual, behavioral, and hormonal problems. Removal of part of the tumor, followed by radiation therapy is a treatment option that can lessen the long-term side effects. Treatment depends upon the location and the size of the tumor, and may include surgery from an intracranial or transphenoidal ap-

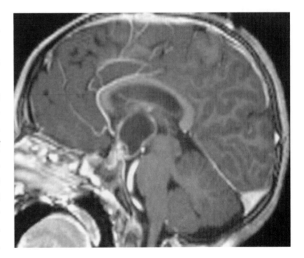

**Fig. 6.15.** Craniopharyngioma

proach, observation, or focused radiation therapy [17,28].

### Germ Cell Tumors

Germ cell tumors typically grow in the pineal or suprasellar regions (Fig. 6.16). There are two types of germ cell tumors: pure germinomas and nongerminoma germ cell tumors. Nongerminoma germ cell tumors secrete substances called tumor markers. Doctors can diagnose these tumors by checking the blood or CSF for two markers: called alpha fetoprotein and beta-HCG. Therefore, diagnosis of a nongerminoma tumor does not require surgery. If the tumor is very large, however, part of it is removed (debulked) if the neurosurgeon feels it can be done with few to no side effects. Treatment for nongerminoma germ cell tumors includes chemotherapy followed by radiation [27].

Pure germinomas are diagnosed by a surgical biopsy. These tumors respond dramatically to radiation and chemotherapy. Radiation therapy is the standard of care for treatment. Recently, physicians have given chemotherapy following surgery, with a reduction in the dose of radiation for those tumors that completely disappear with the chemotherapy. This is an attempt to reduce the dose of radiation needed, possibly reducing long-term side effects. If the tumor disappeared after chemotherapy, the radiation dose is usually reduced [27].

### Choroid Plexus Tumors

Choroid plexus papillomas (slow growing) or choroid plexus carcinomas (fast growing) arise from the cho-

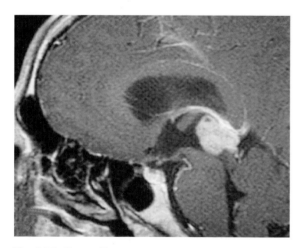

**Fig. 6.16.** Germ cell tumor

roid plexus, which is located in the ventricles. The choroid plexus is the part of the brain that produces CSF. These tumors account for 1–3% of all childhood brain tumors, and most often occur in infants. The tumor is usually diagnosed simultaneously with hydrocephalus. Surgery followed by observation is the treatment for choroid plexus papillomas. Surgery followed by chemotherapy and radiation is the treatment for choroid plexus carcinomas [27].

### Dermoids, Epidermoids, Eosinophilic Granulomas, and Histiocytosis X

Dermoid and Epidermoid cysts/tumors arise from dermal and epidermal tissues. They are benign tumors that can be found anywhere in the CNS. Scalp dermoid and epidermoid tumors can be surgically removed and rarely regrow. Intracranial and intraspinal dermoid or epidermoid tumors are rare, and are treated with maximal surgical removal [17].

Eosinophilic granulomas and histocytosis are tumors that primarily affect the skull or spine. They present as painful lesions and treatment involves surgical removal with margins whenever possible. Bone grafting may be necessary if there is a large bone defect after the lesion is removed. Rarely, recurrent or residual tumors may be treated with low-dose radiation or chemotherapy [17].

### Infant Tumors

Children diagnosed with a CNS tumor in infancy should be discussed separately. These tumors are more difficult to treat because they are often aggressive histologically and any treatment will have an affect on the rapidly developing brain. The most common types of tumors associated with infancy are astrocytomas, PNETs, ependymomas, and choroid plexus tumors. Surgery is the primary treatment for all infant CNS tumors. If adjunctive treatment is necessary, most clinicians advocate utilizing chemotherapy in an attempt to delay radiation therapy. Radiation is recommended for children less than 3 years of age only as a last resort [16].

### Posterior Fossa Syndrome

Posterior fossa syndrome (also called cerebellar mutism) is a complication of posterior fossa (cerebellum or brainstem) surgery. The most common tumors in this area are medulloblastomas, astrocytomas, and ependymomas. Most children wake up from the surgery moving their arms and legs and responding to questions. In some cases, 24 or more hours later, the child stops talking, may develop weakness of arms and legs, and cranial nerve deficits appear. Emotionally, the children seem disconnected from their environment and may respond by simply crying. These symptoms improve over a period of days in the minimally affected child, but improvement may take months in the severely affected child. Physical, occupational, and speech therapy should be started immediately. Children who have severe posterior fossa syndrome require transfer to an inpatient rehabilitation center [13].

## Nursing Care: Overview

Nursing management for the child with a CNS tumor is dependent upon many variables, including age at diagnosis, specific type of tumor, neurological deficits, treatments required, and the individual family dynamics present to deal with the illness. All patients and families have a need for education and emotional support throughout all facets of the illness. The management of children with CNS tumors involves a large multidisciplinary team, including nurses, pediatricians, pediatric neurosurgeons, neurologists, oncologists, endocrinologists, radiologists, social work, Child-Life, and radiation oncologists to name a few. Nurses and nurse practitioners are the healthcare providers who have the majority of contact with the patient and families both in the hospital and as coordinators of outpatient care. Thus, nurses serve as patient advocates, case managers, and educators in a liaison role between patient/family and various members of the medical team throughout the course of the illness. They are also responsible for coordination of re-entry to school and normal life once the acute treatment phase is completed. Nursing intervention is indeed critical at diagnosis and throughout the treatment of pediatric CNS tumors [10,24].

## Developmental Considerations

It is uniformly accepted that children need to be told of their diagnosis and plan of treatment as soon as possible. Delay in providing information only will escalate the child's fears. Parents may delude themselves into thinking that the diagnosis is a secret, but children are very perceptive. Nurses can assist parents in providing developmentally appropriate information to their children. Nurses can also ensure that age-appropriate explanations are provided to patients prior to any procedure or treatment given. Educational materials should be provided for the families whether written, or by video or access to the Internet. The children and families should be encouraged to ask questions and keep a notebook with information regarding the diagnosis and treatment, as well as tests that have been performed and results [27].

## Diagnosis

The nurse's main responsibility during the diagnostic period is to provide the child and family with information about why various tests are being performed and how to prepare their child or each test. Nursing management of the patient undergoing diagnostic studies includes a large amount of patient/family education and coordination of diagnostic activities. Most young children (and older children whose level of consciousness is altered) receive conscious sedation or anesthesia for their MRI scans. The nurse must monitor the child closely for signs and symptoms of increased intracranial pressure and seizures. If the child is not hospitalized during the diagnostic testing phase, instructions should be given to the family regarding the signs and symptoms of increased intracranial pressure and seizure precautions, as indicated. Patient/family education should reinforce information given to the parents, including information on how to contact the medical team with any questions or concerns [24].

Obviously, the acuity of the situation will determine the extent of preparation the nurse can provide for the child and family. A neurologically unstable child may go from the emergency room to the scanner, and then to the operating room. In other situations, the surgery is planned as an elective procedure with the child at home prior to the surgery. Whenever possible, nurses should be present when the physician presents the information about diagnosis and treatment to the child and family. The nurse will be able to reinforce and clarify information communicated as well as answer some of the many questions that will arise later. The nurse can provide preoperative education, including location of the incision, bandages, presence of a drain or shunt postoperatively, and other tubes that may be needed. Diagrams, booklets and other audio-video tools assist in this preparation. Nurses can also refer the child and family to social work and Child-Life teams to reinforce this information [26].

## Surgery

Nursing care of the postoperative pediatric CNS tumor patient depends upon the location of the tumor, the extent of surgical removal, and clinical condition of the patient. Intraoperative guidance systems have dramatically reduced the size of many craniotomies and thus impacted positively on the recovery period for these children. Where children with CNS tumors would spend 2–5 postoperative days in an intensive care setting 10 years ago, today they spend on average 1–4 days. Intensive care monitoring is based upon level of consciousness. Most children are able to maintain their own airway and are extubated at the end of the surgery. For those children, it is a matter of careful hourly assessment for changes in level of consciousness or increased intracranial pressure for the first 24 h postoperatively. Hourly neurological checks and vital signs will allow nurses to alert the physicians of any changes in neurological status. Intracranial pressure monitoring is utilized for operations where the child is neurologically impaired preoperatively, if there is a sudden bleed or change in intracranial dynamics during the operation, or if intraoperative monitoring shows a change in the integrity of the nervous system in a specific region. Intracranial pressure can be monitored from a transducer through an externalized drain or, if no hydrocephalus is present, through an external intracranial pressure monitor, called an intraparenchymal wire, inserted between the bone and the brain tissue [3].

Surgically removing some or all the tumor is the first step in treating increased intracranial pressure. The presence of an external drain to remove CSF allows for further control of the intracranial pressure. Intravenous steroids, most commonly dexamethasone, are used to combat swelling. Further medical management includes the addition of osmotic diuretics such as mannitol, and the utilization of intubation and hyperventilation. The prognosis is poorer if the child requires the latter. As in most positive outcomes with medical management, the least amount of medi-

cal intervention required usually results in the best outcome in terms of long-term survival and ultimate cure [3].

Children are released from the intensive care unit when they are neurologically stable, usually within 24–48 h postoperatively. A steroid taper is begun with the idea of stopping steroids as soon as possible. The long-term side effects of steroids have to be weighed with the side effects of long-term steroid use. These side effects of steroids include increased appetite and weight gain, irritability, difficulty sleeping, and muscle weakness. In addition, long term steroid use can adversely weaken the immune system. It is understood that the use of postoperative steroids makes the examination of a child "better than reality." Steroids are only increased if there is a severe loss of function in a short period of time in a particular patient [3].

The use of postoperative anticonvulsants is necessary for children who presented with seizures preoperatively, or for those who have tumors in areas of the brain where seizures can occur because of location. Intra- or postoperative seizures can occur in an area of the brain prone to epileptic activity that is associated with the removal of the tumor, or associated interference with normal electrical activity in adjacent areas. Pre and postoperative 24-h electrocorticography may be necessary for tumors where removal of the tumor and removal of an adjacent seizure focus is necessary. The recent advances in monitoring activity have resulted in long-term remission from the tumor, as well as eventual cure of a seizure problem, with removal of all anticonvulsants, in a tumor associated with seizures [7].

Patients who have hypothalamic and pituitary tumors are at risk for the development of DI, or syndrome of inappropriate secretion of antidiuretic hormone (SIADH), as a result of the tumor or the surgeon injuring the pituitary stalk. In the normal individual, water balance is controlled by the release of vasopressin from the posterior pituitary gland. The hypothalamus produces and releases the hormone, which travels via the pituitary stalk to the posterior pituitary gland where it is stored. Vasopressin is circulated to the kidney where it controls the amount of water retained or excreted. Vasopressin's hormonal influence controls the salt and water balance within the body. Imbalance in this system secondary to increased or decreased amounts of circulating vasopressin is commonly associated with DI or SIADH. Children with suprasellar, hypothalamic, or pituitary tumors are at risk for primary DI, while SIADH can occur as result of overtreatment of DI, or because of confusion with salt wasting issues, which occur following injury to the posterior fossa and brainstem. Careful monitoring of fluid intake and output, as well as serum and urine sodium levels, is necessary for the regulation of water and sodium balance in the body. DI may be permanent or transient depending on the extent of injury to the pituitary stalk. If resolution of this problem is to occur, it usually will do so in the first 2 weeks after surgery [28]. For nursing management of sodium problems refer to Chap. 7 (Traumatic Brain Injury).

The majority of the suprasellar tumors are approached from an intracranial direction. Some tumors, however, may be approached from a transsphenoidal direction or in a two-step transsphenoidal and intracranial procedure. This approach is utilized in older children whose sphenoid sinuses are large enough to accommodate the approach. Postoperatively, these children must be monitored carefully for leakage of CSF. Often, their noses are blocked for a few days and they are prohibited from nose blowing or sneezing [17].

For those children without significant intracranial pressure, seizure, or hormonal problems, careful monitoring is necessary for 24–48 h. Postoperative imaging is necessary within the first 2 days to determine the extent of tumor resection. For those children requiring sedation or anesthesia, nursing coordination is essential. Physical and occupational therapy is ordered in the immediate postoperative period to begin working with any physical weaknesses that may be evident [3].

Pain management is different depending upon location in the CNS. Brain tumor surgery is generally less painful than spinal cord tumor surgery. Postoperative analgesics for intracranial surgery include a short period of opiates such as morphine, with a rapid switch to codeine or oxycodone, with or without acetaminophen. Nonsteroidal anti-inflammatory drugs such as ketorolac or ibuprofen are often used to potentiate the narcotic effects. Spinal cord operations usually require a longer course of opiates, usually with patient-controlled analgesia. By the 2nd postoperative day, the patient becomes increasingly mobile, with a decrease in intravenous narcotics and an increase in oral drugs. Switching from opioids to nonsteroidal anti-inflammatory medications while the dexamethasone (steroid) is decreased further aids in mobility [3].

Children with severe alteration in intracranial pressure or altered level of consciousness preoperatively, or those who are unstable during surgery, will require longer-term intensive care management postoperatively. Placement in an intensive care unit setting with intensive nursing monitoring is required. Airway, breathing and circulation are the priorities. These are linked closely with intracranial pressure, which must be monitored constantly. Intake and output, management of fluid and electrolytes, especially sodium, and fluid balance, is a key nursing function. Continued interface with the family members by the nurses to keep them up to date on the current clinical situation, as well as providing ongoing education about the illness, is also important. As an individual's clinical condition improves, the patient transitions into a less intensive level of care that focuses on maximal recovery [3].

The goal with all postoperative patients is to minimize the time spent in the intensive care unit and initiate rehabilitative treatments while decreasing steroids and any other pain medications as soon as possible. This goal will allow for maximization of physical function with the least amount of medical support as the next step of the treatment process is identified. Nurses must assist patients and families in participating in physical therapy while minimizing medical support. They must also provide education as to the diagnosis of the tumor and the plan for further treatment [27].

## Observation

For many children with CNS tumors, surgery is the only initial treatment. The next phase of treatment is simply clinical and radiographic observation. Other children get to the observation phase after having any combination of surgery, radiation, and chemotherapy. Whatever the course, families of children with CNS tumors who reach a period of observation do so with a certain amount of fear and anxiety about not having an "active treatment" plan. This period may include treatments that focus on residual clinical issues caused by the tumor and its treatment, such as physical, occupational and speech therapies, seizure medications, or hormonal replacements. MRI scans are needed at specific intervals based upon previous scans [27].

Nurses play a key role in the coordination of care in the observation phase. At this time families often rely on the nurses for emotional support and to answer questions that may arise. They coordinate the scheduling of diagnostic tests and appointments with various medical teams. Nurses educate the parents or caregivers so that they can effectively advocate for their children within the medical and community systems. Education should emphasize return to school and other normal activities as soon as possible. To facilitate this, nurses can provide information and education to the school community regarding the illness and treatment, and the importance of the child returning to school with as few limitations as possible [27].

### Radiation Therapy

Nursing intervention throughout radiation treatment involves coordination of the treatment along with providing education to the child and family regarding the radiation and its potential adverse affects. Coordination of treatment is more complex for younger children, who will require daily anesthesia. Ideally these children should be scheduled in the morning to minimize the time of "nil by mouth" status. Coordination also includes gaining the cooperation of the children to participate in the radiation treatments. Nurses collaborate with Child-Life and Social Work in using play therapy to gain cooperation. Children who require positioning in a mold may be allowed to take it home in the evening to practice with it, thus increasing the child's comfort level. Allowing the child to visit the facility several times before the beginning of treatments will also decrease anxiety and increase cooperation [9, 24].

School age and adolescent patients need support in coping with body issues of hair loss or other physical changes that may occur. While these children may not require sedation or anesthesia for daily treatments, they may need medication to help with the simulation of radiation, a lengthy session, which is the technical planning and measuring session. At this session the child is marked so that he can be aligned in the same position for each treatment. Radiation markings are small ink marks that should not be scrubbed off in the bath. They do fade over time and the technologist will mark over them as needed during the treatment [27].

Nursing intervention throughout radiation treatment involves monitoring the patient for any side effects of radiation, as well as educating patients and families. Patients need to be instructed to watch for signs and symptoms of brain swelling as the treatments begin to take effect. This may include a reappearance of the tumor's presenting symptoms which, when not adequately prepared for, causes much anxiety. If the symptoms are dramatically interfering with the child's activities of daily living, a short course of steroids, or boosting of existing steroid dose with a subsequent taper, may improve things. As with surgical patients, steroids are important to treat acute problems but should be tapered as quickly as possible to prevent side effects [24].

Nutritional support of these children during radiation is important. Nurses should be monitoring for any decreased appetite or weight loss. Some children may experience nausea and vomiting after the treatment. The parents administering antiemetics prior to the treatment each day can prevent this. Children who lose an excessive amount of weight may require enteral feedings. In this situation, nurses must educate the family on how to provide the feedings [21].

Toward the end of treatment and for a few weeks thereafter, it is not unusual for the patient to feel fatigue and increased sleepiness. This is usually short-lived and, as with acute symptoms, severe cases can be treated with a short pulse of steroids. Finally, children who are receiving craniospinal irradiation must have their complete blood count monitored because bone marrow suppression is possible during the spine component of the treatment. Weekly complete blood counts and other appropriate blood tests are performed on children who are receiving chemotherapy at the same time as the radiation [10].

### Chemotherapy

The majority of children who receive chemotherapy will follow some type of treatment protocol. This includes very specific road maps or recipes for timing of drug administration and monitoring for side effects. Nursing care of the child receiving chemotherapy includes the actual administration of the drugs in most cases, but also, as with radiation therapy, involves coordination of care and patient/family education and support. Monitoring for side affects of chemotherapy is another key nursing function. Common chemotherapy drugs and their side effects are listed in Table 6.2 [27].

Nausea and vomiting may occur with some of the chemotherapies. Nursing care includes administration of antiemetics and monitoring for adequate nutrition and hydration. Small, frequent meals may ensure adequate nutrition rather than traditional meal times. Fluid and electrolyte imbalances can occur during administration of chemotherapy and can be intensified in the child with endocrine issues such as DI [25].

Immunosuppression is one of the common side effects of chemotherapy; therefore blood counts are monitored on a frequent basis as per the individual protocol. When blood counts are low, packed red blood cells may be given to treat anemia and platelets given to treat very low platelet levels. Children with decreased white blood cell counts must be isolated from sick people and must be hospitalized if they have a fever or any sign of infection. Some treatment protocols that induce severe immunosuppression advocate the use of marrow stimulants such as neupogin or erythopoetin to increase production of these cells. Immunosuppression is even more pronounced in the patient who has received or is receiving craniospinal irradiation. This radiation can affect the bone marrow's ability to recover following chemotherapy [24, 27].

Several of the commonly used chemotherapies for the treatment of pediatric brain tumors also adversely affect hearing and kidney function. Children are routinely monitored with audiograms to assess for any change in hearing. Changes, if they occur, will do so in the higher frequency sounds first. Kidney function is monitored with blood and urine tests. Dose modifications of the chemotherapy are outlined in the protocols if adverse toxicity occurs. Nurses are responsible for checking these results prior to the administration of chemotherapy, and administering reduced doses as necessary. Peripheral nerve toxicity resulting in pain in the extremities and difficulty walking can also occur with some of the chemotherapies. This is exaggerated in children with CNS tumors who may have weakness from steroids and or surgery. Nurses must ensure that these children are receiving physical and occupational therapy and, if toxicity is severely impairing activities of daily living, a dose modification as per the individual protocol may be required [27].

Nursing care for the child receiving high-dose chemotherapy with peripheral stem-cell reinfusion involves all of the above interventions, with toxicities being expected. Such children have a greater chance at fever and neutropenia admissions, increased transfusion requirements, nutritional issues, and neurological complications. These children also spend more time in the hospital and thus are removed from school and other normal activities [27].

## The multidisciplinary team

Care of children with CNS tumors requires a multidisciplinary approach. These patients are cared for by neurosurgeons, neurologists, pediatricians, nurses/advance practice nurses, radiologists, endocrinologists, dieticians, neuro-ophthalmologists, neuropsychologists, social workers, Child-Life specialists, and psychologists to name a few. Primary responsibility for treatment and coordination of care may shift from one subspecialty to another depending upon whether the child is on active or inactive (observation) treatment. It is essential that the patient and family know which healthcare team(s) is coordinating care at any given time. Communication must exist within and between members of each team. This coordination most often falls to the patient, parents, or caregivers. Nurses and nurse practitioners are instrumental in providing parents with the information and education that they need to advocate for their children. In situations where patients and/or caregivers are unable to coordinate or advocate, the nurse/practitioner can assume that role. Patients and families look to nurses for coordination of diagnostic testing, explanation and reinforcement of all procedures and surgery, and integration of information given to them regarding the treatment plan and side effects. The nurse can coordinate physician-patient-family conferences as necessary to clarify the current plan of care. In addition, the nurse can identify communication inconsistencies between members of consulting teams [26, 29].

## Late Effects of CNS Tumors and Treatment

It is a rare child that manages to complete treatment for a CNS tumor and walk away without some type of late effect. Each child and family will end a treatment phase and need to carve out a new "normal" life pattern. For some, physical changes or handicaps are a constant reminder of the diagnosis and treatment. This new life often includes physical, occupational

and/or speech therapy, and coping with learning issues. Others require hormonal replacement or medications for seizure disorders. All survivors of CNS
tumors are seen periodically for imaging studies and
follow up with their individual physicians, or in a
multidisciplinary follow-up clinic [19, 27].

### School Re-Entry: Physical and Neurocognitive Sequelae

Children with CNS tumors often experience disrup-
tions in their education due to repeated hospitalizations, cycles of treatment and therapy, physical weakness and fatigue, and the cumulative effects of medications, surgery, chemotherapy, and radiation. In
addition, many children also have neurological
changes, including seizures, behavior disorders,
memory problems or visual deficits. For many children, school is a refuge from the life of a CNS tumor
with hospitalizations and procedures. Other children,
especially teenagers or those with visible impairments, may dread returning to school. Finally, subtle
learning issues, when not handled in a sensitive manner, can affect a child's confidence and self-esteem.
All of these issues can be managed with good planning and communication via the parents, educators,
and healthcare providers. Nurses can provide information and guidance, or be an advocate for the parents and/or child. They can also provide the school
professionals with information regarding CNS tumors in general and specific issues related to a given
child's plan of care [27].

It is helpful for children with CNS tumors to maintain some connection to the school throughout the
diagnosis and treatment. Being able to attend school
during windows of no active treatment or even during treatment on "off days" is helpful in maintaining
relationships. Home schooling or tutoring is often
necessary even if the child can attend school some of
the time. The majority of children with CNS tumors
will ultimately have some type of physical or cognitive impairment, and this requires assessment for an
individual education plan (IEP). The extent of the
needs will depend upon the location of the tumor and
treatments utilized. Those children who have received
radiation therapy will have more intensive cognitive
issues, specifically with visual spatial skills, memory,
attention, speed of information processing, and verbal fluency [19].

The IEP mechanism evaluates all aspects of the
individual's learning styles and physical needs, and
then a plan is developed as a collaboration between
parents and professional educators to determine the
curriculum and how it will be taught. It may be focused on preparation for college, vocational training,
or simply independent living skills with education
(special or mainstream), speech therapy, physical and
occupational therapy, and counseling. Nurses, as part
of the healthcare team, can interface with the family
and school and advocate for an IEP to happen [27].

### Ototoxicity

Children who have received cranial radiation or oto-
toxic chemotherapy have a significant risk of hearing
problems that can interfere with their learning potential. High-frequency sounds are the first to be affected, interfering with children's ability to sort out back-
ground noise. In a classroom situation this prevents
children from hearing the teacher above peripheral
noise. Amplification systems for the child in the classroom may help the child with this problem. More severe ototoxicity can result in substantial hearing loss
requiring hearing aids [27].

### Neuroendocrine Late Effects

The most common neuroendocrine effects of CNS tumors and their treatment are hormone deficiencies.
This can happen in children who have midline tumors, but can also happen after treatment with chemotherapy alone and almost always occur in the child
who has received radiation treatments. Endocrine
problems include growth, thyroid, and secondary sex
hormonal deficiencies. An endocrinologist who will
monitor growth rate and pubertal status, as well as
obtain blood tests to check for thyroid and growth
hormone deficiency, must follow all children and adolescents with CNS tumors. Films to determine bone
age are obtained, prior growth curves evaluated, and
linear growth closely monitored. Hormonal replacement is necessary for many of these children, with
thyroid replacement taken by mouth, and growth and
secondary sex hormones given by injection. Nurses
can coordinate follow-up appointments and also can
teach the child and family about the administration
of hormonal replacement [15].

## Psychological/Social

The diagnosis and treatment of CNS tumors can bring with them significant psychological and social sequelae. Body image changes that are visible, such as a hemiparesis, facial weakness, or hair loss, can adversely affect the development of a positive self-esteem. If the child has missed a lot of school or is having educational difficulties, then completing the educational process is difficult. Nurses can play an integral role in mainstreaming children as early as possible, and in connecting these patients with educational specialists and rehabilitation early on to foster as normal a life as possible. As the number of long-term survivors of CNS tumors increases, as has happened with other childhood cancers, there will be a greater need for such specialized clinics and programs, in which nursing can have an integral role [27].

## Secondary Cancers

As the long-term survival for all childhood cancers has increased with improvements in treatment, so has the incidence of second primary cancers as a side effect of chemotherapy, and more commonly radiation therapy. There are reports of secondary meningiomas or cavernomas after whole-brain irradiation. While the overall number of secondary cancers for all childhood cancers is less than 2%, there is not enough data on survivors of pediatric CNS tumors to quantify the risk. This will be followed closely in long-term follow-up clinics and as part of future cooperative group studies [22].

## Recurrence, Death and Dying, and Hospice

Recurrence or progression can happen at any time during treatment or after therapy is completed. When this occurs, the patient's history, clinical information, pathology, and sequential radiology studies are presented at the tumor board and a new treatment plan designed. This may include surgery, radiation (if it hasn't already been given), or chemotherapy. Experimental drugs including new chemotherapeutic drugs may be tried in patients who have undergone multiple previous standard treatment modalities. As with all aspects of care,

nurses can provide education and emotional support to families in this situation [27].

For some children with CNS tumors there comes a time where treatments have stopped working and the tumor continues to grow. Some families want to try every available treatment and exhaust all possible medical remedies. For those who choose to discontinue active treatment, the focus shifts to end-of-life care, either in the hospital setting, at home, in a hospice, or a combination of both. Hospice programs not only assist the child in comfort, but also allow the family to receive support and counseling as their family member dies [27].

## Conclusion

The diagnosis of a CNS tumor in the pediatric population does not always carry the poor prognosis that it did several decades ago. Technology is now available to successfully diagnose, treat, and cure many children with CNS tumors. MRI helps surgeons plan delicate surgeries and radiation treatments that allow newer machines to deliver more focused doses of radiation while (hopefully) minimizing side effects. Chemotherapy has been shown to penetrate the blood–brain barrier, and many drugs have been found to be effective in destroying CNS tumor cells. The enrollment and participation in national clinical trials has significantly impacted our understanding of various subsets of CNS tumors and customizing treatment protocols [27].

We know that each tumor is different and that tumors within the same disease groups may behave differently. Children with tumors that are maximally removed with surgery have a much better prognosis and longer period to progression of disease than do tumors that cannot be removed. Slow-growing tumors may remain dormant for months or years without treatment, and some will shrink in size with chemotherapy treatments. The greatest success in the treatment of malignant CNS tumors comes in the areas of medulloblastoma, PNET, and germ cell tumors. Radiation treatments are withheld in younger children whenever possible, and are delayed in children with slower growing tumors, in an attempt to spare intellectual development. Rehabilitation advances and the existence of special education programs has fostered independent living for long-term survivors of CNS tumors who have neurological impairment.

As technology continues to explode there is good reason to believe that our results in the next generation will continue to improve [27].

The complex issues associated with pediatric CNS tumors demand a multidisciplinary healthcare team to ensure optimal patient/family care. Nurses and advanced practice nurses are the consistent members of the team (along with the parents or primary caregivers), from diagnosis, through various treatment or observation periods through long-term follow-up. Parents or an identified advocate need to be in charge to ensure checks and balances in the system so that optimal care is delivered. Patients and families look to nurses for coordination of diagnostic testing, explanation and reinforcement of all procedures and surgery, integration of information given to them by members of the medical team, education regarding the treatment plan and side effects, discharge teaching and planning, and, most important, caring and support throughout the course of the illness and follow-up. As with most things in life, those with the strongest, consistent, and most cohesive team will win the championship [24, 26].

---

### Pediatric Practice Pearls

- The extent of tumor resection is the most significant factor in predicting long-term outcome.
- New advances in radiology and treatments have changed and will continue to positively impact the prognosis for children with CNS tumors.
- Care of children with CNS tumors requires a multidisciplinary team, with nurses serving in the role of educator, coordinator, and advocate.

---

### References

1. Abbott R, Epstein F, Shiminski-Maher T (1996) Tumors of the medulla: predicting outcome after surgery. Pediatr Neurosurg 25:41–44
2. Albright AL, Sposto R, Holmes E, Zeltzer PM, Finlay JL, Wisoff JH, et al (2000) Correlation of neurosurgical subspecialization with outcomes in children with malignant brain tumors. Neurosurgery 4:879–885
3. Avellino A, Berger M (1997) Intensive care management of children with brain tumors. In: Andrews B, Hammer G (eds) Pediatric Neurosurgical Intensive Care. American Association of Neurological Surgeons, Park Ridge, IL, pp 235–256
4. Benz M, Benz M (2004) Reduction of cancer risk associated with pediatric computed tomography by the development of new technologies. Pediatrics 114:205–209
5. Biagi E, Bollard C, Rousseau R, Brennan M (2003) Gene therapy for pediatric cancer: state of the art and perspectives. J Biomed Biotechnol 1:13–24
6. Black P, Wen P (1995) Clinical imaging and laboratory diagnosis of brain tumors. In: Kaye A, Laws E Jr (eds) Brain Tumors. Churchill Livingstone, Edinburgh, pp 191–214
7. Cataltepe O, Turnanli G, Yalnizoglu D, Topcu M, Akalan N (2005) Surgical management of temporal lobe-related epilepsy in children. J Neurosurg 3:280–287
8. Finlay JL, Wisoff JH (1999) The impact of extent of resection in the management of malignant gliomas of childhood. Childs Nerv Syst 15:786–788
9. Halpern E, Constine L, Tarbell N, Kun L (2004) Pediatric Radiation Oncology. Lippincott Williams and Wilkins, Philadelphia
10. Hickey J (2002) The Clinical Practice of Neurological and Neurosurgical Nursing. Lippincott Williams and Wilkins, Philadelphia
11. Jallo G, Freed D, Epstein F (2004) Spinal cord gangliogliomas: a review of 56 patients. J Neurooncol 68:71–77
12. Khatua S, Jalali R (2005) Recent advances in the treatment of childhood brain tumors. Pediatr Hematol Oncol 5:361–371
13. Kirk E, Howard V, Scott C (1995) Description of posterior fossa syndrome in children after posterior fossa brain tumor surgery. J Pediatr Oncol Nurs 12:181–187
14. Kirsch D, Tarbell N (2004) New technologies in radiation therapy for pediatric brain tumors: the rationale for proton radiation therapy. Pediatr Blood Cancer 42:461–464
15. Lerner SE, Huang GJ, McMahon D, Sklar CA, Oberfield SE (2005) Growth hormone therapy in children after cranial/craniospinal radiation therapy: sexually dimorphic outcomes. J Clin Endocrinol Metab 12:6100–6104
16. Lieberman D, Berger M (2001) Brain tumors during the first two years of life. In: Albright AL, Pollack I, Adelson PD (eds) Operative Techniques in Pediatric Neurosurgery. Thieme, New York, pp 125–129
17. Maher C, Raffel C (2004) Neurosurgical treatment of brain tumors in children. Pediatr Clin North Am 51:327–357
18. Mehta V, Chapman A, McNeely PD (2002) Latency between symptom onset and diagnosis of pediatric brain tumors: an Eastern Canadian geographic study. Neurosurgery 51:365–373
19. Moore IM (1995) Central nervous system toxicity of cancer therapy in children. J Pediatr Oncol Nurs 12:203–210
20. Muszynski C, Constantini S, Epstein F (2001) Intraspinal intramedullary neoplasms. In: Albright AL, Pollack I, Adelson PD (eds) Operative Techniques in Pediatric Neurosurgery. Thieme, New York, pp 193–200
21. Petriccione MM (1993) Central nervous system tumors. In: Foley G, Fochtman D, Mooney KH (eds) Nursing Care of the Child with Cancer. WB Saunders, Philadelphia, pp 239–253

22. Robinson LL (2005) The Childhood Cancer Survivor Study: a resource for research of long-term outcomes among adult survivors of childhood cancer. Minn Med 4:45–9

23. Ryan J, Shiminski-Maher T (1995) Hydrocephalus and shunts in children with central nervous system tumors. J Pediatr Oncol Nurs 12:223–229

24. Shiminski-Maher T (1990) Brain tumors in childhood: implications for nursing practice. J Pediatr Health Care 4:122–130

25. Shiminski-Maher T (1990) Diabetes insipidus and syndrome of inappropriate secretion of antidiuretic hormone in children with midline suprasellar brain tumors. J Neurosci Nurs 22:220–226

26. Shiminski-Maher T (1993) Physician-patient-parent communication complications. Pediatr Neurosurg 19:104–108

27. Shiminski-Maher T, Cullen P, Sansalone M (2002) Childhood Brain and Spinal Cord Tumors: A Guide for Families, Friends and Caregivers. O'Reilly Associates, Sebastopol, CA

28. Shiminski-Maher T, Rosenberg M (1990) Late effects associated with treatment of craniopharyngiomas in children. J Neurosci Nurs 22:220–226

29. Shiminski-Maher T, Shields M (1995) Pediatric brain tumors: diagnosis and management. J Pediatr Oncol Nurs 12:188–198

30. Shiminski-Maher T, Wisoff J (1995) Pediatric brain tumors. Crit Care Clin North Am 7:159–169

31. Yock T, Tarbell N (2002) Technology insight: proton beam radiotherapy for treatment in pediatric brain tumors. Nat Clin Pract Oncol 1:97–103

# Traumatic Brain Injury

7

*Angela Enix, Jodi Mullen, Carol Green, and Sherry Kahn*

## Contents

## Epidemiology

Despite prevention efforts, pediatric head trauma remains the most common cause of serious injury and death in children. Seventy-five percent of children who are hospitalized secondary to trauma, sustain head trauma. Most pediatric head trauma is mild in severity, although central nervous system (CNS) injury is the most common cause of pediatric traumatic death [22]. The overall incidence is 200–300 cases per 100,000 in the population annually. Deaths from severe traumatic brain injury (TBI) occur at an alarming rate of 7,000 annually [20]. This is especially concerning when considering that upwards of 20–40% of the injuries are preventable. The financial burden on individuals and society is immense, and is estimated at $7.5 billion annually in the United States. Many childhood survivors of severe TBI are left with varying degrees of permanent disability.

## Pediatric Anatomy and Physiology in Head Trauma

The adage that "children are not just small adults" holds true when discussing pediatric head trauma. The pediatric craniocerebral anatomy increases the child's vulnerability to head trauma as well as protects them against worsened severity or outcome. In general, children under the age of 2 years or who are nonverbal require a higher level of suspicion for injury, as the assessment is less revealing secondary to the child's developmental age [25].

## Skull

The physically larger and proportionately heavier pediatric cranium, together with the increased laxity of the cervical spine, create a fulcrum leading to an increased propensity for traumatic injury of the head and cervical spine. The skull consists of eight cranial bones, which are separated by sutures until around 18–24 months. Open cranial sutures are protective against gradual increases in intracranial pressure (ICP), for example as a result of tumors or hydrocephalus increased. Rapidly expanding mass lesions, however, are not tolerated and result increased ICP. The head circumference of infants should be measured and recorded on admission and daily, as a rapidly increasing head circumference is indicative of increased ICP. Presence of bulging or firm fontanels, with infant calm and in an upright posture, can also be an indicator of increased ICP. The infant's skull is thinner, softer, and more deformable when fractured, but heals quickly after fracture due to accelerated bone growth. The temporal and parietal regions are the thinnest cranial bones and the most common sites of accidental fracture. The thickest cranial bones are the frontal and occipital. Occipital fractures are related to more serious brain injury due to the increased force necessary to generate a fracture in the thickest bone of the skull [22].

## Brain

The pediatric brain is softer due to a higher water content and less myelination. The subarachnoid space is wider. The thin pediatric skull, soft brain, and large subarachnoid space allow increased movement of the brain within the skull, which makes the child more susceptible to brain injury, including extraparenchymal hemorrhage, shearing or tearing of neuronal processes, and diffuse axonal injury (DAI) [5,19,25,71]. The wider subarachnoid space predisposes the child to tearing of the bridging veins and development of subdural hematomas. In children, the pressure–volume curve is shifted to the left, meaning that children tolerate acute increases in intracranial volume poorly. Children have a smaller intracranial space in which smaller increases in volume produce exponentially larger increases in ICP. The pediatric skull can absorb a significant impact with little external evidence of significant intracranial injury. When evaluating the head-injured child, the nurse must consider all external indications such as bruising, swelling and lacerations, as well as the mechanism of injury and the degree of neurologic deficit.

## Initial Evaluation and Resuscitation

Following traumatic injury involving the head or neck, the child should arrive at an emergency room secured on a backboard and wearing a well-fitted cervical collar. A comprehensive multidisciplinary trauma evaluation should be performed to assess for multiple injuries. Immediate baseline neurologic examination should be carried out simultaneously with evaluation and resuscitation of airway, breathing, and circulation. Neurologic examination should be performed consistently, and be clearly documented on arrival and at frequent intervals. Critical evaluation of trends in the neurologic exam, vital signs, and ICP measurements is the most sensitive method of detecting early neurologic deterioration [4].

Infants and young children are not able to communicate the circumstances of their injuries. Therefore, the caregiver must rely on the report of parents or other custodians regarding previous medical history, baseline neurologic/cognitive/developmental deficits, and vital information to determine the circumstances of the child's injury. The circumstances of the accident or trauma are vital to determine the mechanism of injury and the potential severity of the child's injuries. First responders provide vital information such as a photograph, description of the scene, or a police report. Witnessed loss of consciousness, amnesia before (retrograde) or after (anterograde) the event, posttraumatic seizures (PTSs), initial clinical evaluation (Glasgow Coma Scale, GCS), cardiorespiratory collapse or hypotension, interventions provided, and the patient's response (worsened or improved) should be included in the paramedic's report to the trauma team. Table 7.1 includes elements of the TBI history and physical examination.

## Primary Versus Secondary Mechanism of Injury

Primary injury includes that which is present at impact, to include cortical contusions, lacerations, DAI, and brainstem injury. Secondary injury is that which

**Table 7.1.** Initial history and physical in traumatic brain injury (TBI). *EMT* Emergency medical technician, *LOC* level of consciousness, GCS Glasgow Coma Scale, *CN* cranial nerve, *DTRs* deep tendon reflexes, *PMH* past medical history, *NPO* nil by mouth, IDDM insulin-dependent diabetes mellitus

| |
|---|
| **Subjective:** <br> Witness to mechanism of event (i.e., police, EMT, parent report, photographs), LOC, anterograde or retrograde amnesia, witnessed traumatic seizure, abnormal behavior or vomiting, cardiorespiratory compromise/resuscitation, immobilization of cervical spine, improved or worsened exam after initial resuscitation |
| **Objective:** <br> General survey for multiple traumatic injuries, including spine. Survey for cranial injury: scalp hematoma, laceration, contusion or abrasion, open or penetrating intracranial injury. Evidence of basal skull fracture includes: battle sign, raccoon's eyes, otorrhea, rhinorrhea, and hemotympanum. Facial fractures (Le Fort, orbital rim, or jaw) may indicate serious neurologic injury |
| **Physical examination:** <br> General assessment provides suspicion of location and severity of injury. <br> Vital signs, LOC/mental status, GCS, orientation. <br> **Cranial nerve exam:** <br> Olfactory nerve (CN I). <br> Optic Nerve (CN II) – assess vision (Snellen card, finger counting, hand motion, light perception). Note: may have temporary cortical blindness, 1–2 days, after blow to back of head. <br> Oculomotor Nerve (CN III) – pupillary size and reaction to light, ptosis, abducted gaze. <br> Oculomotor (CN III), trigeminal (CN IV), and abducens (CN VI) nerves – extraocular eye movements. <br> Trochlear Nerve (CN V) – facial sensation, sensory portion of corneal reflex. <br> Facial Nerve (VII) – facial movement, motor portion of corneal reflex. <br> Acoustic Nerve (CN VIII) – hearing. <br> Glossopharyngeal (CN IX) and vagus (CN X) – intact gag and cough. <br> **Motor exam:** <br> cooperative – assess strength ×4 extremities, uncooperative – movement to noxious stimuli, posturing (caution: spinal cord reflexive movement). <br> **Sensory exam:** <br> Cooperative – differentiate tickle and pinch in all extremities, if uncooperative – assess for grimace, vocalization, to central painful stimuli. <br> **Reflexes:** <br> DTRs, Babinski reflex. |
| **History:** Any previous head injury – timing, frequency, severity, other PMH such as bleeding dyscrasias, seizures, medications and allergies, NPO status, alcohol or drug use, metabolic abnormality (e.g., IDDM). <br> Previous developmental or cognitive impairments [22]. |

develops subsequent to the impact. This includes injury from hemorrhage, edema, hypoxemia, and ischemia. All patient management decisions and interventions are directed at preventing secondary injury [22].

## Neurologic Assessment and Deterioration in Pediatric Head Trauma

## General Assessment

Inspection for external trauma, such as scalp or facial swelling, abrasions, laceration, or ecchymosis, can indicate TBI. Palpable step-off or depression indicates skull fracture, which may be associated with contusion of the brain, laceration of the dura or brain, and cere-

brospinal fluid (CSF) leak. Significant scalp swelling in the infant may be indicative of hemorrhage, which can cause anemia with pallor and tachycardia. A basilar skull fracture at the base of the anterior fossa causes "raccoon's eyes," or periorbital ecchymoses and can be associated with rhinorrhea (CSF leak from the nares). Fracture in the base of the middle fossa causes "battle sign," or postauricular ecchymoses, and can be associated with otorrhea (leak of CSF from the ear). Hemotympanum can indicate temporal or basilar skull fracture. Otorrhea indicates disruption of the tympanic membrane related to temporal skull fracture. The cervical spine must be immobilized and protected from spinal cord injury until radiographic clearance is accomplished [19]. The entire spine is immobilized, inspected, and palpated for deformity, swelling, tenderness, and crepitance. Please refer to Chap. 8 (Spine).

## Vital Functions

Every patient assessment must begin with evaluation of adequate airway, breathing, and circulation, which are vital to sustain life. A decreased level of consciousness (LOC) after TBI can interfere with protection of the pediatric airway. Inadequate ventilation results in hypercarbia and hypoxia, which cause vasodilation and secondary ischemic brain injury. Vasodilation and resultant ischemia contribute to further increases in ICP. Vital control centers located within the brainstem regulate respiratory and cardiac functions. Brainstem pathophysiology can be identified by changes in the vital signs. The following abnormal respiratory rate and patterns indicate neurologic dysfunction secondary to progressive brainstem compression as a result of increasing ICP [19,22,30]:

1. Cheyne-Stokes: repeated cycles of breaths that gradually increase and decrease in rate and depth, followed by a respiratory pause – indicates bilateral hemispheric or diencephalic injury.
2. Central Neurogenic Hyperventilation: increased rate and depth of respirations – indicates midbrain/upper pons injury.
3. Apneustic: a pause at full or prolonged (slow and deep) inspiration – indicates injury to the upper pons.
4. Ataxic: no pattern in rate or depth – indicates medulla or lower brainstem dysfunction with impending herniation; injury to the respiratory centers in the medulla (also known as agonal respirations).
5. Apnea: respirations cease.

Following loss of autoregulation (the ability of the brain to maintain perfusion despite changes in systemic perfusion), the cerebral blood flow (CBF) is dependent on systemic blood pressure. Adequate systemic perfusion is critical following pediatric TBI because hypotension causes secondary injury and is associated with a poor outcome [41]. In children, hypotension is a late sign, which indicates compromised systemic and probable cerebral perfusion. Other earlier indications of poor systemic perfusion include tachycardia, decreased LOC, signs of inadequate skin perfusion (capillary refill >2 s), and decreased urine output (less than 1 $cm^3$/kg/h). Hypertension occurs as a compensatory mechanism to maintain cerebral perfusion in the face of increased ICP. The mechanism, known as Cushing's response, is activated by decreased cerebral blood perfusion and includes increased systolic blood pressure, a widened pulse pressure, and bradycardia [30]. Cushing's Triad is a classic presentation of vital signs, including hypertension, bradycardia, and an increasingly abnormal respiratory pattern, which is a late and ominous sign of severe increased ICP and impending herniation [19,22,30].

## Level of Consciousness

The child's LOC, and whether it is worsening or improving, is the most important indicator of neurologic status [19]. The neurologically intact child is awake, alert, and responsive to his/her surroundings. Level of responsiveness varies with the developmental age of the child. Infants should respond to feeding and measures to console them [25]. Toddlers and older children should recognize and respond to their parents. Older children and adolescents should be able to follow commands. Children of all ages should respond to and withdraw from painful stimulus. After neurologic injury, pediatric head-injured victims may have alteration in LOC, first subtly, becoming restless, disoriented, and confused. Further decreases in the LOC leads to somnolence (arouses to full consciousness and resumes sleep if not stimulated), lethargy (requires vigorous stimulation to arouse to full consciousness), stupor (nearly unconscious, may moan or withdraw from pain), and finally comatose (unresponsive) [34]. A worsening LOC suggests neurologic deterioration. Any subtle change from documented baseline, including parent's concern that child is "not acting right," must be taken seriously and reported to the physician.

## Glasgow Coma Scale

The modified Pediatric Glasgow Coma Scale (GCS) score measures the severity of head injury as well as the child's level of responsiveness (Table 7.2). As pediatric responses are different than those of adults, the GCS was modified to allow for consistent, objective, serial measurements of the child's level of neurologic responsiveness following TBI. The scale considers the child's best response following adequate central stimulation to eye opening, motor, and verbal responses, with each assigned a score and the three scores totaled [25]. The scores range from 3 (lowest score indicating

**Table 7.2.** Modified Glasgow Coma Scale for infants and Children [26]

| Response | Child | Infant | Score |
|---|---|---|---|
| Eye opening | Spontaneous | Spontaneous | 4 |
| | Verbal stimuli | Verbal stimuli | 3 |
| | Pain only | Pain only | 2 |
| | No response | No response | 1 |
| Verbal response | Oriented, appropriate | Coos and babbles | 5 |
| | Confused | Irritable cry | 4 |
| | Inappropriate words | Cries to pain | 3 |
| | Incomprehensible words or sounds | Moans to pain | 2 |
| | No response | No response | 1 |
| Motor response | Obeys commands | Moves spontaneously and with purpose | 6 |
| | Localizes painful stimulus | Withdraws to touch | 5 |
| | Withdraws to pain | Withdraws to pain | 4 |
| | Flexion to pain | Decorticate posture (abnormal flexion) to pain | 3 |
| | Extension to pain | Decerebrate posture (abnormal extension) to pain | 2 |
| | No response | No response | 1 |

no response) to 15 (highest score indicating intact neurologic status). A worsening GCS score and decreased level of responsiveness indicates a rise in ICP [19]. A change of two or more points on the GCS score is highly significant and should be reported to the physician immediately.

When assessing responsiveness, it is important for the nurse to use an adequately painful, central stimulus to elicit the child's best response. Application of firm pressure to the mandible, sternum, supraorbital area, or sternocleidomastoid muscle all provide central painful stimulation [25,52]. Peripheral painful stimulation should be avoided, as it can elicit a spinal reflex. The spinal reflex arc is a response to peripheral sensory stimulation, in which the sensory afferent fibers carry stimulation to the dorsal root and spinal cord. The signal synapses in the cord with the motor neuron in the anterior horn. Motor efferent fiber signals travel back to the neuromuscular junction, which elicits a contraction [34]. The spinal reflex should not be confused as a demonstration of cerebral function.

The immediate postresuscitation GCS score modified for Infants and Children is used to rate the severity of pediatric head trauma, as well as to predict outcome. The severity of head trauma is determined by the following:
1. GCS 14–15 = Mild head trauma
2. GCS 9–13 = Moderate head trauma
3. GCS ≤8 = Severe head trauma [22].

Coma is defined as the inability to arouse or interact with the environment. A GCS of 8 or less is considered an operational definition of coma [22].

## Cranial Nerve Evaluation

## Visual Acuity

Following TBI, it is essential to assess for presence of bilateral vision, which is indicative of the eyes innervation by the optic nerve (cranial nerve, CN, II). The presence of a squint to light in an infant indicates intact vision. Vision in older children can be assessed on a continuum progressing from abnormal to normal, including blindness, light perception, hand motion, finger counting, to full baseline vision [88]. The presence of papilledema on a fundoscopic exam indicates the presence of increased ICP. This finding presents 12–24 h after injury, however, and its absence should not delay treatment when other findings are consistent with severe brain injury [19]. The presence of retinal hemorrhages with subdural hematomas is a classic finding in inflicted injury [86], but can also be seen with high-impact accidental injuries.

## Pupillary Response

Pupillary response represents a balance between the sympathetic and parasympathetic systems, and dysfunction in either results in unopposed action of the other [19]. The pupillary response is innervated by CN III. The pupils are normally equal in size, round, and reactive to light and accommodation, thus the acronym PERRLA. When assessing pupillary response, darken the room if possible, bring the light in from the periphery and note the direct (same side) and consensual (opposite side) response to light, repeat with the other eye. Accommodation, assessed by directing the patient's gaze at a distant object, causes the pupils to dilate. Their gaze is then directed to a near object (finger), which causes the pupils to constrict and converge on the near object [34].

Bilateral dilated (mydriatic) and nonreactive pupils, caused by unopposed sympathetic input, indicate an injury to the oculomotor (CN III) nucleus in the midbrain or CN III injury due to trauma or increased ICP [19]. Unilateral mydriasis in TBI suggests either direct orbital trauma, transtentorial (uncal) herniation, or an expanding mass hemorrhage on the same (ipsilateral) side as the dilated pupil. A new finding of pupillary inequality, even if only 1 mm, must be taken seriously and reported to the physician. Bilateral mydriasis can also occur following seizure or medications that mimic the sympathetic response, such as atropine. A pharmacologically dilated pupil is very large (7–8 mm), whereas mydriasis due to CN III compression is typically 5–6 mm [22]. The nurse should be aware of what medications are given and notify other caregivers of the iatrogenic pupillary dilation.

Miosis (pupillary constriction) occurs with injury to the pons or carotid artery, and with administration of narcotics or other miotic drugs. Hippus is a spasmodic, rhythmic pupillary response to light manifested as alternating dilation and constriction [22]. Hippus can be a normal variant or indicate increasing pressure on CN III, with impending transtentorial herniation [30]. Anisocoria (inequality of the pupil size) is a variant of normal in approximately 20% of the population [22]. Physiologic anisocoria is a pupillary difference of <1 mm. Common causes of pathologic anisocoria include CN III palsy or compression caused by transtentorial herniation, Parinaud's syndrome, and Horner's syndrome. Parinaud's syndrome, caused by a lesion (tumor) or pressure (increased ICP or hydrocephalus) exerted on the tectum of the midbrain, results in impaired upgaze ("sunsetting"), impaired convergence, dilated and fixed pupils, and lid retraction. Horner's syndrome occurs with interruption of sympathetic input to the eye and face, resulting in a reactive miotic pupil, ptosis, and lack of perspiration (anhydrosis) on the affected side of the face. Abnormal mydriasis is caused by unopposed sympathetic input, whereas miosis is due to unopposed parasympathetic input [22].

### Extraocular Eye Movements

Eye position and movement are controlled by CN III (oculomotor), CN IV (trochlear), and CN VI (abducens), as well as the cerebral hemispheres and the brainstem. Extraocular eye movements are assessed by having the conscious child follow the examiner's finger in the pattern of an "H" (cardinal fields of gaze). CN injury following TBI is manifested as extraocular eye muscle weakness, resulting in abnormal eye position in the conscious or unconscious child. CN III innervates four of the six ocular muscles, which control all directions of gaze except down and in (CN IV) and lateral (CN VI). When control of eye movements in one direction is lost, there is overcompensation of positioning of the eye in the opposite direction. Table 7.3 gives a limited review of abnormal eye position and related etiology (localization of injury) [19,87]. Saccadic eye movements (rapid, voluntary movements to search a field) are controlled by the frontal gaze centers, where injury causes deviation toward the lesion. Pursuit movements (slow, involuntary movements keeping the eyes fixated on a moving target) are controlled by the occipital gaze centers.

### Brainstem Reflex Exam

The CNs originate in the brainstem, with CNs I–IV from the midbrain, CNs V–VIII from the pons, and CNs IX–XII from the medulla. Evaluation of CN and brainstem function is valuable for locating neurologic injury. The trigeminal nerve (CN V) innervates the sensory portion of the corneal reflex, where stimulation of blowing into the child's eye elicits eye closure. The motor response of blinking is innervated by CN VII. A unilateral facial (CN VII) weakness or hearing loss (CN VIII) can occur with a basilar skull fracture. The integrity of the vestibular function (CN VIII) is assessed by performing oculovestibular and oculocephalic testing, which indicates the presence or absence of brainstem function in the comatose patient (Table 7.4) [22,88]. Intact gag and cough reflexes as-

**Table 7.3.** Etiology of abnormal eye position in pediatric head trauma. *ICP* Intracranial pressure

| Location of lesion | Eye deviation | Hemiparesis | Other |
|---|---|---|---|
| Frontal lobe injury | Toward lesion | Opposite | |
| Expanding mass hemorrhage | Toward lesion | Opposite | |
| Occipital injury | Toward lesion | | Hemianopsia (contralateral loss of vision) |
| Seizure | Away from lesion | Same side | |
| CN III (oculomotor) | Down and out (exotropia). Also causes: ptosis, dilated pupil, unable to accommodate | Uncal herniation: contralateral hemiparesis or motor posturing | Uncal herniation: unitalateral fixed, dilated pupil (↑ICP causes pressure on CN III nucleus) |
| CN IV (trochlear) | Elevates (inability to look down or in; causes double vision | | CN IV injury (rare) |
| CN VI (abducens) | Loss of lateral gaze; inability to abduct | | ↑ICP secondary to trauma, skull (clivus) fracture |
| | Causes double vision with lateral gaze to affected side; squint and head tilt | | Originates in pons; Prone to injury from longest intracranial course |
| Parinaud's syndrome | Convergence and accommodation lost; upward gaze palsy (sunsetting sign); pupils fixed, dilated | | Elevated ICP, hydrocephalus; mechanism is pressure on the tectum of brainstem |
| | Infants unable to fix/follow | | |

**Table 7.4.** Brainstem (*BS*) reflexes: assess BS function between the pons and the oculomotor (CN III) nuclei in the midbrain. *HOB* Head of bed, *TM* tympanic membrane, *COWS* cold opposite, warm, same

| Brainstem reflex | Awake | Comatose | Brain death |
|---|---|---|---|
| Oculovestibular (cold calorics) **Caution: must have intact TM** Elevate HOB, 60–100 ml ice water instilled into ear | Awake or obtunded with intact brain stem – slow ipsilateral gaze; then rapid contralateral nystagmus "COWS." Refers to direction of nystagmus | Comatose – conjugate, tonic eye deviation toward stimulus; no nystagmus | Brain death – no eye movement |
| Oculocephalic (doll's eyes) **Caution: Do not perform unless C-spine clearance obtained** | Awake – eyes move with or away from (contraversive to) lateral head rotation | Comatose with intact BS – contraversive conjugate eye movement (positive doll's eyes) | Brain death – no eye movement |

sess continuity of the glossopharyngeal (CN IX) and vagus (CN X) nerves [19,88].

### Motor Exam

The infant should have dominant flexor tone, but relax to easily perform full range of motion. The child's ability to follow commands should be assessed by asking them, for example, to hold up two fingers.

Note whether the child initiates movement spontaneously, or what stimulus is required to elicit movement. Note the symmetry and quality of strength using the following scale: 0 – no muscle contraction; 1 – palpation of trace contraction; 2 – movement without gravity; 3 – movement against gravity, but not resistance; 4 – movement against some resistance; 5 – movement against full resistance. Unilateral or generalized hypotonia, weakness, or flaccidity are abnormal and indicate localized or generalized brain trauma [25].

Abnormal flexion or extension posturing indicates severe TBI. Posturing indicates neurologic activity (or inactivity) secondary to brainstem compression and impending herniation in comatose patients [90]. Deterioration of neurologic status occurs in a rostral (head) to caudal (tail) progression. This is true of CN and brainstem dysfunction with impending herniation. Decorticate posturing implies a more rostral lesion and a better prognosis [22]. Decorticate posture is abnormal flexion of the upper extremities with extension of the lower extremities and is indicative of disinhibition of the corticospinal pathways above the midbrain. Decerebrate posturing implies further deterioration and impending herniation as it indicates disinhibition of the pons and medulla. Decerebrate posturing includes abnormal extension of the upper and lower extremities (Fig. 7.1). Posturing may be reversible or may represent impending brain death. Progression from decorticate to decerebrate indicates worsening brainstem function, where progression from decerebrate to decorticate indicates improvement. Figure 7.2 illustrates the brainstem centers that are compressed by downward herniation, progressing from decorticate to decerebrate posturing, and finally herniation (brain death) [90]. Posturing may be reversible, but it is associated with a more ominous outcome.

### Reflexes

A reflex is an automatic nervous system motor response to stimulation [57]. The stimulus (striking tendon) travels via sensory (afferent) fibers to the dorsal ganglion and anterior horn of the spinal cord. The ventral horn relays the motor (efferent) signal back to the muscle, causing a reflexive contraction. This chain of events is referred to as the reflex arc. Deep tendon reflexes (DTR), or muscle stretch reflexes, are assessed to determine the presence and location of nervous system dysfunction in both conscious and unconscious children. Injury can occur to the CNS – brain and spinal cord (upper motor neurons) or the peripheral nervous system (PNS; lower motor neurons, LMN).

With upper motor neuron (UMN) injury, signals (both excitatory and inhibitory) from the cortex are diminished, or cut off, causing the spinal cord to become hyperreflexic. Hyperreflexia indicates injury to the CNS corticospinal tract with resultant irritability

in the spinal cord. UMN injury is associated with increased tone, spasticity, clonus (muscle spasm with forceful dorsal flexion of the ankle), and a present Babinski sign. Unilateral hyperreflexia indicates a CNS injury, such as an expanding mass hemorrhage on the opposite side of the brainstem or cerebral cortex, resulting in increased ICP. Injury to the PNS, or LMN, is associated with hyporeflexia or areflexia (loss of efferent motor fibers), as well as muscle weakness, flaccidity, and atrophy [22,30,90]. Hypotonia and atrophy occur due to the loss of LMN, which innervate muscles and maintain normal tone [90]. Preserved reflexes in a flaccid limb indicate CNS (UMN) injury, not a PNS (LMN) injury. Injury to the cerebellum causes hyporeflexia, as well as ataxia, hypotonia, and dysarthria [63].

The Babinski sign is present when stroking the plantar surface of the foot results in dorsiflexion of the great toe and fanning of the other toes. This is a primitive reflex seen normally in infants, and usually disappears by 10 months (range 6–12 months) [22]. The presence of a Babinski sign after age 6 months in TBI is pathologic and indicates injury to the corticospinal tract at any level [30].

### Supratentorial Versus Infratentorial Injury

The tentorium cerebelli is a fold of the dura mater that separates the cerebral hemispheres from the cerebellum and brainstem. The "tent" is an important landmark, as assessment or deterioration of neurologic status differs based on whether the injury is above the tentorium (supratentorial), or below the tentorium (infratentorial). The tentorium also contains the notch through which the brainstem herniates as a result of increased ICP. Bilateral supratentorial lesions, which cause mass effect and increased ICP, progress in a rostral (head) to caudal (tail) progression with impending herniation of the brainstem through the tentorial notch (see previous discussion of CNs and brainstem reflexes).

A primary infratentorial injury occurs with either a tear of the dural sinuses (rare in children) or as a primary injury (hemorrhage) in the brainstem or cerebellum, which affects the reticular activating system (consciousness) directly. Coma does not progress in a rostral–caudal progression. Deterioration with an infratentorial lesion is marked by pathologic alteration in vital signs. More often, posterior fossa lesions in

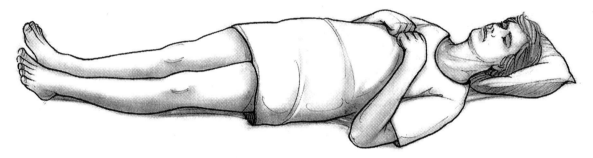

**A. Decerebrate : upper and lower limbs extend**

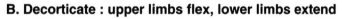

**B. Decorticate : upper limbs flex, lower limbs extend**

**Fig. 7.1 a, b. a** Abnormal posturing indicates brainstem compression in the comatose patient. **b** Decerebrate posturing with abnormal upper extremity (UE) and lower extremity (LE) extension (late). Decorticate posturing with abnormal UE flexion and LE extension (early). Reprinted with permission from Young and Young (1997) [90]

**Fig. 7.2.** Brainstem compression occurs in a rostral (head) to caudal (toe) progression. This is a median view of the brainstem showing levels of impairment associated with abnormal posturing. Decorticate indicates a more rostral lesion (above the red nucleus), Decerebrate indicates a more caudal lesion (midbrain or pons). Reprinted with permission from Young and Young (1997) [90]

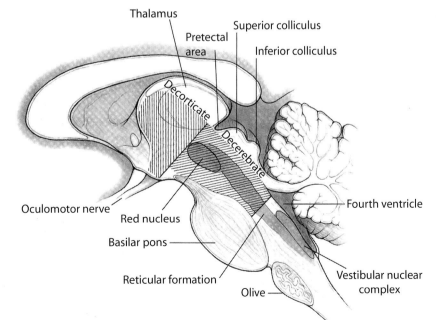

children show progressive deterioration, with or without development of hydrocephalus, and present with rostral-caudal deterioration or CN deficits. Ataxia (decreased muscle coordination) is noted with cerebellar injury (see Chap. 1, Neurological Assessment of the Neonate, Infant, Child and Adolescent).

## Radiographic Imaging in Pediatric Head Trauma

For the purpose of this chapter, traumatic intracranial injuries are discussed individually, but in reality any combination of lesions can and do occur. The noncontrast head computerized tomography (CT) is the initial study of choice in pediatric head trauma. Obtaining CT imaging is fast and allows for ease of monitoring of the unstable child with moderate to severe TBI. The CT scan is sensitive to hemorrhage, mass effect, and skull fractures. Magnetic resonance imaging (MRI) is more useful in the subacute or chronic stage of injury and should also be considered if CT scan findings do not fully explain the extent of neurologic deficit. Be aware that CT scans do expose the child to radiation, and order them wisely. See Table 7.5 for a comparison of modalities for neuroimaging. Skull radiographs are minimally useful. When obtained in the presence of scalp swelling or other injury, x-rays can reveal skull fractures or intracranial air, which may indicate more serious intracranial injuries. Ultrasound can be useful in neonates and infants with open fontanels as a screening tool for hemorrhage, although it is limited to allow imaging of the full periphery of the brain. Cerebral ultrasound is useful in identifying the presence of intracerebral hemorrhage and intraventricular hemorrhage, as well as assessment of ventricular size if there is hydrocephalus. The neuroimaging modality of choice will be discussed in greater detail with each classification of pediatric head trauma [5].

## Types of TBI

### Birth-related TBI

Traumatic injury to the brain may occur during the birth process. Infants with greater risk for birth-related injuries include those above the 90th percentile for weight. The rate of birth injury is higher in infants weighing more than 4500 g. Birth injuries may also be related to the infant's position during labor and delivery (e.g., breech presentation, cephalopelvic disproportion, where the mother's pelvis size or shape is not adequate for vaginal birth, difficult labor or delivery, prolonged labor, fetal anomalies, and very low birth weight or extremely premature infants). Some of the more common birth injuries to the neonatal head and brain include extracranial hemorrhage (caput succedaneum, subgaleal hemorrhage, or cephalohematoma), skull fracture, and intracranial hemorrhage (epidural, subarachnoid, subdural, or intracerebellar hemorrhage).

Caput Succedaneum, a common finding in the newborn, involves soft tissue swelling of the presenting part of the head in a vertex (head first) delivery. The scalp edema consists of serum or blood, or both, and may have ecchymosis (bruising), petechiae or purpura. Caput succedaneum may occur after spontaneous delivery due to pressure of the fetal head against the uterine wall, the cervix, or the vaginal wall, or after use of a vacuum extractor. The scalp edema may cross over suture lines, and does not continue to increase in size after delivery. It heals in hours to days and rarely has complications. Nursing care involves parent education about the cause of the tissue swelling and/or discoloration [28,73].

Subgaleal hemorrhage is much less frequent than caput succedaneum. It occurs below the epicranial aponeurosis (connective tissue over the brain) and may spread beneath the entire scalp and down the subcutaneous tissue in the neck. There is a strong association between vacuum extraction and subgaleal hemorrhage. The hemorrhage may be from suture diastasis (separation), linear skull fracture, or fragmentation of the superior margin of the parietal bone. Subgaleal hemorrhage presents as a firm fluctuant mass, crosses suture lines, and may increase in size after birth. Blood loss can be significant, requiring urgent blood transfusion and contributing to hyperbilirubinemia [87]. Early detection is vital. Nursing measures include serial measurements of head circumference, inspection of the back of the head and neck for increasing edema, observation of the ears being pushed forward and lateral, and monitoring for changes in LOC and decrease in hematocrit [6]. Parent teaching includes preparing them for the swelling and discoloration of the face, head, and neck. Lesser lesions resolve in 2–3 weeks [87]. Moderate to severe

**Table 7.5.** Comparison of neuroimaging modalities in pediatric TBI. *CT* Computed tomography, *MRI* magnetic resonance imaging, *ICP* intracranial pressure, *IICP* increased ICP, *EDH* epidural hemorrhage, *SDH* subdural hemorrhage, *SAH* subarachnoid hemorrhage, *IVH* intraventricular hemorrhage, *ICH* intracerebral hemorrhage, *MRA* magnetic resonance angiogram

|  | X-ray | Ultrasound | CT scan | MRI |
|---|---|---|---|---|
| Timing | Early, especially if scalp swelling, trauma is present | Useful with open fontanel; Portable | Fast, immediate post-trauma imaging | Subacute or chronic imaging |
| Type of Injury Identified | – Skull fracture<br>– Pneumocephalus<br>– Foreign body<br>– Split cranial sutures with increased ICP | – Hemorrhage<br>– Ventricular size: (hydrocephalus or small, obliterated ventricles with IICP)<br>– Cranial Doppler for vasospasm secondary to SAH | – Scalp swelling<br>– Skull fracture<br>– Pneumocephalus<br>– Extraparenchymal hemorrhage:<br>(EDH, SDH, SAH, IVH)<br>– Intraparenchymal hemorrhage:<br>(ICH, hemorrhagic contusion)<br>– Mass effect: (obliteration of ventricles and cisterns, poor gray-white differentiation, splitting cranial sutures)<br>– Hydrocephalus | – Nonhemorrhagic contusion<br>– Diffuse axonal injury<br>– Early ischemic injury (cerebral infarct)<br>– CT scan does not explain neurologic deficit<br>– Injury dating in child abuse<br>– MRA: (posttraumatic aneurysm) |

lesions may require intensive care and up to 25% of these babies may die [18].

Cephalohematoma is a subperiosteal collection of blood secondary to the rupture of blood vessels between the skull and the periosteum. It is usually over the parietal bone, and is usually unilateral, but can occur bilaterally. Cephalohematoma is seen most often in male infants after a prolonged, difficult, or forceps-assisted delivery. The characteristic finding is a firm, tense mass that does not cross the suture lines. It may enlarge slightly by 2–3 days of age, and takes weeks to months to resolve, occasionally with residual calcification. The calcified "lump" gradually subsides as bones grow and reshape. Approximately 10–25% of cephalohematomas have an underlying linear skull fracture [87]. Rarely, the cephalohematoma may contain enough blood to affect hematocrit and bilirubin levels. Nursing care involves monitoring and parent teaching about hyperbilirubinemia. Anemic infants should also be evaluated for symptoms of intracranial hemorrhage. Generally, there are no long-term sequelae from a cephalohematoma.

### Neonatal Skull Fracture

Skull fractures, both depressed and linear, are occasionally seen in the newborn. The fetal skull is flexible, malleable, and poorly ossified when compared to the adult skull, and thus is often able to tolerate mechanical stressors relatively well. Skull fractures can occur in utero, during labor, and forceps delivery (Fig. 7.3), or during a prolonged or difficult labor. The fetal skull can be compressed against the maternal ischial spines, sacral promontory, or symphysis pubis. Cerebral injury should be suspected when neurological signs are apparent and there is a history of a difficult delivery. Skull x-rays or CT are used to confirm the fracture and identify cerebral contusion or hemorrhage. CT is preferred as it identifies space-occupying hematomas and injury to the underlying brain (Fig. 7.3).

Depressed skull fractures (which are not really fractures, but an indentation of bone) are usually seen after forceps delivery, but occasionally are seen after a spontaneous vaginal or cesarean delivery [81]. A depressed skull fracture is a visible and palpable dent in the skull, usually over the right parietal bone, and does not cross suture lines. There may be no other symptoms unless there is an underlying cerebral con-

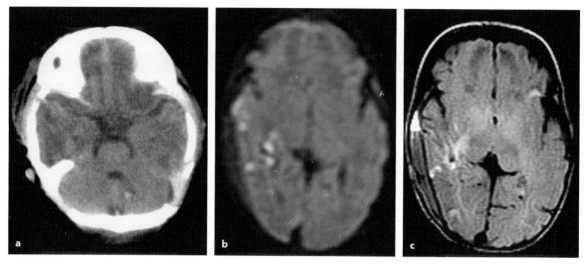

**Fig. 7.3 a–c.** Neonate with significant birth trauma after vaginal delivery with forceps. **a** Infant sustained a right parietal depressed skull fracture, scalp swelling (caput succedaneum), bilateral extra-axial hematomas (subdural hemorrhage, SDH), right temporal and left cerebellar hemorrhage as seen on computed tomography (CT) images. Subarachnoid hemorrhage was also seen on the tentorium and at the vertex (not shown). **b** Diffusion-weighted magnetic resonance imaging (MRI) scan on DOL 7 shows brain contusion with injury in the right temporal lobe and corpus callosum (not shown). **c** Fast fluid-attenuated inversion-recovery (FLAIR) MRI reveals right temporoparietal SDH and scattered white-matter hemorrhage bilaterally (right temporal, bilateral occipital, and left frontal). The infant was treated with observation only; the lesions resolved, and the child did well, without development of hydrocephalus

tusion or hemorrhage. A depressed skull fracture may be referred to as a "ping-pong" lesion, as it resembles a dent in a ping-pong ball. The uncomplicated depressed fracture can be manually elevated if it does not occur spontaneously in the first few days [59]. Manual elevation becomes more difficult later on. Methods to elevate the fracture include gentle pressure, use of a breast pump, or use of a vacuum extractor. Surgical intervention is necessary when the depressed fracture cannot be elevated manually, when bone fragments are in the cerebrum, if neurological deficits exist, or if ICP is increased. If there is CSF leakage, antibiotics may be prescribed for prophylaxis. Some infants will require treatment for shock and hemorrhage.

Linear skull fractures are usually seen in the frontal and parietal bones, and are often associated with extracranial hemorrhage, such as cephalohematoma. These fractures are diagnosed with skull x-rays and are usually asymptomatic. The exact incidence is unknown as routine x-rays in otherwise healthy newborns are uncommon. Linear fractures are rarely complicated by intracranial hemorrhage [12]. Linear skull fractures in infants may heal in 6 months [6]; they heal spontaneously with no sequelae, unless a dural tear allows the leptomeninges to protrude into the fracture site (i.e., growing fracture of childhood). A cyst may form and grow, causing the fracture to enlarge. Leptomeningeal cyst is rare, occurring in less than 1% of linear fractures in children under age 3 years [22]. Depressed fractures that are small or treated early have a good prognosis. Larger fractures have a greater risk of sequelae, especially if treatment is delayed. Sequelae are related to the cerebral injury, either from dural hemorrhage or a hypoxic event, or both, not from the fracture itself [12].

Nursing assessment involves supportive care and monitoring of the infant for signs of neurological dysfunction (increased ICP from hemorrhage, seizures, apnea, and meningitis). Parents may be concerned about brain damage and their infant's appearance if there is a depressed fracture. Parents should be educated to observe their infant for and report signs of increased ICP (irritability, poor feeding, vomiting, hypersomnolence) and growing fracture (growing bulge at fracture site) to the physician. They should be instructed to have the fracture site examined at each newborn visit.

## Intracranial Hemorrhage

Intracranial hemorrhage may occur in the neonate secondary to trauma or hypoxia in the perinatal period (epidural hemorrhage - EDH, primary subarachnoid hemorrhage - SAH, subdural hemorrhage - SDH, intracerebellar hemorrhage), or due to immature structures and hemodynamics in the premature infant (periventricular/intraventricular hemorrhage - P/IVH), especially those under 32 weeks gestational age at birth. The pathophysiology of P/IVH involves disruption to the autoregulation of CBF, which is affected by hypoxia and acidosis, leaving the germinal matrix area vulnerable to systemic blood pressure changes. Systemic blood pressure changes may be caused by handling, suctioning, positive-pressure ventilation, hypercapnia, and rapid volume expansion [12].

## Epidural Hemorrhage

EDH is a rare occurrence and may be associated with cephalohematoma. It refers to blood collection above the dura mater and below the periosteum (inner surface of the skull). Most cases are associated with a linear skull fracture. Nearly all affected infants have a history of difficult delivery. Signs of increased ICP, including a bulging fontanel, may be apparent in the first hours of life. An emergent CT scan should be performed. Surgical evacuation may be required. Aspiration of the accompanying cephalohematoma has been reported as a means of reducing the epidural lesion [61]. Untreated lesions may result in death within 48 h.

Nursing care involves prompt recognition and reporting, timely preparation and transport for CT scan, transfer to the appropriate facility, and preparation for surgery. Postoperative nursing care includes supportive care for oxygenation, ventilation, thermoregulation, fluids and nutrition, pain management, and monitoring of neurological signs. Parents will need support and teaching to understand their infant's condition and participate in the treatment plan. Complications range from none to permanent neurological deficits and/or seizures.

## Subarachnoid Hemorrhage

Primary SAH is the most common intracranial hemorrhage in the neonate. SAH occurs in full- and preterm infants, but is more common in the premature infant. Primary SAH consists of venous bleeding into the subarachnoid space (arterial bleeding is usually the cause of SAH in older children and adults.) The usual site in the neonate is over the cerebral convexities, especially in the posterior fossa [87].

Trauma causing increased intravascular pressure and capillary rupture is associated with SAH in the full-term infant. Asphyxia may cause SAH in the premature infant. Risk factors for SAH include birth trauma, prolonged labor, difficult delivery, fetal distress, and perinatal asphyxia.

The most common presentation of SAH is the asymptomatic premature infant with a minor SAH. The SAH is discovered accidentally with a bloody lumbar puncture during a sepsis work-up or cerebral ultrasound to rule out intraventricular hemorrhage. Another presentation of SAH occurs in a full-term or preterm infant who presents with seizures or apnea at 2–3 days of age. Between seizures, the infant appears healthy. Infants with a massive SAH (quite rare) associated with birth trauma and severe asphyxia have a rapid and fatal course [12,87].

Ultrasonography or CT is useful to confirm the diagnosis of SAH. If the infant has seizures, other causes of seizures must be eliminated. Blood in the CSF on lumbar puncture may be from a SAH or from a bloody tap. Rarely a severe, acute SAH may require a craniotomy. Infants with minor or asymptomatic SAH survive and generally have good developmental outcomes. Up to half of infants with symptomatic SAH, with sustained traumatic and hypoxic injury, have neurological sequelae. Occasionally, SAH results in hydrocephalus due to CSF obstruction by adhesions. Periodic cerebral ultrasound evaluation for ventricular size may be indicated. Nursing care involves assessment for seizures and other neurological signs. Parents will need support and teaching about SAH, so they can understand the needs of their infant.

## Subdural Hemorrhage

SDH is not unusual after vaginal delivery. Small posterior fossa SDHs are common after uncomplicated vaginal deliveries [6]. The most likely site for hemorrhage is over the cerebral hemispheres. Significant bleeding over the posterior fossa causes compression of the brainstem, as do dural tears near the great vein of Galen. SDH affects full-term infants more often than preterm infants, usually as a result of a precipitous, prolonged, or difficult delivery, use of forceps, cephalopelvic disproportion, breech delivery, or large infant [81,87].

Excessive head molding results in stretching of the falx (folds of dura mater that separate the two cerebral hemispheres and the two cerebellar hemispheres) and tentorium (dura mater between the cerebrum and cerebellum), and venous sinuses, with tearing of the vein of Galen or cerebral or cerebellar veins [50]. As with SAH, SDH diagnosis depends upon the history and presentation of the infant. If seizures are present, other causes must be excluded. SDH can occur along with SAH, cephalohematoma, subgaleal, subconjunctival, and retinal hemorrhages, skull fractures, and bracheal plexus and facial palsies. An MRI or CT scan will help to confirm the diagnosis. Ultrasound is less reliable. Clinical signs are related to the site and severity of the bleeding. There are three patterns of presentation in infants with bleeding over the cerebral hemispheres [86]. The most common presentation is seen in infants with a minor hemorrhage. They are asymptomatic or have minor signs such as irritability and hyperalertness. The second presentation pattern involves seizures in the first 2–3 days of life. The seizures are usually focal, and other neurological signs may or may not be present: hemiparesis, unequal or sluggish pupils, full or tense fontanel, bradycardia, and irregular respirations. The third pattern of presentation is seen in infants who had no or nonspecific signs in the neonatal period, and present at 4 weeks–6 months of age with increasing head size as a result of continued hematoma formation, poor feeding, failure to thrive, altered LOC, and occasionally, with seizures due to chronic subdural effusion [87].

If the posterior fossa SDH is small, there may be no signs for 3–4 days. As the subdural clot enlarges, signs of increased ICP appear and the infant's condition deteriorates. Infants with significant posterior fossa SDH have abnormal neurological signs from birth, including stupor or coma, eye deviation, asymmetric pupil size, altered pupillary reaction to light, tachypnea, bradycardia, and opisthotonos (prolonged, sustained posture with leg extension, trunk arching, and variable arm posture, often extended). As the clot enlarges, there is rapid deterioration with signs of shock in minutes to hours. The infant becomes comatose, with fixed, dilated pupils, altered respirations and heart rate, and finally respiratory arrest.

Care is primarily supportive, including oxygenation and perfusion, thermal management, fluids and nutrition. Surgical evacuation of bleeding over the temporal convexity with increased ICP may be necessary for infants who can not be stabilized neurologically. Massive posterior fossa hemorrhage requires neurosurgical intervention. Infants at risk for SDH should be monitored for 4–6 months for head size, growth, feeding, activity, LOC, and seizure activity. Aside from supportive nursing care, nurses provide parents with education about the cause and prognosis for their infant. Referral to early intervention services is recommended at discharge.

Prognosis varies with the size and severity of the hemorrhage. Infants with SDH who are asymptomatic or have transient seizures in the neonatal period do well if there is no associated cerebral injury. Minor posterior fossa hemorrhages rarely have clinical significance [6]. Early diagnosis of large posterior fossa hemorrhage with MRI and CT has improved the outcome for those infants. Most infants with massive bleeding over the tentorium or falx cerebri (near the great vein of Galen) die. Those who survive usually have hydrocephalus and neurological sequelae.

## Intracerebellar Hemorrhage

Intracerebellar hemorrhage is more common in preterm than full-term infants. Although rare, it is generally associated with hypoxia in the preterm infant, and associated with trauma in the full-term infant.

Intracerebellar hemorrhage may be caused by intravascular factors (vitamin K deficiency, thrombocytopenia), vascular factors (damage due to hypoxia, followed by hypertensive spikes; e.g., from too rapid intravenous colloid infusion), and extravascular factors (mechanical deformation of the occiput during forceps or breech delivery in the full-term infant, compression of the compliant skull during care-giving, or the use of constrictive bands around the head, especially in the preterm infant) [50,87]. Intracerebellar hemorrhage may be a primary bleed or extension of a hemorrhage into the cerebellum.

Infants with intracerebellar hemorrhage either present critically ill from birth, with apnea, a declining hematocrit, and death within 24–36 h, or present less ill with symptoms developing at up to 2–3 weeks of age. Clinical signs include apnea, bradycardia, hoarse or high-pitched cry, eye deviations, facial paralysis, opisthotonos or intermittent tonic extension of the limbs, seizures, vomiting, hypotonia, diminished or absent Moro reflex, and hydrocephalus [12,87].

A high index of suspicion is important. Cranial ultrasound and/or CT scan are used for diagnosis. Lack of echogenicity of the cerebellum may be an important finding [50]. Intracerebellar hemorrhage is frequently diagnosed at autopsy. Treatment is primarily supportive. Surgery may be indicated, including hematoma evacuation or ventriculoperitoneal shunt for hydrocephalus. Nursing care involves supportive care for the infant, and care and comfort for the parents/family, including referral for early intervention services after discharge. Prognosis is poor in preterm infant survivors. Full-term infants have more favorable outcomes, but generally with subsequent neurological deficits, especially motor and variable involvement of intellect. About half of the infants have hydrocephalus [87].

## Pediatric TBI

## Concussion

Among the many definitions of concussion, there is consensus that concussion is a transient alteration in the level of alertness, assessed either by the affected person or an observer. Children experiencing concussion have an altered level of mental status, ranging from a period of confusion or amnesia to a loss of consciousness. Concussion produces brief, nonfocal clinical findings (Table 7.6), which often resolve completely over time.

Concussion is generally associated with a normal neurologic examination and normal neuroimaging [20,22]. Imaging is recommended for severe grades of concussion, symptoms lasting greater than 1 week, and for clearance to play after the second or third concussion in the same season. Alterations in LOC are thought to be secondary to a transient disturbance in neuronal function.

There is experimental evidence that biochemical changes involving alterations in neurotransmitters, (glutamate), metabolic substrates (ATP, $N$-acetylaspartate), and electrolytes (calcium), among others, produce a metabolic state of vulnerability. Greenberg [22] cites research that reveals evidence of increased levels of glutamate (an excitatory neurotransmitter), which results in a hypermetabolic state in the brain for up to 7–10 days postinjury. Vagnossi et al. [83] utilized a rat model where ATP and $N$-acetylaspartate levels were measured following repetitive mild TBI at varying intervals. Two consecutive mild TBI occurring within 3 days produced the same biochemical damage as a severe TBI. After 5 days, however, the two mild TBIs acted as two independent events. The conclusion was that the interval of time between injuries is important because the brain is metabolically vulnerable to repeat injury. Guidelines for return to play are crucial to prevent more severe injury or sudden death caused by second-impact syndrome. This occurs when the vulnerable brain sustains a second in-

**Table 7.6.** Early and late symptoms of concussion

| Symptoms of concussion (early) | Symptoms of concussion (late) |
|---|---|
| Headache | Persistent low-grade headache |
| Dizziness or vertigo | Light-headedness |
| Lack of awareness of surroundings | Poor attention and concentration |
| Nausea or vomiting | Memory dysfunction |
| Dazed or amnesia | Easily fatigued |
| | Irritable or frustrate easily |
| | Intolerance to bright lights (blurred vision) or noise (ringing in ears) |
| | Anxiety or depression |
| | Sleep disturbance |
| | Cognitive, behavior, emotional changes |

jury, resulting in swelling due to dysautoregulated cerebral perfusion, and most often results in death [22].

There is no consensus on grading the severity of concussion or guidelines for when an athlete should return to sports participation following concussion. Many concussion grading scales exist, the most well known of which are the Cantu, Colorado, and American Academy of Neurology (AAN) Guidelines (Tables 7.7 and 7.8). All of the guidelines assess grade of severity and number of concussions, and include recommendations for evaluation, management, and return to activity. All agree that the athlete must be symptom free even with exertion prior to returning to the game [20,22,36,83]. The most current recommendation is that no child should be allowed to return to play on the same day in which the concussion occurs [56].

**Table 7.7.** American Academy of Neurology (AAN) Concussion Grading Scale. Permission to reprint obtained from the American Academy of Neurology [36]

| AAN Concussion Grading Scale | |
| --- | --- |
| Grade 1: | 1. No loss of consciousness<br>2. Symptoms last less than 15 min |
| Grade 2: | 1. No loss of consciousness<br>2. Symptoms last more than 15 min |
| Grade 3: | Any loss of consciousness |

The recommended treatment for concussion is rest and slow return to normal activity. Recurrence of symptoms with exertion are indicative of continued brain injury. Over-the-counter analgesics such as acetaminophen can be employed to treat headache. The duration of postconcussive symptoms is unpredictable and not related to the grade or severity of injury [31]. Although most have resolution of symptoms within days to weeks following injury, some have persistent cognitive impairment, behavioral issues, or emotional lability, whether the original symptoms have cleared or not. This phenomenon is known as postconcussive syndrome. These children benefit from formal neuropsychological testing and often require Individualized Education Plans, either on a temporary or permanent basis to assist them with school performance.

## Skull Fractures (Pediatric)

The pediatric skull provides a protective box, which houses the brain. Forces exerted on the skull are absorbed initially in a centrifical configuration, then directed inward toward the brain. Fractures occur when the skull cannot withstand the force of impact. As mentioned previously, the pediatric skull is thinner and more flexible when compared to the adult skull, which predisposes the child to significant TBI without the presence of a skull fracture. A higher de-

**Table 7.8.** AAN recommendations. Permission to reprint obtained from the American Academy of Neurology [36]

| AAN assessment and management recommendations | | Recurrent injuries | |
| --- | --- | --- | --- |
| Grade 1: | 1. Remove from play<br>2. Examine every 5 min<br>3. May return to play if symptoms resolved within 15 min (with and without exertion) | Grade 1: | same day, out of play that day |
| Grade 2: | 1. Remove from play for the entire day<br>2. Requires physician clearance prior to return to play, minimum 1 week after clearance of symptoms (with and without exertion)<br>3. CT or MRI scan recommended for persistent symptoms | Grade 2: | any time, remove from play for two weeks minimum |
| Grade 3: | 1. Transport athlete to healthcare facility<br>2. Professional neurological examination and indicated neuroimaging<br>3. Hospital admission for persistent symptoms or abnormal findings on examination/imaging<br>4. For seconds of loss of consciousness, may return to play after 1 week of being asymptomatic<br>For minutes of loss of consciousness, may return to play after 2 weeks of being asymptomatic | Grade 3: | remove from play for one month minimum |
| | | **Note:** Any abnormality on CT or MRI – athlete should be removed from play for remainder of season.<br><br>**Assumption:** based on highest grade, regardless of sequence | |

gree of suspicion should be maintained in the decision-making for obtaining radiographic imaging based on the reported mechanism of injury. Twenty percent of children presenting with head trauma will have a skull fracture. Of these, most do not require surgical intervention. The initial focus in the management of skull fractures is the identification of serious underlying acute hemorrhage or brain injury. Skull fractures are classified by their location, type, and associated complications [22,46].

The linear nondepressed skull fracture, which is most common in children, heals rapidly without intervention. The most common site for linear skull fractures is the parietal bone, which is the thinnest of the cranial bones and is most frequently the site of impact in pediatric falls. The frontal and occipital, which are the thickest, require a more severe impact to cause fracture, and therefore, are associated with a higher degree of brain injury. Ping-pong skull fractures occur in newborns and young infants due to the thin, pliable skull, and resemble a depression in a ping-pong ball. Most heal well without surgical injury and do not require surgical intervention unless there is underlying brain injury. Open, depressed, or comminuted skull fractures may require surgical intervention and are more frequently associated with underlying hemorrhage or brain injury. An underlying brain contusion secondary to skull fracture can cause PTSs.

Basilar skull fractures occur in the anterior, middle, or posterior fossa at the base of the skull. Temporal bone fractures are classified as transverse (extending across the petrous portion) or longitudinal (extending lateral to medial). The middle meningeal artery is housed in a groove of the temporal bone, causing serious life-threatening epidural hematoma formation and the need for emergent surgical intervention following temporal bone fracture. Complications associated with transverse temporal bone fracture include sensorineural hearing loss (CN VIII) and facial nerve dysfunction (CN VII), whereas longitudinal temporal fracture can cause hemotympanum, torn tympanic membrane, CSF leak, and conductive hearing loss secondary to bony disruption. In most cases, the hearing loss resolves, but it can be permanent.

The nursing assessment should include inspection and gentle palpation of the scalp to assess for findings consistent with a skull fracture. External evidence of skull fracture includes contusion, laceration, depression, and hematoma on the scalp. Basilar skull fractures are identified by external clinical findings. Basilar fracture of the temporal bone results in "battle sign," which is postauricular ecchymoses and can be associated with CSF otorrhea. A frontal basilar fracture results in "raccoon's eyes," which is periorbital ecchymoses. CSF rhinorrhea can result secondary to frontal basilar fracture. The majority of CSF leaks resolve within 7 days without surgical intervention. Nursing care of the patient with CSF leak includes elevation of the head of the bed, restriction of nose blowing, if possible, and to report fever or other signs of meningitis. The neurosurgeon may need to place a lumbar drain, so the leak can seal. Check with the neurosurgeon before placement of a nasogastric tube, as a frontal fracture through the cribiform plate can allow placement of the catheter into the brain.

## Extraparenchymal Hemorrhage

There is a lower incidence of mass hemorrhage in infants and children than in adults. The anatomy of the pediatric brain and skull dissipates the impact of traumatic injury in this population. The protective features include the thin deformable skull, wider CSF spaces, and softer brain. This is true until 4 years of age, at which time the child's skull is a closed, rigid box. Interestingly, the anatomical differences that are protective against mass hemorrhage also predispose the pediatric patient to shearing injuries and subarachnoid hemorrhage. Extra-axial hemorrhages are defined by the location in which they occur in relationship to the meninges. The presentation and acuity level varies based on the child's age, as well as location and size of the hemorrhage. Small hemorrhages with minimal or no clinical deterioration may be observed with close monitoring and radiographic follow-up, whereas hemorrhages with significant mass effect and a deteriorating or comatose patient require emergent craniotomy and surgical decompression [71].

## Epidural Hemorrhage

EDH is less common in infancy, and steadily increases in incidence with age. Outcome following EDH is improved in children when compared to adults. EDHs can be either venous or arterial in origin. In neonates and infants, EDH is usually venous, secondary to tearing of the dural veins (see Birth-Related TBI, above). More commonly, especially in older children, EDH results from a tear of the middle meningeal artery, which is housed within a groove of the temporal and parietal bones. This artery is lacerated by a sharp bone edge when a skull fracture is sustained. Regardless of the origin, the bleeding creates a space between the dura mater and the periosteum (or inside) of the skull. The frontal, temporal, and parietal regions are typical locations for EDH. Infratentorial (or posterior fossa) EDHs occur, but are less common in older children [71].

Clinical presentation of EDH in pediatrics can be delayed due to the plasticity of the child's skull. The hallmark "lucid interval" following EDH may differ in that the child only appears stunned, while the older child or adult will have loss of consciousness. The volume of a rapidly expanding mass lesion (or hemorrhage), however, is not well tolerated even in the more plastic pediatric cranium. The increased intracranial volume results in general increased ICP. Nursing care and assessment is dependent on the location of the hemorrhage, being either supratentorial or infratentorial (above or below the tentorium cerebelli). The clinical presentation and indications of neurologic deterioration with expanding mass lesions vary based on this important landmark. Surgical management may be indicated if the patient has a focal neurologic exam, increasing drowsiness, midline shift, herniation, fracture transversing a major dural vessel, or concomitant intraparenchymal lesion. Nonsurgical management may be considered if the patient is only experiencing symptoms such as headache, nausea, vomiting, and irritability [71].

Radiographic evaluation of EDH is best accomplished with a CT scan, which reveals a lentiform, hyperdense (bright white), extraparenchymal fluid collection that is contained within the cranial suture lines (Fig. 7.4). The blood is contained within the sutures because of the attachment of the dura to the periosteum. EDHs are often also associated with CT scan findings of scalp swelling and the presence of a skull fracture in the frontal, temporal, or parietal regions [5]. Common practice is to repeat the radiographic imaging within 24 h for small, nonsurgical EDHs.

### Subdural Hemorrhage

The incidence of SDH is opposite to that of EDH, in that they are more common in infants and less common in older children. There is more often underlying brain injury associated with SDH than with EDH. Common etiologies for SDH in children include birth trauma, accidental falls, and child abuse. This type of hemorrhage is due to stretching and tearing of the bridging veins in the subdural space. The subdural space is located below the dura mater and above the arachnoid membrane. Hemorrhage in this space is not limited to the suture lines, and therefore can result in large, bilateral blood collections over the entire convexity (Fig. 7.4).

Large expanding mass lesions of subdural origin significantly increase intracranial volume, and therefore ICP. Infants with SDH present with seizures, irritability, lethargy, vomiting, and increased head circumference. Older children have a decreased LOC, pupil asymmetry, and hemiparesis. Severely increased ICP results in an irregular respiratory pattern, hypertension, and bradycardia, also known as "Cushing's Triad." (see section on Collaborative Management of Intracranial Hypertension). Expansile subdural collections require emergent craniotomy and evacuation to prevent herniation and death. In contrast, a small SDH in a child with minimal neurologic deficits can

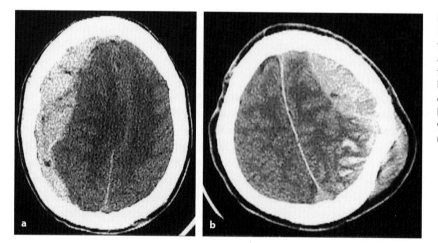

**Fig. 7.4 a, b.** Extraparenchymal hemorrhage. **a** Subdural hematoma appears on CT scan as an acute, crescent-shaped collection that crosses suture lines. **b** Epidural hematoma is seen on the CT scan as a hyperdense, lentiform collection, contained within the suture lines. Also note significant scalp swelling

be observed closely with follow-up imaging. Needle aspirations can be performed in infants with an open fontanel to temporarily relieve ICP.

The presence of blood in the subdural space is well visualized on CT scan. Subdural hematomas appear as acute, crescent-shaped, extraparenchymal blood collections, which crosses the suture lines. It is important to determine the severity of a SDH based on its size, location, and the presence of mass effect. The mass effect with any intracranial lesion is manifested as a right or left shift of the cerebral hemispheres, effacement (compression) of the ventricles, displacement of the brainstem, and obliteration of the sulcal pattern, indicative of increased ICP. There may also be underlying brain injury, which is less visible until the clot is surgically decompressed (Fig. 7.5). MRI can be useful to determine the timing (acute versus chronic) of SDHs, which can be helpful in an investigation for child abuse (see section on Inflicted TBI, below).

### Subarachnoid Hemorrhage

Intraparenchymal injury is often associated with the presence of hemorrhage in the subarachnoid space [5]. The subarachnoid space is located between the arachnoid and the pia mater, which is a thin membrane that is adhered to the brain's surface. CSF is made primarily in the ventricles and then circulates around the brain within the subarachnoid space. Circulation of CSF allows delivery of metabolic substrates, cushions the brain from trauma, and removes waste products. On CT scan images, SAH appears bright white and is seen within the gyral and sulcal pattern on the brain's surface, in the interhemispheric fissure, along the tentorium, and within the cisterns.

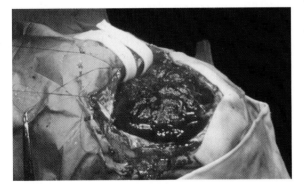

**Fig. 7.5.** Intraoperative photograph demonstrating a large open craniotomy after severe head trauma. Note the large SDH clot on the surface of the brain

Clearance of subarachnoid blood is fairly rapid as the blood is "washed out" with the circulation of CSF. MRI is not useful to identify SAH, but should be considered in a child with SAH and severe neurologic deficits. MRI can be useful to identify nonhemorrhagic intraparenchymal lesions, which are often associated with SAH.

The child with SAH should be observed for irritability, headache, stiff neck, and other signs of irritation to the meninges, similar to the presentation of meningitis. Children can develop posttraumatic hydrocephalus, especially when SAH or intraventricular hemorrhage is present. The presentation of hydrocephalus is identical to that of increased ICP. Development of hydrocephalus can be seen on CT scan and, when present, requires CSF diversion to prevent increased ICP and possible herniation. Temporary CSF diversion techniques include drainage via a ventriculostomy, and transfontanel tap in an infant with an open fontanel. Permanent CSF diversion requires placement of a shunt, consisting of a ventricular catheter, a one-way pressure-regulated valve, and a distal catheter to divert CSF to the peritoneum, pleural space, or right atrium.

### Parenchymal Injury

Following severe head trauma, children have generalized brain swelling. This is thought to occur due to edema and a process of dysautoregulation. The cerebrovascular resistance decreases significantly, which results in vasodilation and cerebral edema. Neuroimaging with a CT scan completed 12 h after the injury appears normal, whereas repeat imaging at 24 h postinjury reveals poor gray–white matter differentiation with compressed or absent ventricles and sulcal pattern. This is the typical picture of increased ICP, or what is referred to as a "tight" brain (Fig. 7.6).

The mass effect following parenchymal injury can be compartmentalized or global. The mass effect secondary to the hemorrhage and surrounding cerebral edema, when confined to the temporal (middle) cranial fossa, is concerning and can lead to transtentorial (or uncal) herniation. Surgical intervention becomes necessary to prevent impending or uncal herniation, or other neurologic deterioration. The child with an expanding contusion or mass lesion on the right side, with pending uncal herniation, will present with a right unilateral dilated pupil and contralateral motor weakness or posturing. The goal of neurosurgical intervention is to remove the hemorrhage, as well as the

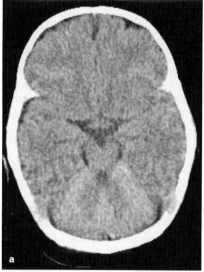 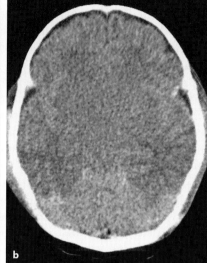

Fig. 7.6 a, b. a Severe traumatic brain injury (TBI). Early CT scan without evidence of injury, cisterns and normal extra-axial fluid are maintained. b Follow-up CT scan taken on day 2 showing what is referred to as a "tight" brain; with generalized edema, poor gray-white differentiation, and obliteration of the ventricles, cisterns, and sulcal pattern

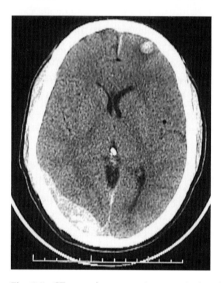

Fig. 7.7. CT scan demonstrating a typical surface contusion in the left frontal lobe, which was likely a contrecoup injury. Note right posterior SDH. The ventricles are asymmetric secondary to the mass effect of the SDH

## Contusion

A contusion is a focal bruise to the surface of the brain, which, depending on the location, can cause neurologic deficits, seizures, local mass effects, and increased ICP resulting in herniation. Contusion occurs when the skull impacts a stationary object with sudden deceleration, causing the brain to collide with the bony prominences of the frontal, temporal, or occipital skull. The point of initial impact of the brain on the internal skull is referred to as the "coup" injury. The brain, being suspended in fluid, then strikes the opposite side of the skull, which can cause a "contrecoup" injury. The French meaning of the word contrecoup is "counter blow" [22]. Contrecoup injuries are less common in young children, occurring with a frequency of less than 10% at ages 0–3 years, and 25% at ages 3–4 years.

Only hemorrhagic contusions are visible on CT Scan (Fig. 7.7). The CT may also reveal any accompanying extra-axial hemorrhage or intracranial air, also known as pneumocephalus [5]. It is a hallmark for contusions that enlarge subacutely and, therefore, require repeat CT imaging within 12–24 h of the injury [5,19,20,22,25]. Close observation and repeat imaging is required, but contusions typically coalesce and resolve without surgical intervention. Following resolution of a contusion, encephalomalacia (or "dropout") of the brain can occur, with the space then being filled with CSF [5].

The child with a focal contusion in an eloquent area of brain, such as speech or motor centers, will likely have worsening of their neurologic function

injured portion of the brain to decompress the compartment and reduce related volume and, therefore, pressure. It is paramount for the nurse to prevent secondary injury due to fluid overload, hyponatremia, hypercapnea, hypotension, and to prevent life-threatening edema or herniation [20]. Any deterioration in the child's LOC indicates increasing ICP and should be reported to the physician immediately, and documented (see the Collaborative Management of Intracranial Hypertension section).

specific to the area of injury as the contusion enlarges. Nurses should be aware of the location of injury and anticipate what deficits may develop. Any change in neurologic function should be reported to the physician immediately. The family should also be warned that the deterioration is likely to occur [22].

## Posttraumatic Seizures

PTSs are much more common in young children than in adults [14,19,20,25,32], and occur in 10% of children following head trauma. The majority of early pediatric PTSs occur in the first 24 h postinjury. Studies have indicated that children who experienced PTS after blunt head trauma, with a nonfocal neurologic exam and a negative CT scan, can safely be discharged to home. Holmes et al. [32] prospectively observed a cohort study of 63 children under 18 years with blunt head trauma. A head CT was obtained on all of the children. Ten children had findings on CT scan and were admitted to the hospital, three underwent craniotomy, and two had further seizures. The remaining 52 with negative CT imaging were either observed in the hospital or discharged to home. Follow-up revealed that none of the 52 patients with normal CT scan results had further seizures or required neurosurgical intervention.

Use of antiepileptic medications is controversial in either early (occurring within 7 days) or late (occurring 7 or more days postinjury) PTS. The Guidelines from the Society of Pediatric Critical Care Medicine [14] could not find conclusive evidence to determine that antiseizure medication should be a standard of care in head trauma, but did recommend antiseizure therapy as an option to prevent PTSs in young pediatric patients at high risk for seizures following head injury. Practice varies among physicians, but most utilize prophylactic anticonvulsant therapy for 7 days after a significant intracranial injury. Visible intracranial injury, including brain swelling, SDH, depressed skull fracture, and penetrating injuries, especially with lower GCS scores, carry a higher risk for early and late PTSs, and often require prolonged anticonvulsant therapy for 6–12 months [19]. Seizures must be prevented following severe TBI, as they result in increased brain metabolism and increased ICP, and can cause secondary brain injury.

## Diffuse Axonal Injury

A decreased LOC and generalized increased ICP are more likely to happen with DAI. DAI occurs when the pediatric skull is subjected to rotational forces during an acceleration or deceleration injury. The mechanism of DAI in children varies with age, with older children and adolescents involved in motor vehicle accidents (MVA) and bicycles versus MVA. Younger children are often pedestrians versus MVA. DAI is rare in infants. The softer, more plastic pediatric brain moves within the skull. This movement is further facilitated by the wider subarachnoid space found in children. Neuronal injury occurs when the axons are stretched until there is sufficient strain to cause the axons to fracture [5,20].

DAI typically occurs at the junctions of gray and white matter, the corpus callosum, the basal ganglia, and the brainstem. The hallmark presentation for DAI is immediate loss of consciousness that often lasts more than 6 h. Abnormal flexion (decorticate) posturing, or extension (decerebrate) posturing can accompany loss of consciousness, as well as a variation in the GCS score on serial assessments. Children may also have pupillary and other CN dysfunction, and brainstem abnormalities, which will be reflected in assessment findings. The typical triad of pediatric DAI is hypertension, hyperhydrosis (perspiration), and brainstem abnormalities.

CT is not sensitive enough to diagnose DAI. MRI is most sensitive to shearing injury and should be considered if the CT scan does not reveal injury sufficient to explain the degree of neurologic deficit (Fig. 7.8). The T2- and gradient-echo-weighted MRI sequences are very sensitive to DAI. Follow-up CT scan should be obtained in the face of DAI with significant sudden increase in ICP, to assess for an expanding mass lesion [5].

There is no treatment for DAI. Children with severe TBI (GCS 3-8) should be monitored and treated for increased ICP. The presentation and management of increased ICP is discussed elsewhere in this chapter. Pure DAI is associated with mild increased ICP. Greatly increased ICP in children with DAI requires repeat imaging with CT scan for suspected expanding mass lesion (hemorrhage). Recovery from DAI is a slow and gradual process, and can continue for weeks or months following DAI. The typical progression of assessment findings and recovery is as follows:

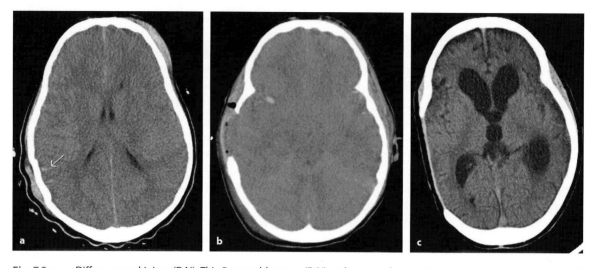

**Fig. 7.8 a–c.** Diffuse axonal injury (DAI). This 5-year-old was struck by a van, sustaining severe closed head injury. **a** CT scan taken on the day of the injury, shows a depressed right parietal skull fracture, with overlying soft tissue swelling. The child also sustained right temporal and orbital fractures. Multiple punctuate hemorrhages consistent with DAI are seen adjacent to the fracture (*arrow*). **b** An intracranial pressure (ICP) monitor was placed. Due to uncontrollable elevated ICP, an emergent decompressive craniectomy was performed (see absent bone flap). Multiple small parenchymal hemorrhage (DAI) at the gray-white matter junction can be seen on the CT scan. Also note that brain is "tight," with poor gray-white matter differentiation and complete effacement of the ventricles and sulci. **c** Cerebral atrophy and ventriculomegaly are seen on the CT scan performed 6 months after injury. The child survived his injury but is functionally wheelchair bound with severe morbidity. Films compare the CT scan, where the DAI is not apparent, and MRI performed due to neurologic impairment, which was not explained on CT scan

1. Teeth grinding, chewing motions, eyes open but not responsive with persistent posturing.
2. Periods of agitation with arms flailing.
3. Return of ability to localize painful stimulus.
4. Ability to follow commands, which represents the end of coma [20].

## Penetrating Craniocerebral Injury

Penetrating craniocerebral injuries (PCIs) are less common, but more often fatal in children, accounting for 12% of all pediatric TBI deaths [19]. Causes of PCI include accidental falls, impalement with sharp objects, accidental and nonaccidental gunshot wounds, and suicide [55]. Injuries may be sustained to the face, scalp, skull, and brain (Fig. 7.9). High-velocity PCI is associated with skull fractures, which can be severely depressed and comminuted (multiple fragments), causing further brain injury. Low-velocity PCI is associated with an increased (43%) risk of infection or brain abscess within the path of the projectile [55]. It is important to note location of the foreign missile because, if it is transventricular and crosses the midline, outcomes are extremely poor. Most neurosurgeons

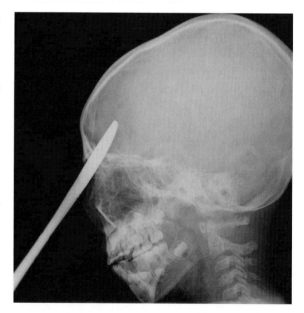

**Fig. 7.9.** Skull x-ray reveals a penetrating cerebral injury, after a 3-year old fell and was impaled onto a butter knife

will treat with broad-spectrum prophylactic antibiotics, although the majority are *Staphylococcus*-related infections. Clinical findings of infection or brain abscess include fever, new focal neurologic deficits, and change in mental status. The protruding object must be secured and left in place by the nurse until evaluation and surgical removal by the neurosurgeon. Hemorrhage, cerebral edema, severe increased ICP, and herniation are likely to occur with PCI. Goals of surgical intervention include removal of the object without causing further injury, debridement of necrotic brain tissue, evacuation of blood, and placement of an ICP monitor (see the Collaborative Management of Intracranial Hypertension section). Surgery is contraindicated if removal of the object would cause further injury [55]. Incidence of PTSs following PCI has been found to be as high as 50% [22]; therefore, treatment with antiseizure medications is recommended. MRI is contraindicated if none or a portion of the foreign body can be removed (i.e., bullet fragment).

### Inflicted TBI

Child abuse, both common and severe, is a leading pediatric health problem in the United States. In the year 2003, 1,500 children died of abuse and neglect, and were known to child protective service agencies [82]. More than three-quarters of the children that die are younger than 4 years of age, with 89% being under the age of 1 year, and infant males having the highest rate of death [82]. Inflicted TBI (ITBI) results in the occurrence of more frequent deaths than any other type of abusive injury, as well as morbidity of serious neurological sequelae [35,62]. ITBI is frequently misdiagnosed. In a retrospective study by Jenny et al. [35] at Denver Children's Hospital, 54 (31%) of 173 children with inflicted head injury were misdiagnosed, resulting in 5 deaths, and 15 (27.8%) being reinjured.

The mechanism of ITBI is well described, including violent shaking, which is often associated with an impact causing sudden deceleration of the head and brain. Common clinical findings include scalp or skull injury, SDH, retinal hemorrhage (RH), and other fractures or injuries. The acute and long-term clinical outcome of ITBI ranges from mild to severe, with a varied spectrum from full recovery to death or permanent disability. The neuroscience nurse must be knowledgeable of, and suspicious for, indicators of ITBI. As healthcare professionals, nurses are mandated to report any suspicion of child maltreatment. A multidisciplinary plan for treatment and investigation is paramount in treating the child with ITBI.

### Pathophysiology

The considerable force of ITBI causes focal and diffuse brain injury. Violent shaking causes rotational acceleration-deceleration of the child's head [13], and is often associated with impact of the child's head [20]. Anatomic differences between small children and older children or adults predisposes them to significant brain injury, including a proportionally larger head, weak neck muscles [13], less myelinated (softer) brain, wider subarachnoid space [25], and susceptibility of the white matter in a developing brain [74]. Impact injury may cause focal swelling or contusion of the scalp, although external findings are rare or difficult to appreciate [86]. Skull fracture may be seen in as many as half of inflicted TBI cases and is most easily detected on skull radiographs [15]. The skeletal survey may also reveal rib or other skeletal fractures.

SDH, unilateral or bilateral, is frequently associated with ITBI. Vinchon et al. [86] found that SDH was present in 81% of child abuse cases, with ITBI accounting for 64% of all traumatic SDH in infants. Movement of the brain within the skull causes bridging veins within the subdural space to tear, creating a SDH. Acute SDHs may resolve or become walled-off by a membrane, which can chronically rebleed [15]. If inflicted TBI occurs repeatedly, the child may have hemorrhages of different ages. CT scan is the initial study of choice, although MRI is useful to reveal multiple ages of injury and membranes associated with chronic SDH [5]. SDH may be mild, requiring only observation, or can cause a significant mass effect and require neurosurgical intervention, such as serial transfontanel taps and placement of a subdural drain or subdural shunt. DAI is created by severe ITBI and includes axonal shearing, diffuse swelling, global hypoxic-ischemic injury, and vascular injury [22,47]. The hallmark presentation of DAI is decreased LOC (see Diffuse Axonal Injury, above) [20]. Outcome after DAI is generally poor as many remain in a persistent vegetative state indefinitely. Significant recovery more than 1 year posttrauma is rare [76].

RH occurs in both accidental and ITBI. Vinchon et al. [86] found that severe RH (grade 2 or 3) was 100% specific for the diagnosis of child abuse. It is requisite that grading of RH be determined by a trained ophthalmologist to assure a correct diagnosis and prevent misdiagnosis.

## Clinical Presentation

Children with ITBI most commonly present with seizures, RH, or apnea [20,29,86]. Findings of altered sensorium, nausea, vomiting, irritability, tense fontanel, and focal deficit are less common [71]. Pallor, tachycardia, or poor perfusion may indicate anemia secondary to intracranial hemorrhage. Children may present with minimal or no external signs of ITBI, despite significant neurologic sequelae. External findings may include ecchymosis in the pattern of finger marks on chest or elsewhere. It is essential to obtain a detailed history of the child's condition from the parent or guardian. It is important to determine the timing of the onset of symptoms and who was responsible for the child's care at or around those times. Inquire specifically about any history of trauma, which may have caused the injuries. Symptoms are often reported with no history of trauma, or with a history of minor trauma not consistent with the extent of the child's injury [20]. Inconsistencies in the history between caregivers, or from the same caregiver on separate occasions, is concerning for ITBI [29]. Multidisciplinary team members (e.g., Child Abuse Physician, Social Worker, Children's Service Board, and law enforcement) will interview the family as part of a detailed investigation for ITBI. Input from other physicians, the neurosurgeon, the ophthalmologist, the radiologist, and the nurse is critical to the investigation.

## Management

Medical care begins with the emergency medical technician (EMT)/paramedics arrival at the scene or upon the child's arrival to the emergency room. It is important to stabilize the patient's cardiorespiratory status rapidly to prevent further injury. Once the emergency room physician has suspicion of ITBI, the remainder of the multidisciplinary team should be involved. The neurosurgeon must evaluate the child to determine whether urgent surgical intervention is warranted.

## Outcomes

In the acute stage of ITBI, the full extent of brain injury on the child's development may not be visible. Imaging 1-year postinjury may show extensive atrophy to the brain tissue despite improvement in the patient's neurologic deficits, due to the ability of the brain to reassign functions to healthy brain tissue [7]. Research shows that chronic changes, such as cerebral atrophy and ex vacuo (brain dropout), are present in 40–45% of ITBI cases (Fig. 7.10) [15].

Information is limited regarding the long-term outcome of ITBI. Barlow [7] studied survivors for 59 months, proving that 68% of the sample had developmental delays at the initial follow-up visit (16% with mild delays, 16% with moderate delays, 36% with severe delays). Study results indicated 60% had motor deficits, 48% visual deficits, 20% seizures, 64% speech and language deficits, and 52% behavioral difficulties. Outcomes of ITBI, in addition to developmental or cognitive delays, may include seizure disorder, blindness, cerebral palsy, hydrocephalus, and emotional or behavioral problems; 40% have deficits severe enough to impair their life-long ability to live independently [7].

## Case Study

A 5-month old female was brought to the emergency room by emergency medical services (EMS) for decreased responsiveness. The mother stated that the

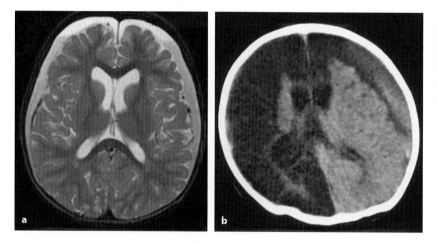

**Fig. 7.10 a, b.** Inflicted TBI. **a** Bilateral SDH seen on MRI, which reveals two different densities, implying acute and chronic injury. Subdural membranes are present. **b** Severe cerebral atrophy 3 months after infant was shaken

child fell from a changing table a week prior onto a hardwood floor, cried, and vomited. The mother allegedly called 911 for advice. The child had continued vomiting, fever, and diarrhea, and was diagnosed by her primary care physician with "stomach flu".

The child was brought to the emergency room by the EMS after parental concern of decreased responsiveness. The mother denies that the child suffered any trauma other than the fall the week before, but did state that the sibling (age 4 years) was "rough" with the child. The child is otherwise healthy and there is no family history of abnormal bleeding. The mother is the primary caregiver, the father works.

### Exam Findings

**General:**   Irritable cry, pale, bulging fontanel.

**Head/ears/eyes/nose/throat:**   Pupils sluggish reaction, right gaze preference.

**Lungs:**   Respiratory rate 28–32/min.

**Cardiovascular:**   Heart rate 135 beats/min, (ST), blocked premature atrial contractions, capillary refill <2 s.

**Abdomen:**   Soft, nontender, no organomegaly or palpable masses.

**Extremities:**   Limbs normal, painless to palpation. Symmetric, full range of movement.

**Neurologic:**   Child has frequent thrusting movements of the tongue, no tonic-clonic movement to extremities, stiff neck, global hypotonia.

**Skin:**   Faint blue bruise to left inferior periorbital area. Mucous membranes moist.

### Diagnostic Findings

**MRI:**   Bilateral frontal extra-axial fluid collections (chronic SDH) and an acute interhemispheric bleed. Figure 7.10 shows bilateral subdural hematomas with formed membranes secondary to ITBI.

**Skeletal survey:**   Split sutures, no fractures.
**Ophthalmology:**   Bilateral RH.
**Lumbar puncture:**   Red blood cell count 1580.

### Discussion

Multidisciplinary team investigates possible nonaccidental trauma (NAT). Admit to pediatric intensive care unit for observation. Bilateral subdural drains placed with resolution of SDH. Discharged to foster home. Investigation failed to prove NAT and she was returned to her biological Mother. Presented 1 year later with inflicted trauma (2 months after placement with biological parents). Injuries this admission included:

- Left distal radius fracture
- Proximal left tibia fracture
- Right distal radius fracture
- Left distal ulna fracture
- Bilateral optic edema, with RHs
- Increased SDH, with mass effect
- Multiple ecchymosis throughout the body, bite marks throughout integument
- Increased bone scan activity, ribs (10 and 11) and left scapula

Child is currently doing well after adoption by foster family. Has mild developmental delay and behavioral issues, requiring Early Intervention and rehabilitation therapies.

### Conclusion

Current research continues toward development of a diagnostic screening tool, utilizing serum and/or CSF, biochemical markers (neuron-specific enolase and myelin-basic protein) to evaluate the infant that presents with nonspecific symptoms such as vomiting or fussiness, or acute life-threatening event, enabling them to have additional evaluation (a head CT, head ultrasound, MRI) to facilitate correct diagnosis of ITBI [9]. The future of research for ITBI is looking toward prevention, and transplantation of stem cells and progenitor cells. Additional strategies for the future treatment of TBI includes the use of growth factors to treat head injuries, or a combination of promoting a stimulating environment to release transplant friendly growth factors and treatment with cell transplants [43,79,80].

The future of children's safety is partially influenced with the choices we, as healthcare providers, make. Being able to recognize the characteristic features of inflicted injury, having a better understanding of the pathophysiology, morbidity, and mortality of ITBI, and understanding human behaviors and emotions, places us in the unique position to assist with prevention of child abuse.

# Concepts of Cerebral Physiology

## Intracranial Dynamics

The skull forms a protective vault, which houses the brain and other cerebral structures. The protection offered by the cranial vault is not infinite. Severe TBI results in cerebral edema, increased intracranial volume, and eventual increased ICP, leading to decreased perfusion, decreased oxygen delivery, and cell death.

The Monroe-Kellie Doctrine recognizes that the skull is a rigid structure and that the total intracranial volume is finite. Intracranial components consist of brain (80%), CSF (10%), and blood (10%) within the cerebral vasculature. The ICP is determined by the total intracranial volume and intracranial compliance (the change in pressure that results from a change in volume). When any of the components increases in volume, there must be a compensatory decrease in the others to maintain equilibrium and to prevent an increase in ICP.

## Compensatory Mechanisms

The brain is incapable of a decrease in volume. The CSF and the blood compartments can compensate to a point. Following TBI, an accumulation of CSF, also known as hydrocephalus, may further increase ICP. The CSF is most easily displaced from the ventricles and cerebral subarachnoid space into the thecal, or spinal subarachnoid spaces. The CSF can also decrease in volume of production and increase in rate of absorption. The intracranial CSF volume can be decreased therapeutically via an external ventricular drain (EVD), or, if the ventricles are compressed and the basal cisterns are patent, a lumbar drain [44]. With severe increased ICP, the CSF ventricles and cisterns are easily compressed and are absent on neuroimaging. Cerebral blood volume can increase secondary to increased CBF, decreased venous return, or the presence of a mass hemorrhage. Increased intracranial volume is transmitted to the low-pressure cerebral venous system, causing increased cerebral venous pressure and eventually decreased CBF.

## Intracranial Compliance

Cerebral compliance is defined as the change in pressure that results from a change in cerebral volume. Compliance is a measure of the brain's tolerance of increases in the ICP. Compliance is limited in that ICP will rise once the compensatory mechanisms are exhausted. The pressure–volume curve (Fig. 7.11) demonstrates that initial increases in intracranial volume are tolerated with little increase in pressure, indicating that intracranial compliance is high. Further increases in volume, however, result in poor compliance and ICP rises quickly. After compliance is lost, progressively smaller increases in intracranial volume are associated with significant increases in ICP [25]. The normal ICP waveform depicts P1 (the percussion wave) as the initial sharp peak, which indicates cardiac ejection. The tidal wave, or P2, is the second, lower and rounded peak, which reflects intracranial compliance. A progressive rise in P2 indicates rising ICP and poor compliance as increased ICP is transmitted to the low-pressure venous system. The nurse should monitor the ICP waveform for worsening intracranial compliance or intolerance of nursing interventions.

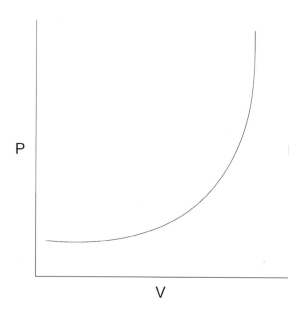

**Fig. 7.11.** Pressure-volume curve. With expanding mass lesions (hemorrhage) in TBI, intracranial volume (*V*) rises. Pressure (*P*) rises once compensatory mechanisms fail (pressure-volume curve)

## Cerebral Blood Flow

Maintenance of CBF and oxygen delivery is critical to maintain normal cerebral metabolism and to prevent neuronal injury and ischemic cell death. In children, the brain receives 25% of the total cardiac output and consumes 20% of the total oxygen content. The brain rapidly becomes ischemic if CBF is decreased or compromised [30]. Autoregulation is a protective mechanism, which balances vasoconstriction and vasodilation, to maintain homeostasis (constant CBF) despite changes in systemic circulation. Failure of autoregulation renders the cerebral circulation completely dependent on the mean arterial blood pressure (MAP) and the cerebral perfusion pressure (CPP).

Dysautoregulation occurs secondary to vasomotor dysfunction following TBI in children. The delicate balance between vasoconstrictor and vasodilator substances is upset, leading to vasomotor dysfunction and cerebral ischemia [37]. Abnormal hypoperfusion or hyperperfusion can decrease CBF and oxygen delivery, resulting in ischemia and secondary brain injury [8,30,85]. Adelson et al. [1] demonstrated that hypoperfusion occurs in the first 24 h, when cerebral metabolic demand is highest, and is associated with poor outcome after pediatric TBI. Hypotension must be treated aggressively to prevent secondary ischemic injury.

Hyperperfusion, also known as hyperemia, is defined as CBF in excess of metabolic demand [8]. Hyperemia following pediatric TBI increases the risk of intracerebral hemorrhage and further increases ICP, causing secondary ischemic injury. A prospective cohort study by Vavilala et al. [85] measured cerebral autoregulation with transcranial Doppler ultrasonography in 36 children and found that impaired cerebral autoregulation was greater after moderate to severe TBI in children and was associated with poor outcome. Hyperemia was associated with impaired cerebral autoregulation and poor outcome. There is a flurry of current research for the treatment of dysautoregulation related to hyperemia, which focuses on manipulation of endogenous vasoreactive substances such as nitric oxide and endothelin-1 [8,37].

CBF is also affected by changes in the partial pressures of carbon dioxide ($P_aCO_2$) and oxygen ($P_aO_2$), by chemical changes in electrolytes and pH balance, and by increased metabolism with seizure activity or fever. The physiologic mechanism underlying this is a change in the tone or resistance of cerebral arteries, due to local tissue biochemical responses. Hypercarbia is the most potent vasodilator, followed by hypoxia, when $P_aO_2$ falls below 50%. A low body pH, or acidosis, also causes vasodilation. Presence of fever and seizure activity increases cerebral metabolism and produces vasodilation to meet the increased metabolic demand. Vasodilation increases intracranial blood volume and, after compliance is lost, increases ICP.

CBF is also affected by decreased venous return. Venous return decreases due to increased ICP, as pressure is transmitted to the low-pressure venous system. Improper positioning of the child's neck in a rotated position impedes venous return by compression of the internal jugular vein. Decreased cerebral venous return increases cerebral blood volume and ICP. The child's head should be positioned in the midline with the head of the bed elevated to 30°. Increased intrathoracic pressures secondary to high positive end-expiratory pressure with mechanical ventilation can also impede cerebral venous return.

## Cerebral Metabolism

The brain is dependent on glucose for energy. The neurons utilize glucose in the Kreb's cycle to produce ATP to meet metabolic demand and maintain aerobic metabolism. Without glucose for energy, the Kreb's cycle is not able to function properly, leading to anaerobic metabolism. Anaerobic metabolism produces excess lactate and pyruvate, which contributes to tissue acidosis, decreased ATP, decreased energy, and cell death. Administration of barbiturates decreases the cerebral metabolic rate [25]. A hypermetabolic state exists after TBI due to the release of excitatory neurotransmitters (glutamate and aspartate) and the liberation of intracranial calcium [8].

## Pathophysiology of Intracranial Hypertension

Primary TBI is caused by an impact that directly disrupts brain tissue. Secondary injury is caused by inflammation and other factors (increased metabolism, dysautoregulation, neuroexcitation, and calcium dysregulation), which form a complex cascade of responses that are each affected by the others [37]. Cerebral metabolism and dysautoregulation were discussed earlier. The majority of our knowledge about increased ICP and the treatments employed are directed at reducing cerebral inflammation and cerebral blood volume.

## Cerebral Edema

Children have generalized cerebral inflammation after TBI, which can develop or worsen with incurred secondary injury. Cerebral swelling occurs due to a combination of cerebral edema and, as previously discussed, increased cerebral blood volume secondary to dysautoregulation [25,30]. Both result in increased intracranial volume, which increases ICP and contributes to ischemic injury.

Cerebral swelling is defined as an increase in CBF from regional or generalized hyperemia, or CBF in excess of metabolic demand, which peaks at 24–48 h postinjury. Cerebral edema is an increase in brain volume, either local or generalized, due to increased intracellular or extracellular water content [25]. There are three types of cerebral edema.

1. Vasogenic: Extracellular edema of the white matter. Diffuse injury produces an alteration in the permeability of the blood–brain barrier, which is more vulnerable to disruption in the pediatric brain, allowing plasma and protein to leak into the extracellular space [8]. The cellular membrane potential is also altered by: ischemia, free oxygen radicals, and other toxic mediators.

2. Cytotoxic: Increased intracellular swelling as a result of failure of the ATP-dependent sodium–potassium pump, allowing fluid and sodium to accumulate in the cells. Cytotoxic edema results in diffuse brain swelling in both the gray and white matter. Cytotoxic occurs after hypoxic-ischemic injury and in conditions of hypo-osmolality, such as hyponatremia and syndrome of inappropriate secretion of antidiuretic hormone (SIADH). Edema secondary to hypoxic-ischemic injury peaks at 48–72 h or longer after injury. Vasogenic and cytotoxic injury occur within hours of injury [22] and often coexist after TBI [30]. The use of osmotic diuretics (mannitol) is useful in the acute treatment of vasogenic and cytotoxic edema.

3. Interstitial: Occurs in severe hydrocephalus where the CSF, which is under pressure, crosses the ependymal tissue, out of the ventricle, and into the periventricular white matter.

## Intracranial Hypertension

ICP is the pressure exerted on the intracranial content. Normal fluctuations of the ICP occur with any mechanism that increases cerebral venous pressure, such as coughing, crying, and the Valsalva maneuver. The normal value for ICP ranges from 0 to 10 mmHg, and varies with age in children: in infants it lies in the range 1.5–6 mmHg, in children 3–7 mmHg, and in adolescents it is less than 10 mmHg. Intracranial hypertension in the adult is defined as ICP sustained greater than 20 mmHg. Because ICP is normally lower in children, neurosurgeons may initiate measures to treat increased ICP at 15 mmHg in children, or 10 mmHg in an infant [18].

## Cerebral Perfusion Pressure

CPP is an estimated measure of the adequacy of cerebral perfusion. CPP is the difference between the MAP required to perfuse the brain and the opposing ICP (thus CPP = MAP – ICP). CPP, however, may or may not reflect an accurate estimate of cerebral perfusion. Low CPP is worrisome, while a normal CPP may not be reassuring [25]. Although the minimal CPP necessary to provide adequate CBF has not been clearly established for children, the general guideline is >50–60 mmHg for children and >40–50 mmHg for infants and toddlers [25,52]. Fluid volume or vasopressor administration, as well as measures to decrease ICP can improve the CPP.

## Cerebral Herniation Syndromes

The brain is not acutely compressible, but it will shift within the cranium. Excessive pressure gradients between compartments lead to herniation, where part of the brain is herniated into an adjacent compartment (i.e., supratentorial, infratentorial) or into the spinal column [25,52]. It is important to consider the anatomic landmarks that separate the intracranial compartments. The tentorium cerebelli is a tent-like partition between the cerebrum and the cerebellum. The space above the tentorium is referred to as the supratentorial space, where the space below the tentorium is referred to as the infratentorial space. The foramen magnum is the opening at the base of the skull through which the brainstem and spinal cord are connected. There are two types of cerebral herniation syndromes (Fig. 7.12), including uncal and central herniation, which are significant in head trauma. Uncal herniation occurs when the uncus, or medial, inferior portion of the temporal lobe herniates downward through the incisura of the tentorium. Central herniation occurs when excessively increased ICP in the supratentorial space causes herniation of the cerebellar tonsils and brainstem through the foramen magnum into the spinal column, causing cessation of CBF and brain death.

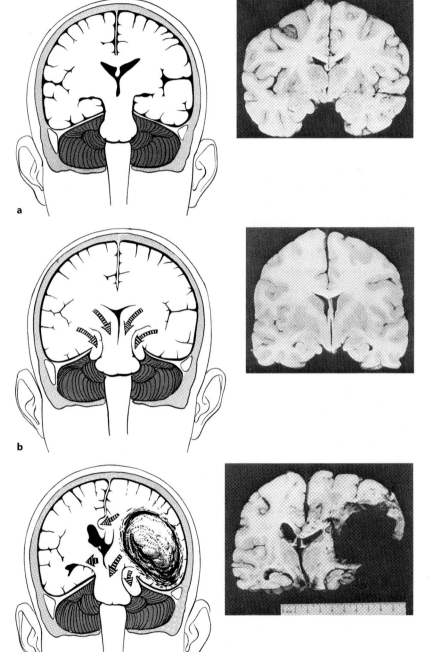

**Fig. 7.12 a–c.** Cerebral herniation syndromes. **a** Coronal view: normal relationship of the supratentorial and infratentorial compartments. **b** Central herniation occurs when excessive increased ICP in the supratentorial space causes herniation of the cerebellar tonsils and brainstem through the foramen magnum into the spinal column, causing cessation of cerebral blood flow and brain death. **c** Uncal herniation occurs when the uncus, or medial, inferior portion of the temporal lobe herniates downward through the incisura of the tentorium. Reprinted with permission from Plum and Posner (1982) [68]

## Collaborative Management of Intracranial Hypertension

Treatment of the child with a TBI focuses on preventing secondary insults and optimizing functional outcomes. Maintaining CBF, and optimizing oxygen and substrate delivery and utilization, while preventing or effectively managing intracranial hypertension, accomplishes these goals. Additionally, the child needs to have adequate airway support, effective oxygenation and ventilation, and good perfusion. When these fundamental needs are addressed, the child's chances of meaningful recovery and effective brain injury management are improved.

The main focus of management is to prevent or minimize secondary injuries, such as cerebral ischemia, cerebral edema, and neurochemical alterations. Since hypoxia and hypotension are known to worsen secondary injury by causing cerebral vasodilation, care must be taken to quickly recognize and treat these mitigating factors [67]. In general, the goal of treatment is to maintain an ICP at <20 mmHg, along with age-appropriate CPP. ICP management interventions include therapies to decrease cerebral volume, control CSF volume, control cerebral blood volume, and decrease cerebral metabolic rate. Because there exists a lack of data from well-designed and controlled pediatric studies to direct the treatment of children with brain trauma, recent guidelines have been released that assimilate the research results that are available and provide expert consensus on therapies [14]. In addition, children with severe TBI are more likely to survive when they are transported to a pediatric trauma center if one is available or an adult trauma center with added capabilities to treat children [70].

## Initial Resuscitation

Prehospital care of the child with TBI begins at the scene with rapid assessment and support of airway, breathing, and circulation. Supplemental oxygen should be administered and hypoxia (oxygen saturation <90% or $P_aO_2 < 60$ mm Hg) avoided. In general, if the GCS is ≤8, endotracheal intubation should be considered, although there is no research evidence that supports endotracheal-tube intubation over bag-valve-mask ventilation for prehospital management [14]. Upon arrival at a medical center, rapid-sequence intubation should be performed if the CT scan demonstrates diffuse cerebral edema, or if there is risk of neurological decompensation, respiratory instability, or loss of protective airway reflexes [48]. The intubation procedure should include medications to facilitate the process that do not further increase ICP, such as thiopental, lidocaine, and a short-acting, nondepolarizing neuromuscular blocking agent [3]. Normoventilation ($P_aCO_2$ 35–40 mmHg) should be ensured during initial resuscitation.

Hypotension has been shown to increase the morbidity and mortality of traumatically brain-injured children [41]. Because hypotension is a serious and potentially preventable secondary insult, signs of inadequate perfusion should be recognized and treated aggressively. Cerebral perfusion is partially dependent on an adequate MAP; therefore, age-appropriate blood pressure must be maintained to ensure adequate end-organ perfusion, CPP, and to prevent ischemia and resultant infarction. The following formula is used to determine median blood pressure (50th percentile) for children greater than 1 year of age: 90 + (2 × age in years) [3]. Table 7.9 shows ranges for median to 90th percentile age-related blood pressures in children. Children can be severely hypovolemic without demonstrating decreased blood pressure, and so rapid fluid volume resuscitation should occur both at the scene and upon arrival at the hospital. If appropriate amounts of fluid volume resuscitation do not improve signs of inadequate perfusion, vasopressor support should be initiated [52].

## Intensive Care Management

The child with TBI should be initially evaluated in the emergency room and then taken to the medical imag-

Table 7.9. Normal blood pressure in children (50th–90th percentile) [33]

| Age | Systolic pressure (mmHg) | Diastolic pressure mmHg |
|---|---|---|
| Birth (3 kg) | 50–70 | 25–45 |
| Neonate (96 h) | 60–90 | 20–60 |
| Infant (6 months) | 87–105 | 53–66 |
| Toddler (2 years) | 95–105 | 53–66 |
| School age (7 years) | 97–112 | 57–71 |
| Adolescent (15 years) | 112–128 | 66–80 |

ing department for further evaluation. Radiographic testing may include cervical spine evaluation, CT scan, and possible MRI. From there, the child may proceed to the operating room for removal of expanding lesions, control of hemorrhage, evacuation of significant hematomas, insertion of an ICP catheter or catheter for extraventricular drainage, or decompressive craniectomy. Although randomized controlled trials of the safety and efficacy of decompressive craniectomy in pediatric patients with severe brain injury have not been undertaken, there are instances when this procedure may lower ICP and improve outcomes. Table 7.10 lists criteria to guide the practitioner in determining whether the child is a candidate for decompressive craniectomy. After determining if any surgical intervention is necessary, further head injury management then generally takes place in the intensive care unit.

### ICP Monitoring

The ability to identify rapidly increasing pressure is crucial in the treatment of severe TBI and in the prevention of cerebral ischemia and infarction. ICP monitoring is recommended for the child with a TBI that has a GCS ≤8 [14]. It should be noted that the presence of an open fontanel does not negate the utility of ICP monitoring or preclude the development of intracranial hypertension. In addition, a monitor may be placed in the child who has clinical signs of increasing ICP, after major neurosurgical procedures, or when serial neurological assessments may be masked by sedation, neuromuscular blockade or anesthesia.

Either a fiberoptic-tipped wire or fluid-filled catheter system can be placed in the intracranium, which allows for the continuous measurement of ICP. While fiberoptic-tipped devices can be placed in the intraventricular, parenchymal, and less often in the epidural, subdural, and subarachnoid spaces, fluid-filled ICP catheters are generally placed in the intraventricular space, particularly if CSF drainage is desired. Table 7.11 lists potential complications associated with the use of intracranial catheters.

A fiberoptic-tipped catheter is zeroed before insertion and requires a monitoring unit supplied by the manufacturer for ICP readings. Alternatively, a fluid-filled ventriculostomy catheter system can be set up to allow for the continuous drainage of CSF. This system contains an external strain-gauge transducer that is coupled to the patient's intracranial space through a fluid-filled line. The transducer must be secured at a fixed reference point, usually the level of the lateral ventricle, which can be approximated by positioning the transducer at the level of the external auditory meatus. The system must be zeroed to atmospheric pressure and leveled to ensure accuracy of the ICP data. Nursing care of the patient with an ICP monitor is outlined in Table 7.12.

**Table 7.10.** Criteria for decompressive craniectomy*

| |
|---|
| 1. Severe TBI |
| 2. Refractory intracranial hypertension |
| 3. Diffuse cerebral edema on CT imaging |
| 4. Within 48 h of injury |
| 5. No episodes of sustained ICP >40 mmHg prior to surgery |
| 6. GCS ≥4 at any point prior to surgery |
| 7. Secondary clinical deterioration |
| 8. Evolving cerebral herniation syndrome |

*some or all may be present [14]

**Table 7.11.** Potential complications associated with ICP-monitoring catheters. *CSF* Cerebrospinal fluid

| |
|---|
| Hemorrhage |
| Infection |
| Overdrainage of CSF |
| Catheter misplacement |
| Catheter migration |
| Catheter obstruction |

**Table 7.12.** Nursing priorities for the child undergoing ICP monitoring. *CPP* Cerebral perfusion pressure

| |
|---|
| 1. Keep the ICP monitoring system operational and intact, ensuring that all connections are secure |
| 2. Prevent strain on the tubing and cables, particularly during patient repositioning and transport. |
| 3. Zero and level the system according to manufacturer's recommendations. |
| 4. Ensure the transducer of a fluid-filled system is leveled at the appropriate anatomical location, especially after patient repositioning and transport. |
| 5. If draining CSF, maintain the drainage chamber at the level ordered. |
| 6. Empty the drainage chamber regularly, recording the amount of CSF output. |
| 7. Do not allow the air filter of the drainage chamber to get wet. |
| 8. Document ICP and CPP readings. |
| 9. Note child's ICP response to interventions and ICP trends over time. |
| 10. Maintain a dry sterile dressing around the insertion site as per hospital policy. |
| 11. Monitor for and notify the neurosurgeon of CSF leakage around the insertion site, other drainage, and signs of infection. |

Intracranial hypertension is defined as an ICP $\geq 20$ mmHg and treatment designed to reduce ICP and improve cerebral perfusion should be initiated at this point. Prolonged periods of increased ICP and dramatic elevations in ICP are associated with poor outcomes in the pediatric patient [2]. Although there are no pediatric studies to document what target CPP is needed to improve outcomes, depending on the child's age, CPP should be maintained between 40 and 65 mmHg at all times during head injury management [2]. In addition to ICP data, evidence of intracranial hypertension should be corroborated by frequent patient assessment, other physiologic parameters, and cranial imaging studies.

### Jugular Venous Oxygenation Saturation Monitoring

Continuous measurement of venous saturation can be obtained using a fiberoptic catheter placed retrograde into the jugular vein. This monitoring technique can provide information on cerebral oxygen delivery and consumption, and the effectiveness of therapies. Because most of the cerebral circulation drains into one jugular vein, oxygen saturation is measured after cerebral perfusion has occurred. Normal jugular venous oxygen saturation ($S_{jv}O_2$) values are 55–70%. Values below 55% indicate inadequate oxygen delivery or utilization within the injured brain. Conditions that decrease $S_{jv}O_2$ are hypoxia, hypotension, increased ICP, and hypocarbia. $S_{jv}O_2$ monitoring provides a global picture of CBF and metabolic need, but does not provide any information about oxygen consumption at the site of injury.

### Monitoring Partial Pressure of Oxygen

$P_{bt}O_2$ is a measure of cerebral (brain tissue) oxygenation. A microprobe is inserted into uninjured parenchymal brain tissue, or the area of primary injury (penumbra) of an intracerebral lesion. While placing the microprobe into uninjured brain tissue will more closely assess global cerebral oxygenation, placement in an intracerebral lesion will provide data regarding cerebral oxygenation in an area most at risk [24]. Either method should give an indication of cerebral oxygenation and ischemia. Normal values for noninjured brain tissue range from 20 to 35 mmHg. In-

stances that can decrease $P_{bt}O_2$ are hypocarbia, hypoxemia, hyperthermia, decreased CBF and ischemia, decreased CPP, and elevated ICP [45]. Treatment interventions to improve cerebral oxygenation should begin when $P_{bt}O_2$ values are <15 mmHg [84]. Values below this have been associated with poor outcomes and death.

### CSF Drainage

External ventricular drainage of CSF is a common management therapy that is often used in conjunction with ICP monitoring. The CSF is drained to reduce intracranial fluid volume, and thus decrease ICP. Drainage can be continuous or intermittent, depending on the child's situation and the neurosurgeon's preference. For instance, drainage may be ordered any time the ICP is above a preselected value for a specified time. Moving the CSF collection device up or down in relation to the reference level point will control the amount of drainage. The higher the drain is above the reference level, the higher the ICP must be for CSF to flow into the collection device. Conversely, lowering the drain will cause CSF to flow at a lower ICP. Care must be taken when draining CSF to treat elevated ICP, as excessive drainage of CSF may cause the lateral ventricles to collapse. In addition, excessive CSF output may lead to hyponatremia, which is corrected with intravenous fluid administration designed to replace the CSF fluid volume.

The use of lumbar CSF drainage has occasionally been reported in pediatric patients with ICP refractory to other management therapies [44]. The lumbar drain is used simultaneously with a functioning ventricular catheter when the basilar cisterns are open. Patients for whom lumbar drainage is contraindicated include those with intracranial masses or shifts, because transtentorial herniation could result.

### Analgesia, Sedation, and Neuromuscular Blockade

Analgesia and sedation are important adjuncts to other treatments for the brain-injured child. Because pain and anxiety contribute to increased ICP and the cerebral metabolic rate, it is imperative to provide relief from pain, anxiety, and agitation. Additionally, the use of these agents can also facilitate the child's tolerance of other therapies, such as mechanical ventilation and suctioning, intradepartmental transport, and monitoring devices. The nurse is in a vital position to assess, advocate for, and effectively manage the child's level of sedation and analgesia. Depending on practitioner preference, common agents used are opiates, benzodiazepines, and barbiturates. Although routinely used in the adult with TBI, the use of continuous infusions of propofol has recently been determined by the Food and Drug Administration to be contraindicated in pediatric patients with TBI, as it has been associated with fatal metabolic acidosis, rhabdomyolysis, and hypoxia [64].

While the use of short-acting neuromuscular blockade agents may facilitate intubation and the tolerance of therapies, the patient's neurological exam is blunted. Therefore, these agents are generally used only when the child's agitation and increased ICP persist despite adequate doses of sedation and analgesia. The paralytic agent is generally allowed to wear off at intervals to allow for a complete neurological examination. Neuromuscular blocking agents should never be used without the concomitant administration of a sedative or analgesia.

## Hyperosmolar Therapy

Osmotic diuresis for the treatment of the head-injured child is accomplished through the use of mannitol and/or hypertonic saline (HS). While mannitol has been the mainstay of therapy for many years, a few recent studies using HS in children with intractable intracranial hypertension have demonstrated a decrease in ICP and subsequent increase in CPP [21,38,65,77]. The nurse should keep in mind that the overall goal is euvolemia (fluid balance); therefore, hyperosmolar therapy may be contraindicated in the presence of hypotension.

After mannitol administration, an osmotic gradient between the plasma and parenchymal tissue develops, drawing fluid from brain tissue into the vascular space. Osmotic diuresis then occurs, which results in a net reduction of brain water content. Further, because of fluid movement, mannitol reduces hematocrit and blood viscosity, improving CBF and reducing blood vessel diameter. ICP and cerebral blood volume decrease almost immediately. Therefore, because of its rapid onset of action, a 20% mannitol solution is usually administered as a bolus dose of 0.25–

1 g/kg body weight [14]. The nurse should be aware that mannitol may crystallize, so an in-line filter should be used to prevent the administration of any crystals. Serum osmolarity must be monitored when using hyperosmolar therapies. The maximum recommended serum osmolarity when using mannitol is 320 mOsm/l. Because mannitol is excreted unchanged in the urine, renal failure can result with a higher serum osmolarity. With chronic administration, mannitol may cause rebound cerebral edema because it is believed to disrupt the blood–brain barrier and accumulate in the interstitial space of the brain parenchyma, causing a reverse osmosis [14]. An additional side effect of mannitol therapy is dehydration and hypotension following overly effective osmotic diuresis.

Hypertonic saline works by increasing serum sodium and serum osmolarity, creating an osmotic gradient to pull water from the intracellular and interstitial compartments of the brain, reducing cerebral edema and ICP. Sodium chloride creates a driving force to bring water from the brain into the intravascular compartment in regions with intact blood–brain barrier, thus reducing water content, mass effect, and ICP. In addition, intravascular volume expansion occurs after administration of HS solutions. While there is no change in systemic vascular resistance, MAP increases because of increases in cardiac output and intravascular volume. This increase in MAP can further improve CPP. Although pediatric studies of HS have not reported any, possible side effects include central pontine myelinolysis, which involves demyelination, primarily of the pons, which can be seen clinically by the onset of lethargy and quadriparesis. Other possible side effects of the use of HS include coagulopathy and rebound rises in intracranial hypertension. HS can be administered via continuous infusion at a dose of 0.1–1 ml/kg/h, as needed, to maintain ICP at <20 mmHg [65]. An osmolarity up to 360 mOsm/l has been well tolerated in children receiving HS [14]. Additional side effects of HS therapy include electrolyte imbalance and the risk of phlebitis if the solution is administered via a peripheral vein.

## Hyperventilation

During hyperventilation, $P_aCO_2$ decreases, resulting in cerebral vasoconstriction and a reduction in cerebral blood volume. Although ICP rapidly decreases in this situation, cerebral perfusion is compromised and ischemia can result [78]. Because of these concerns, prophylactic hyperventilation and hypocarbia should be avoided. Mild hyperventilation ($P_aCO_2$ 30-35mm Hg) may be instituted when other therapies such as adequate sedation and analgesia, neuromuscular blockade, hyperosmolar therapy, and CSF drainage have not been effective in correcting intracranial hypertension [14]. Depending on physician preference, aggressive hyperventilation may be used in the event of acute brain herniation or significant ICP elevation. In this instance, $P_{bt}O_2$ and/or $S_{jv}O_2$ may be monitored to allow for immediate detection of cerebral ischemia.

## Temperature Regulation

Hyperthermia is known to increase cerebral metabolic rate and ICP, and should be avoided in the traumatically brain-injured child. Core body temperature may be measured via the bladder or rectal route, or through a pulmonary artery catheter. Brain temperature can also be assessed during both $P_{bt}O_2$ and $S_{jv}O_2$ monitoring. Because core body temperature measurement may be lower than actual brain temperature [27], the nurse may need to institute treatment for fever at a rectal temperature of 37.5°C, instead of the usual 38.5°C. Fever can be treated with antipyretics and external cooling devices, although shivering must be avoided because it will further increase cerebral metabolic rate and ICP. Furthermore, it is important to identify and treat the cause of the elevated temperature. Some common causes of fever after a TBI include atelectasis, infection, cerebral irritation from hemorrhage, and injury to the hypothalamus.

Mild to moderate hypothermia (32–34ºC) as a treatment for intracranial hypertension has recently been considered in both adults and children, although the results do not yet provide clear direction for treatment [11,53,69,75]. The goal of hypothermia therapy is to slow the body's metabolic processes. In addition, induced hypothermia may improve ICP, increase the oxygen supply to areas of ischemic brain, and help prevent seizures [10]. The sequelae of induced hypothermia include increased risk of acquired infection, lactic acidosis, sludging blood flow, cardiac arrhythmias, and seizures.

## Barbiturate Therapy

Barbiturates (e.g., pentobarbital) have been used for many years as a therapy for intracranial hypertension that is not responsive to other treatments. Despite this history of use, limited clinical trials have been performed in children, and other studies in adults have not consistently demonstrated improved outcomes. However, in the pediatric patient with a potentially recoverable brain injury who has elevated ICP that is not responsive to other management strategies, barbiturate coma therapy may be used [14].

Barbiturates decrease the cerebral metabolic requirements of the brain with a resultant decrease in ICP. As a side effect, barbiturate therapy causes myocardial depression and vasodilation, which results in hypotension. The child who is receiving barbiturate therapy should have cardiovascular parameters, including blood pressure and central venous pressure monitored continuously. The nurse should be prepared to administer fluids and inotropic agents as needed during barbiturate therapy. Continuous electroencephalogram (EEG) monitoring is needed to evaluate burst suppression. The barbiturate is administered via continuous intravenous infusion following a loading dose. The infusion is titrated based on the patient's ICP response and EEG tracing.

## Hydration and Nutrition

During the first 48–72 h, the child with a TBI should receive intravenous fluid therapy to maintain a euvolemic state. Fluid boluses, including blood products as indicated, may be administered to maintain adequate perfusion, age-appropriate blood pressure, central venous pressure, and urine output. A bladder catheter is essential for monitoring accurate urinary output. The intravenous fluid of choice is usually normal saline, lactated Ringer's, or hypertonic saline. Hypotonic fluids should be avoided and hyponatremia prevented, since both contribute to cerebral edema.

Research results are beginning to demonstrate that hyperglycemia may be detrimental to the child with a TBI [16]. In adult studies, the harmful effects of hyperglycemia on the traumatically brain-injured patient have been repeatedly verified [42,72,89]. Because of this, glucose-containing parenteral fluids are normally not used during the first 48 h after injury. Serum glucose must be monitored and appropriate glucose correction therapy initiated in the event that the patient becomes hypoglycemic (serum glucose <75 mg/dl) during this time.

Meeting nutritional requirements is of utmost importance. The child with a TBI requires 130–160% of their basal metabolic expenditures [66]. Enteral feedings should begin by 72 h after injury, with full feeds established within 7 days. Nutritional formula appropriate for age and caloric requirements is administered via a gastric or transpyloric tube, which can be inserted by the nurse at the bedside. In cases where enteral feeding cannot be initiated, total parenteral nutrition should be started. In addition, because the patient is likely to be immobile and receiving opiates, a bowel regimen should be established early, which may include a stool softener.

### Additional Nursing Care

The nurse at the bedside caring for the traumatically brain-injured child has the important role of preventing secondary injury and optimizing outcomes. The nurse must also balance the care needs of the patient with the requirement not to further increase ICP. Vigilance to proper patient positioning is necessary. The head of the bed should be elevated 30°. Moreover, the patient's head should be maintained in a midline position to prevent obstruction of venous outflow, which can further worsen intracranial hypertension. The nurse should check that the cervical collar or tracheostomy ties are not so tight that they constrict venous outflow. Complications from immobility should be assessed and prevented. The child will need to be repositioned as tolerated, keeping the head in midline with the body. The risk of skin breakdown should be assessed and skin integrity routinely monitored [17]. Preventive measure for deep vein thrombus, such as passive range of motion or sequential compression devices, should be initiated as indicated based on the child's age and body size.

Depending on the child's response to stimuli, the environment should be quiet and free from extraneous noise. The nurse will need to determine if the child will tolerate the clustering of care activities, or if care needs must be met in increments with rest periods between activities. The child's response, vital signs, and ICP and CPP parameters should be monitored during care activities. For instance, if the ICP

rises significantly during care, the nurse may need to cease care and allow the ICP to return to baseline for a period of time before meeting further care needs. Also, the nurse should assess the child's need for additional analgesia or sedation during care activities that must take place.

Because this child is likely to be intubated and ventilated, the nurse should institute measures to prevent ventilator-associated pneumonia, such as oral care and head of bed elevation. Endotracheal tube suctioning should be initiated based on the child's clinical assessment and not performed on a scheduled basis if the patient does not demonstrate the need for suctioning. Coughing during suctioning can increase ICP. Endotracheal lidocaine may need to be administered before endotracheal tube suctioning to blunt the gag and cough response. Preoxygenation is necessary during the suctioning procedure so that hypoxia can be avoided.

During this time of intensive care, the child's family will need much support and education. They are likely to experience uncertainty and fear about their child's recovery and future. The nurse will need to describe the equipment surrounding the child, and should provide the family with anticipatory guidance on what to expect during the child's initial care and recovery. The family may need to be given direction on the role they can assume in the intensive care unit. A family-centered intensive care unit environment that establishes a partnership between the family and the healthcare team is vital. The family may be encouraged to interact with their child and touch the child as appropriate. The nurse should observe the patient's response to this interaction, including ICP response. Research has demonstrated that family presence and interaction are not detrimental, and actually may decrease ICP [26,58].

### Endocrine Complications

### Diabetes Insipidus

Diabetes insipidus (DI) can occur after a traumatic head injury or intracranial surgery because of damage to the cells in the hypothalamus that produce antidiuretic hormone (ADH). DI can also occur after injury to the posterior pituitary gland, whereby the injured gland does not release ADH. When there is not enough ADH present, the collecting ducts and the

**Table 7.13.** Selected laboratory values associated with diabetes insipidus (*DI*), syndrome of inappropriate secretion of antidiuretic hormone (*SIADH*), and cerebral salt wasting (*CSW*)

|  | DI | SIADH | CSW |
|---|---|---|---|
| **Urine** | | | |
| Specific gravity | <1.005 | >1.020 | >1.010 |
| Osmolality | <250 | >500 | >300 |
| Urine output | >3 ml/kg/h | <1 ml/kg/h | ≥1 ml/kg/h |
| Sodium | <40 mEq/l | >60 mEq/l | >120 mEq/l |
| **Serum** | | | |
| Osmolality | >305 | <275 | <275 |
| Sodium | >150 | <130 | <130 |

distal tubules of the kidneys do not reabsorb free water, which results in intravascular volume depletion. Signs and symptoms of DI include large amounts of very dilute urine, severe dehydration, thirst, hypernatremia, and elevated serum osmolality. Excessive thirst in an alert child may also be indicative of DI, and often is an effective mechanism to prevent severe dehydration. Table 7.13 lists laboratory values associated with DI.

The treatment for DI includes frequent assessment of laboratory values, as well as accurate calculation of fluid administration and urine output. Fluid resuscitation with isotonic solutions may be needed initially to treat severe volume depletion. After stabilization, fluid volume deficits and ongoing urine volume losses are replaced hourly. An intravenous infusion of vasopressin may become necessary if fluid replacement therapy alone is unsuccessful. The infusion is titrated to maintain a urine specific gravity greater than 1.010. For chronic management of DI, desmopressin acetate is administered via the nasal route or, less often, the oral route.

## Syndrome of Inappropriate Secretion of Antidiuretic Hormone

SIADH involves overproduction or release of ADH from the pituitary. This excess ADH increases the permeability of the collecting ducts and the distal tubules of the kidneys, causing water to be retained. The child can become fluid overloaded and fluid can further shift from the intravascular to interstitial spaces, worsening cerebral edema. Clinically, the child will demonstrate decreased urine output, nausea and vomiting, dilutional hyponatremia with the risk of seizures, and mental status changes. Table 7.13 lists laboratory values associated with SIADH.

The treatment for SIADH, like that for DI, also includes frequent assessment of laboratory values, and accurate calculation of fluid administration and urine output. Fluid restriction therapy is usually initiated. The child is also monitored frequently for changes in mental status and seizures. Severe hyponatremia, especially when associated with seizures, is treated with 3% hypertonic saline via the intravenous route. Rapid correction of sodium levels should be avoided because this can cause CNS demyelination.

## Cerebral Salt Wasting

Cerebral salt wasting (CSW) is a condition characterized by true loss of body sodium through natriuresis, which is caused by release of atrial (cardiac) natriuretic factor. SIADH differs, in that it results in dilutional hyponatremia. The exact mechanism by which CSW occurs remains unclear. This sodium loss results in decreased plasma volume, increased concentration of nitrogen (in the form of urea) in the blood, and a negative salt balance. Treatment of this condition involves first distinguishing it from SIADH. Fluid and sodium replacement therapies are then initiated, along with ongoing monitoring of serum sodium levels. Table 7.13 lists laboratory values associated with CSW.

## Postoperative Nursing Care and Complications

Surgical interventions for pediatric head trauma have been discussed earlier in this chapter, and include placement of an ICP monitor and EVD, elevation of depressed skull fractures, evacuation of hematomas, and decompressive craniectomy. Postoperative nursing care following neurosurgery includes observation of the vital signs, baseline and frequent ongoing neurologic assessments, monitoring for postoperative complications, and good general postoperative care to include pain management, prevention of infection, nutritional status, and psychosocial support of the child and family [25].

## Preoperative Baseline

The preoperative assessment is a good baseline for comparison when assessing for postoperative deterioration or complications. For consistency, it is ideal for the same nurse to care for the child before and after neurosurgery. When this is not possible, the nurse assuming care should seek knowledge of the preoperative assessment from the previous caregiver, surgeon, anesthesiologist, postanesthesia care unit nurse, the medical record, and the parents, in order to recognize and anticipate changes in the child's postoperative neurologic assessment.

## Assuming Postoperative Nursing Care

Report of the operation should include location and type of neurosurgical procedure, intraoperative complications, anesthetic and analgesic agents used, fluid/electrolyte status, intraoperative laboratory values, and the postoperative physician's orders. Appropriate monitoring equipment should be attached and may include any or all of the following: cardiorespiratory monitor, mechanical ventilation, pulse oximetry, end-tidal carbon dioxide, arterial line, central venous line, ICP monitor, EVD, $S_{jv}O_2$, and $P_{bt}O_2$ monitoring.

## Vital Functions

Vital signs should be recorded frequently, according to your institution's policy. Normothermia should be maintained as infants can become cold-stressed very quickly. Fever should be avoided as it increases cerebral metabolic demand. Postoperative tachycardia is expected secondary to the stress response, but can also indicate anemia, hypovolemia, cardiorespiratory distress, fever, or pain. Bradycardia is very concerning in the child and may indicate increased ICP or hypoxemia, which requires immediate evaluation and treatment. The nurse should maintain euvolemia by calculating the intake and output totals from surgery, alerting the physician of indications of hypovolemia, hypotension, poor perfusion, and decreased urine output ($<1$ $cm^3$/kg/h). Administration of fluid boluses and vasopressors may be necessary to prevent hypotension, which is a known cause of secondary brain injury and ischemia, resulting in further increased ICP and poor outcome. Cushing's response is a late

ominous sign of impending cerebral herniation and includes: hypertension, bradycardia, and apnea [25].

Protection of the pediatric airway following neurosurgery is paramount, whether the child is extubated immediately following neurosurgery or remains intubated and on mechanical ventilation. The nurse should monitor for signs of respiratory distress, and assist with bag-valve-mask breathing and reintubation if required. Possible causes of airway or ventilatory deterioration include tube displacement, tube obstruction, pneumothorax, and equipment failure [25]. Inadequate ventilation results in hypoxia and hypercarbia, which cause increased CBF, ischemia, and increased ICP.

## Neurologic Function

A full discussion of neurologic assessment and management of increased ICP precedes this section. The general neurologic assessment includes assessment of LOC and responsiveness (GCS), pupillary and CN assessment, and the motor exam. For the purpose of this section the discussion of the postoperative neurologic assessment will focus on the operative region, supratentorial versus infratentorial, and potential complications.

Complications related to supratentorial neurosurgery include hemorrhage, cerebral edema, and cerebral ischemia secondary to increased ICP. Clinical indications of supratentorial complications include symptoms of increased ICP (headache, nausea, vomiting, decreasing LOC), signs of rostral-caudal deterioration, focal motor deficits, and seizures. Complications following infratentorial neurosurgery are acute hydrocephalus, bleeding or clot formation, cerebral edema or swelling, and ischemia. Clinical indications of infratentorial (below the tentorium) neurosurgical complication include headache, bradycardia, hypertension, and abrupt loss of consciousness [22,25].

## General Postoperative Nursing Care

Good general postoperative care includes pain management, prevention of infection, nutritional status, and psychosocial support of the child and family. Multiple scales exist for assessment of pediatric pain (see Chap. 1). One such scale should be used consistently to assess pain in the postoperative neurosurgery patient. Pain physiologically increases ICP and should be adequately controlled with administration of analgesics in the postoperative period. It is important to note that administration of narcotics will decrease the patient's LOC and responsiveness, interfering with performance of the neurologic assessment.

The surgical site should be evaluated for presence of bleeding, dehiscence, wound infection, and CSF leak, all of which should be reported to the neurosurgeon. Enteral nutrition should be started as early as possible, to promote wound healing.

The conscious child should be prepared for the operative experience in a developmentally appropriate manner. Reassure the child that they will remain asleep and unable to feel pain during surgery, and awaken afterwards to see their parents. Educate them that pain is expected and that medications will be available to alleviate their pain. Advise them to anticipate a large number of people and equipment to help take the best care of them when they awaken. Parents need to be prepared for the appearance of the child postoperatively with a head turban dressing, ICP/EVD monitor, multiple intravenous lines, monitors, and possible endotracheal tube and ventilator [25].

## Postoperative Complications

Postoperative deterioration, including worsening neurologic status compared to preoperative assessment, requires emergency evaluation, with repeat CT scan and treatment as indicated [22]. Worsening neurologic assessment in the postoperative period warrants repeat imaging with CT scan to rule out hematoma formation, worsening cerebral edema, and acute hydrocephalus

### Intracranial Hypertension

Increased ICP can develop or become worse during neurosurgery or in the postoperative period. ICP and calculated CPP values must be monitored and recorded, with deterioration reported to the physician immediately. CSF can be drained via the EVD and ICP monitor, either intermittently or continuously, as ordered, to therapeutically lower ICP. See the previous section for full discussion of the pathophysiology, assessment, and management of increased ICP.

### Seizure

The incidence of seizures following TBI in children is 10% and can occur during or following neurosurgery. Seizure activity increases cerebral metabolic demand and must therefore be prevented or treated immediately. Prophylactic administration of antiepileptic medications is controversial (see section on posttraumatic seizures). Management of postoperative seizures must include intubation if the child is unconscious or unable to protect their airway. An immediate CT scan should be done to rule out postoperative development of a hematoma [22]. Administration of anticonvulsants following severe head trauma or craniotomy may be indicated for as long as 6 months. Seizure should be considered as a potential cause of increasing or refractory ICP in the unconscious patient if it is associated with pupil dilation and tachycardia or bradycardia [25].

### Complications After Posterior Fossa Craniotomy

Postoperative complications after posterior fossa, or infratentorial craniotomy deserve further discussion. Complications include respiratory arrest, hypertension, posterior fossa edema or hemorrhage, and CSF fistula. The first indication of posterior fossa complications is often respiratory arrest, prompting many neurosurgeons to delay extubation in the postoperative period for 24–48 h [22]. Hypertension after posterior fossa craniotomy can cause hemorrhage from tenuous vessels, and precipitates the postoperative use of antihypertensives. The child's blood pressure should be monitored closely, with any sudden increases reported to the neurosurgeon immediately.

The posterior fossa is a physically small compartment that contains important structures such as the cerebellum and the brainstem. A small amount of mass effect from edema or postoperative hematoma can be rapidly fatal, secondary to brainstem compression. Increased pressure in the posterior fossa can cause obstruction of the outlet of the fourth ventricle, resulting in acute hydrocephalus. Increased pressure in the posterior fossa is associated with rapid change is respiratory pattern and hypertension. Pupillary reflexes, LOC, and ICP are not affected until late. An immediate reoperation is indicated to prevent cerebral herniation, and is often not delayed to obtain neuroimaging or transport the patient to the operating room [22].

CSF fistula occurs in 5–17% of posterior fossa craniotomies and is evidenced by a persistent leak of clear fluid from the wound, the nose (rhinorrhea), or the ear (otorrhea). Most CSF leaks resolve spontaneously within a few days with the head of the bed elevated and lumbar drainage. CSF leak is a potential source for infection or meningitis. Prophylactic treatment with antibiotics is controversial, with most surgeons agreeing that it does not prevent meningitis, and selects out more potent organisms. Surgical correction of a persistent CSF leak is rare [22].

## Outcomes

Outcomes for children with TBI can be difficult to predict. Children tend to have better outcomes, especially as compared to adults, except that outcomes are far worse for children under the age of 2 years [49,51]. Children with more severe injuries have higher mortality rates. Other factors associated with increased mortality include arriving at the hospital comatose and remaining in that state for at least 6 h [51]. It is also known that the presence of hypotension and the number of hypotensive episodes have an effect on outcome [39,41,67]. Additionally, in one study, the inability to maintain CPP ≥50 mmHg during the first 24 h after injury and the presence of bradycardia in the emergency room were factors associated with mortality [23]. Finally, the child who experiences brain ischemia and hypoperfusion is more likely to have a poor outcome [40].

It has been reported that over 40% of traumatically injured children experience some level of impairment in functional status postinjury [60]. Children with TBI tend to have more impairment. Because of this, rehabilitation must begin early in the recovery period, ideally in the intensive care unit. An interdisciplinary team that includes the child's family is necessary to coordinate treatment. Physical, occupational, and speech therapists should participate in the child's care as soon as possible. Families will need anticipatory guidance about potential impairments and disabilities their child may experience, as well as about behaviors the child may display. They will also need to develop strategies to advocate for their child's maximal recovery and ongoing needs. Because the child's brain is still developing, it is difficult to predict final functional outcome. Children may experience neurocognitive delays or may never reach milestones related to visual-motor abilities, language, cognition, intelligence and school achievement, and behavior [54]. A structured rehabilitation program will provide the child with the best opportunity to meet his or her potential following a TBI.

## Prevention Efforts

Major prevention efforts have included reduced speed limits, seatbelt laws to include a lap and shoulder harness, proper use of child safety seats, and use of safety helmets for bicycling and other activities on wheels. Many local communities and states are passing mandatory bike helmet laws. The difficulty for law enforcement officials becomes how to enforce the law and what if any penalty or reward should be placed on the minor and their guardian. Nurses should take an active interest in lobbying legislators to continue head trauma prevention efforts, and encourage parents to use seatbelts and other safety devices.

### Pediatric Practice Pearls

- Due to their developmental age, young children are more difficult to assess than older children and adults. Young children may have significant intracranial injury with little external evidence, secondary to the more flexible pediatric skull.
- Accidental head injury is uncommon under the age of 2 years. In the face of inadequate mechanism of injury, or a change in the explanation of injury, assess for inflicted injury.
- Establish baseline neurological assessment and communicate clearly and objectively at change of shift. Report any and all changes/deteriorations to the physician immediately.
- Minimal stimulation must not prevent a good assessment and intervention when necessary; base interventions on patient's response, ICP value, and waveform.
- When evaluating a child for causes of increased ICP, assure that the head of the bed is elevated 30° with the head midline, that adequate sedation and analgesia are provided as ordered, and that the ventilator and EVD/ICP monitor are functioning appropriately, prior to calling the physician.

## References

1. Adelson PD, Clyde B, Kochanek PM, Wisniewski SR, Marion DW, Yonas H (1997) Cerebrovascular response in infants and young children following severe traumatic brain injury: a preliminary report. Pediatr Neurosurg 26:200–207

2. Adelson PD, Bratton SL, Carney NA, Chestnut RM, Coudrey HE, Goldstein B, et al (2003) Guidelines for the acute medical management of severe traumatic brain injury in infants, children, and adolescents. Pediatr Crit Care Med 31:S488–491

3. American Heart Association (2002) Pediatric Advanced Life Support. American Heart Association, Dallas

4. Andrews BT, Hammer GB (1997) The neurological examination and neurological monitoring in pediatric intensive care. In: Andrews BT, Hammer GB (eds) Pediatric neurosurgical intensive care. The American Association of Neurological Surgeons, Park Ridge, IL, pp 1–11

5. Barkovich AJ (2000) Pediatric neuroimaging (3rd edn). Lippincott, Philadelphia

6. Barkovich AJ (2005) Pediatric neuroimaging (4th ed). Lippincott, Philadelphia

7. Barlow KM, Thomson E, Johnson D, Minns RA (2001) Late neurologic and cognitive sequelae of inflicted traumatic brain injury in infancy. Pediatrics 116:174–185

8. Bayir H, Kochanek PM, Clar RSB (2003) Traumatic brain injury in infants and children: Mechanisms of secondary damage and treatment in the intensive care. Crit Care Clin 19:529–549

9. Berger RP, Dulani T, Adelson PD, Leventhal JM, Richichi R, Kochanek PM (2006) Indentification of inflicted traumatic brain injury in well-appearing infants using serum and cerebrospinal markers: a possible screening tool. Pediatrics 117:325–332

10. Bernard SA, Buist M (2003) Induced hypothermia in critical care medicine: a review. Crit Care Med 31:2041–2051

11. Biswas AK, Bruce DA, Sklar FH, Bokovoy JL, Sommerauer JF (2002) Treatment of acute traumatic brain injury in children with moderate hypothermia improves intracranial hypertension. Crit Care Med 30:2742–2751

12. Blackburn ST (2003) Assessment and management of the neurologic system. In: Kenner C, Lott JW (eds) Comprehensive neonatal nursing: a physiologic perspective (3rd edn). Saunders, Philadelphia, pp 650–651

13. Caffey J (1974) The whiplash shaken infant syndrome: manual shaking by the extremities with whiplash-induced intracranial and intraocular bleedings, linked with residual permanent brain damage and mental retardation. Pediatrics 54:396–403

14. Carney NA, Chesnut R, Kochanek PM et al. (2003) Guidelines for the acute medical management of severe traumatic brain injury in infants, children, and adolescents. Pediatr Crit Care Med 4:S1–S75

15. Cobbs-Ewing L, Kramer L, Prasad M, Canales DN, Louis PT, Fletcher JM, Vollero H, Landry SH, Cheung K (1998) Neuroimaging, physical, and developmental finding after inflicted and noninflicted traumatic brain injury in young children. Pediatrics 102:300–307

16. Cochran A, Scaife E, Hansen KW, Downey ED (2003) Hyperglycemia and outcome from pediatric traumatic brain injury. J Trauma 55:1035–1038

17. Curley MAQ, Quigley SM, Lin M (2003) Pressure ulcers in pediatric intensive care: incidence and associated factors. Pediatr Crit Care Med 4:284–290

18. Davis JD (2001) Neonatal subgaleal hemorrhage: diagnosis and management. CMAJ 164:1452–1453

19. Dias MS (2004) Traumatic brain and spinal cord injury. Pediatr Clin N Am 51:271–303

20. Duhaime AC (1999) Closed head injury without fractures. In: Albright AL, Pollack IF, Adelson PD (eds) Principles and Practice of Pediatric Neurosurgery. Thieme, New York, pp 799–811

21. Fisher B, Thomas, D, Peterson B (1992) Hypertonic saline lowers raised ICP in children after head injury. J Neurosurg Anesthesiol 4:4–10

22. Greenberg, MS (2001) Handbook of Neurosurgery (5th edn). Thieme, New York

23. Hackbarth RM, Rzeszutko KM, Sturm G, Donders J, Kuldanek AS, Sanfilippo DJ (2002) Survival and functional outcome in pediatric traumatic brain injury: a retrospective review and analysis of predictive factors. Crit Care Med 30:1630–1635

24. Haitsma IS, Mass AIR (2002) Advanced monitoring in the intensive care unit: brain tissue oxygen tension. Curr Opin Crit Care 8:115–120

25. Hazinski MF (1999) Manual of Pediatric Critical Care. Mosby, St Louis

26. Hendrickson SL (1987) Intracranial pressure changes and family presence. J Neurosci Nurs 19:14–17

27. Henker R, Brown S, Marion D (1998) Comparison of brain temperature with bladder and rectal temperatures in adults with severe head injury. Neurosurgery 42:1071–1075

28. Hernandez PW, Hernandez JA (1999) Physical assessment of the newborn. In: Thureen PJ, Deacon J, O'Neill P, Hernandez JA (eds) Assessment and Care of the Well Newborn. Saunders, Philadelphia, pp 114–162

29. Hettler J, Greenes DS (2003) Can the initial history predict whether a child with a head injury has been abused? Pediatrics 111:602–607

30. Hickey JV (2003) The Clinical Practice of Neurological and Neurosurgical Nursing (5th edn). Lippincott, Philadelphia

31. Hinton-Bayre AD, Geffen G (2002) Severity of sports-related concussion and neuropsychological test performance. Neurology 59:1068–1070

32. Holmes JF, Palchak MJ, Conklin MJ, Kuppermann N (2004) Do children require hospitalization after immediate posttraumatic seizures? Ann Emerg Med 43:786–790

33. Horan MJ (1987) Report of the Second Task Force on Blood Pressure Control in Children – 1987. Task Force on Blood Pressure Control in Children. National Heart, Lung, and Blood Institute, Bethesda, Maryland. Pediatrics 79:1

34. Jarvis C (1996) Pocket Companion for Physical Examination and Health Assessment (2nd edn). Saunders, Philadelphia

35. Jenny C, Hymel KP, Ritzen A, et al (1999) Analysis of missed cases of abusive head trauma. JAMA 281:621–626

36. Kelly JP, Rosenberg JH (1997) The diagnosis and management of concussion in sports American Academy of Neurology practice parameter. Neurology 48:575–585

37. Kennedy CS, Moffatt M (2004) Acute traumatic brain injury in children: exploring the cutting edge in understanding, therapy, and research. Clin Pediatr Emerg Med 5:224–238

38. Khanna S, Davis D, Peterson B, Fisher B, Fung H, O'Quigley J, et al (2000) Use of hypertonic saline in the treatment of severe refractory post traumatic intracranial hypertension in pediatric traumatic brain injury. Crit Care Med 28:1144–1150

39. Klauber MR, Marshall LF, Luerssen TG, Frankowski R, Tabaddor K, Eisenberg M (1989) Determinants of head injury mortality: importance of the low risk patient. Neurosurgery 24:31–36

40. Kochanek PM, Clark RS, Ruppel RA, Adelson PD, Bell MJ, Whalen MJ, et al (2000) Biochemical, cellular, and molecular mechanisms in the evolution of secondary damage after severe TBI in infants and children: lessons learned from the bedside. Pediatr Crit Care Med 1:4–19

41. Kokoska ER, Smith GS, Pittman T, Weber TR (1998) Early hypotension worsens neurological outcome in pediatric patients with moderately severe head trauma. J Pediatr Surg 33:333–338

42. Lam AM, Winn HR, Cullen BF, Sundling N (1991) Hyperglycemia and neurological outcome in patients with head injury. J Neurosurg 75:545–551

43. Leker RR, McKay RDG (2004) Using endogenous neural stem cells to enhance recovery from ischemic brain injury. Curr Neurovasc Res 5:421–427

44. Levy DI, Rekate HL, Cherny WB, Manwaring K, Moss SD, Baldwin HZ (1995) Controlled lumbar drainage in pediatric head injury. J Neurosurg 83:453–460

45. Littlejohns LR, Bader MK, March K (2003) Brain tissue oxygen monitoring in severe brain injury: research and usefulness in critical care. Crit Care Nurs 23:17–25

46. Luerrsen TG (1999). Skull fractures after closed head injury. In: Albright AL, Pollack IF, Adelson PD (eds) Principles and Practice of Pediatric Neurosurgery. Thieme, New York, pp 813–829

47. Luerrsen TG (2001) Acute traumatic cerebral injury. In: McLone DG, Marlin AE, Scott R, Steinbok P, Reigel DH, Walker ML, Cheek WR (eds) Pediatric Neurosurgery (4th edn). Saunders, Philadelphia, pp 601–619

48. Luerssen TG, Wolfla CE (1997) Pathophysiology and management of increased intracranial pressure in children. In: Andrews BT, Hammer GB (Eds) Pediatric Neurosurgical Intensive Care. American Association of Neurological Surgeons, Park Ridge, IL, pp 37–56

49. Luerssen TG, Klauber MR, Marshall LF (1988) Outcome from head injury related to patient's age. A longitudinal prospective study of adult and pediatric head injury. J Neurosurg 68:409–416

50. Lynam L, Verklan MT (2004) Neurological disorders. In: Verklan MT, Walden M (eds) Core curriculum for neonatal intensive care nursing (3rd edn). Saunders, Philadelphia

51. Mamelak AN, Pitts LH, Damron S (1996) Predicting survival from head trauma 24 hours after injury: a practical method with therapeutic implications. J Trauma Injury Infect Crit Care 41:91–99

52. Marcoux KK (2005) Management of increased intracranial pressure in the critically ill child with an acute neurological injury. AACN Clin Issues 16:212–231

53. Marion DW, Penrod LE, Kelsey SF, Obrist WD, Kochanek PM, Palmer AM, et al (1997) Treatment of traumatic brain injury with moderate hypothermia. New Engl J Med 336:540–546

54. Massagli TL, Jaffe KM (1994) Pediatric traumatic brain injury: prognosis and rehabilitation. Pediatr Ann 23:29–36

55. Maugans TA, McComb JG, Levy ML (1999) Penetrating craniocerebral injuries. In: Albright AL, Pollack IF, Adelson PD (eds) Principles and Practice of Pediatric Neurosurgery. Thieme, New York, pp 831–847

56. McCrory P, Johnston K, Meeuwisse W, Aubry M, Cantu R, Dvorak J, et al (2005) Summary and agreement statement of the second International Conference on Concussion in Sport, Prague 2004. Clin J Sport Med 15:48–55

57. Miller BF, Keane CB (1987) Encyclopedia and Dictionary of Medicine, Nursing, and Allied Health (4th edn). Saunders, Philadelphia

58. Mitchell PH, Habermann-Little B, Johnson F, VanInwegen-Scott D, Tyler D (1985) Critically ill children: the importance of touch in a high-technology environment. Nurs Admin Q 9:38–46

59. Moe P, Paige PL (1998) Neurologic disorders. In: Merenstein G, Gardner S (eds) Handbook of Neonatal Intensive Care (4th edn). Mosby, St Louis,

60. National Pediatric Trauma Registry Biannual Report (1999) Tufts University School of Medicine. New England Medical Center, Boston

61. Negishi H, Lee Y, Itoh K, Suzuki J, Nishino M, Takada S, Yamasaki S (1989) Neurosurgical management of epidural hematoma in neonates. Pediatr Neurol 5:253–256

62. Parker RS (2001) Concussive Brain Trauma – Neurobehavioral Impairment and Maladaptation. CRC Press, Boca Raton, Florida, pp 99–115

63. Patten J (1980) Neurological Differential Diagnosis. Springer-Verlag, New York

64. Pediatric Exclusivity Labeling Changes (2005, July 7) Retrieved August 23, 2005 from http://www.fda.gov/cder/pediatric/labelchange.htm

65. Peterson B, Khanna S, Fischer B, Marshall L (2000) Prolonged hypernatremia controls elevated ICP in head-injured pediatric patients. Crit Care Med 28:1136–1143

66. Phillips R, Ott L, Young B, Walsh J (1987) Nutritional support and measured energy expenditure of the child and adolescent with head injury. J Neurosurg 67:846–851

67. Piqula FA, Wald SL, Shackford SR, Vane DW (1993) The effect of hypotension and hypoxia on children with severe head injuries. J Pediatr Surg 28:310–316

68. Plum F, Posner JB (1982) The Diagnosis of Stupor and Coma (3rd edn). FA Davis, Philadelphia

69. Polderman KH, Joe RTT, Peerdeman SM, Vandertop WP, Girbes ARJ (2002) Effects of therapeutic hypothermia on intracranial pressure and outcome in patients with severe head injury. Intens Care Med 28:1563–1573

70. Potoka DA, Schall LC, Gardner MJ, Stafford PW, Peitzman AB, Ford HR (2000) Impact of pediatric trauma centers on mortality in a statewide system. J Trauma 49:237–245

71. Ritter AM, Ward JD (1999). Mass lesions after head injury in the pediatric population. In: Albright AL, Pollack IF, Adelson PD (eds) Principles and Practice of Pediatric Neurosurgery. Thieme, New York, pp 849–859

72. Rovlias A, Kotsou S (2000) The influence of hyperglycemia on neurological outcome in patients with severe head injury. Neurosurgery 46:335–343

73. Sansoucie DA, Cavaliere TA (2003) Newborn and infant assessment. In: Kenner C, Lott JW (eds) Comprehensive Neonatal Nursing: a Physiologic Perspective (3rd edn). Saunders, Philadelphia, pp 650–651

74. Shaver E, Duhaime AC, Curtis M, Gennarelli LM, Barrett R (1996) Experimental acute subdural hematoma in infant piglets. Pediatr Neurosurg 25:123–129

75. Shiozaki T, Hayakata T, Taneda M, Nakajima Y, Haskiguchi N, Fujimi S, et al (2001) A multi-center prospective randomized trial of the efficacy of mild hypothermia for severely head injured patients with low intracranial pressure. J Neurosurg 94:50–54

76. Shipley C (2006) Traumatic brain injury. Retrieved: March 25, 2006, www.trialimage.com

77. Simma B, Burger R, Falk M, Sacher P, Fanconi S (1998) A prospective randomized, and controlled study of fluid management in children with severe head injury: lactated ringer's solution versus hypertonic saline. Crit Care Med 26:1265–1270

78. Skippen P, Seear M, Poskitt K, Kestle J, Cochrane D, Annich G, et al (1997) Effect of hyperventilation on regional cerebral blood flow in head-injured children. Crit Care Med 25:1275–1278

79. Society for Neuroscience (2005) Traumatic brain injury and transplants. Retrieved from the Internet March 31, 2006, www.apu.sfn.org

80. Tatsumi K, Haga S, Matsuyoshi H, Inoue M, Manabe T, Makinodan M, Wanaka A (2005) Characterization of cells with proliferative activity after brain injury. Neurochem Int 46:381–389

81. Towbin A (1998) Brain Damage in the Newborn and its Neurologic Sequels. PRM Publishing, Danvers, MA

82. U.S. Department of Health and Human Services: Administration for Children, Youth and Families, Child Maltreatment (2003) (Washington, DC, U.S. Government Printing Office, 2005). Retrieved March 2006, http://www.acf.hhs.gov/programs/cb/publications/

83. Vagnozzi R, Signoretti S, Tavazzi B, Cimatti M, Amorini AM, Donzelli R, Delfini R, Lazzarino G (2005) Hypothesis of the postconcussive vulnerable brain: experimental evidence of its metabolic occurrence. Neurosurgery 57:164–171

84. Valadka AB, Gopinath SP, Contant CF, Uzura M, Robinson CS (1998) Relationship of brain tissue PO2 to outcome after severe head injury. Crit Care Med 26:1576–1581

85. Vavilala MS, Lee LA, Boddu K, Visco E, Newell DW, Zimmerman JJ, Lam AM (2004) Cerebral autoregulation in pediatric traumatic brain injury. Pediatr Crit Care Med 5:257–263

86. Vinchon M, Dhellemmes SD, Desurmont M, Dhellemmes P (2005) Accidental and nonaccidental head injuries in infants: a prospective study. J Neurosurg Pediatr 102:380–384

87. Volpe JJ (2001) Neurology of the Newborn (4th edn). Saunders, Philadelphia

88. Wilson-Pauwels L, Akesson EJ, Stewart PA, Spacey SD (2002) Cranial Nerves in Health and Disease (2nd edn). BC Decker, Hamilton, Ontario

89. Young G, Ott L, Dempsey R, Haack D, Tibbs P (1989) Relationship between admission hyperglycemia and neurologic outcome of severely brain injured patients. Ann Surg 210:466–473

90. Young PA, Young PH (1997) Basic Clinical Neuroanatomy. Lippincott, Baltimore

# Spine

**8**

*Laurie Baker, Suzan R. Miller-Hoover,*
*Donna C. Wallace, and Sherry Kahn*

## Contents

## The Pediatric Spinal Column

The immature pediatric spinal column has unique features that increase the spinal cord's susceptibility to injury without obvious evidence of abnormality in alignment or bony integrity. The pediatric spine does not reach adult characteristics until after the age of 8 years and may not reach full maturity until age 16–18 years [8, 21]. The anatomic features of the immature pediatric cervical spine increase the mobility of the spinal column, causing it to be hypermobile and susceptible to flexion and extension type injuries. The vertebral bodies are wedge-shaped, allowing for slippage of the vertebral bodies anteriorly during flexion. The facet joints are much more horizontally oriented in the pediatric spine in comparison to the adult spine. This again allows for translation of the vertebral bodies as the spine is flexed forward or extended back. The uncinate processes, which serve to limit spinal mobility, particularly with lateral and rotational movements, are flat in the pediatric spine rather than projecting upward and outward, articulating with the vertebral level above as they do in the adult spine. In addition, the interspinous ligaments are quite elastic in the pediatric population and the paraspinous musculature is undeveloped. Both of these factors allow hypermobility of the pediatric spine, thereby increasing the stress on the spinal cord itself [12, 36, 48]. The disproportionate size of the infant head also contributes to the risk of spinal cord injury in the young child. The large head is not well supported because the neck muscles are not adequately developed and lack the ability to support the head and neck. This puts the child at risk for flexion- and extension-type injuries [21, 32, 34, 49, 56].

# Traumatic Spinal Cord Injuries

## Etiology

Spinal cord injuries (SCIs) are rarely found in children [41]; however, because the patient may be treated by neurosurgeons or orthopedic surgeons, the statistics vary on the number and types of injuries. While neurosurgeons more often treat injuries of the cervical spine and orthopedic surgeons usually treat injuries of the lower spine, their practices often overlap. This explains why the statistics for each injury or age population vary. While it is important that the SCI statistics be reviewed, the caregiver must be cognizant of these differences and what they may mean to the patient population being studied. Neurosurgeons note that 42% of pediatric SCIs are in the cervical region, 31% are in the thoracic region, 23% are in the thoracolumbar region, and 27% occur in the lumbar region (L2–S1) [25].

Accidental SCIs are the fourth leading cause of death in the country in all age groups [66]. These injuries are found predominantly in males in their late teens and early twenties. However, in children under the age of 5 years, the incidence in females equals that in males. Before puberty, the unique physical and developmental characteristics of children predisposes them to SCI from lap-belt injuries, injuries related to birth, child abuse, delayed onset of neurologic deficits, and high cervical injuries [66]. Approximately 29% of all patients in all age groups with SCI die prior to reaching the hospital. Of the children with SCI who reach the hospital, survival is determined by the severity of the neurologic injury. The severity of SCI is a function of age and the mechanism of injury. Children of 12 years and younger are more likely to have complete injuries resulting in paraplegia than the older teen. One-half the injured adolescents are expected to have paraplegia and the other half complete injuries, such as tetraplegia. Adolescents who have tetraplegia are usually injured at the C5–C8 level [66]. Quality of life and ability to function in society may be severely affected, especially in those patients who suffer cervical spine (C-spine) injuries. The cost of treating traumatic spinal cord injuries in the pediatric patient is estimated to be $5.6 billion per year [43].

# Injury Classifications

## Spinal Cord Injury Without Radiographic Abnormality

SCI without radiographic abnormality (SCIWORA) is a syndrome of traumatic SCI without evidence of bony injury such as fracture or dislocation on plain radiographs, computerized tomography (CT) or myelogram [18]. This phenomenon was first described before the advent of magnetic resonance imaging (MRI) in older patients with significant spondylitic changes of the spine resulting in a narrowed central spinal canal. In this population, a hyperextension-type injury often resulted in an acute central cord syndrome without evidence of spinal fracture or dislocation. It is rare to see SCI without bony abnormality in patients older than 16 years because of the anatomic and biomechanical differences of the spinal column [48]. MRI imaging has demonstrated that even though there may not be evidence of bony injury, there may or may not be evidence of soft tissue injury such as ligamentous injury or injury to the spinal cord itself.

SCIWORA is most commonly seen in the cervical spine region but it has also been documented in other areas of the spine [13]. Traumatic events such as the application of traction to the neonatal spinal column during delivery, child abuse, falls, sports injuries, or motor vehicle accidents may result in this SCI [9, 48]. This injury may occur when the spinal column deforms elastically when excessive traction is applied to the spinal column, stretching it beyond its limits. The spinal column returns to its normal anatomic alignment without bony injury but with evidence of SCI. The elasticity of the ligaments of the pediatric spine contributes to this laxity of the spinal column. Studies have shown that the infantile spine can be stretched up to two inches before the integrity of the ligaments and spinal column is disrupted. The spinal cord, however, is not so elastic and can sustain damage or even rupture after only a few millimeters of stretch [8, 18, 34]. Another injury that may occur without bony injury due to the elasticity of the spinal column is a concussive injury resulting from a transmission of kinetic energy or concussive force applied to the spine [8, 18].

### Symptomology

SCIWORA usually presents with symptoms immediately; however, symptoms may be delayed for up to 4 days following the initial injury [21]. Patients who experience delayed onset of SCIWORA have usually noted transient symptoms at the time of injury. These symptoms include parasthesias, numbness, or a subjective feeling of weakness [18, 34, 48, 49]. This may then be followed by a period of time where the child appears to be normal but then develops overt signs of SCI, which could progress quite rapidly to complete paralysis. This latent period between time of initial injury and the development of signs of neurological dysfunction is thought to be due to repetitive injury to the spinal cord as a result of occult instability [21]. Recurrent SCIWORA has been documented in cases where stabilization or recovery of the injury has occurred. The child sustains a second injury often due to a low energy mechanism and then redevelops neurological deficits. This seems to occur most often in older children [8].

### Prognosis

The prognosis for recovery following a SCIWORA injury is dependant on the severity of injury at the time of presentation. Incomplete injuries have the best prognosis for a good recovery, whereas complete injuries have the worst prognosis [8, 21]. The patterns of SCI in SCIWORA are similar to those with associated bony injury.

### C-Spine Injuries

In children, C-spine injuries occurring in the upper C-spine account for more than 60% of all spinal injuries [25, 65]. C-spine injuries may be caused by motorcycle crashes, pedestrian accidents, sports activities, bicycle accidents, falls, and motor vehicle accidents. It is estimated that 25–50% of all SCIs have a related severe head injury [65]. Whenever a head injury is suspected, both prehospital and hospital personnel should have a high diagnostic suspicion for C-spine injury, as the risk of C-spine injuries is 8.5 times greater with a head injury than without [17, 43]. C-spine injuries, which alter or sever the communication between the brain and sympathetic nervous sys-

tem in the cord, may lead to hypotension, bradycardia, and/or death [38]. The most common level of injury will change with the age of the child (Table 8.1). The most important intervention provided by prehospital and hospital personnel, is stabilization of the spine or C-spine precautions. Stabilization of the spine at the scene of the accident has been shown to reduce the extent of complete SCIs by 10% [17, 38].

### C-Spine Precautions

C-spine precautions (stabilization) help prevent further spinal cord and vertebral column damage as well as ensure an adequate airway, ventilation, and perfusion. Immobilization of the spine in the neutral position is the goal of this treatment. To achieve neutral positioning in children, allowances for physical differences due to age and physical maturity must be considered. For children under the age of 8 years, one must consider that the head is larger than the torso, resulting in spinal flexion when the body is positioned on a hard surface. It is recommended that for children under the age of 8 years that the torso is elevated or an occipital recess be created to achieve a more normal positioning (alignment of the auditory canal with the shoulders) for spinal stabilization. This position aligns the C-spine and avoids anterior displacement and forward flexion (Fig. 8.1). A rigid collar, a modified half-spine board, and tape were found to be the most effective method to immobilize the spine for transport. Two points of concern should be noted when initiating C-spine precautions. First, the collar should never be used alone. Secondly, the use of tape to secure the torso to the back board has been shown to reduce forced vital capacity by 41–96% (mean, 80%), thus interfering with the child's ability to breathe effectively [6, 26].

It is also important to consider how to secure a patient's airway while maintaining C-spine stabilization. The "jaw-thrust method" is used to open the airway while maintaining C-spine stabilization. This

**Table 8.1.** Age-related injuries and symptoms. Adapted from Dziurzynski et al. (2005) [20]

| Age | Level of injury | Symptoms |
|-----|-----------------|----------|
| All-age children | Occiput-C2 | Respiratory arrest, quadriplegia |
| Infants and Toddlers | C1 to C2 or C2 to C3 | Respiratory arrest, quadriplegia |
| Children 3–8 years | C3 to C5 | Respiratory arrest, quadriplegia |
| Children 9–15 years | C4 to C7 | High injuries: respiratory arrest, quadriplegia<br>Low injuries: some spontaneous respirations and some upper extremity movement may persist |

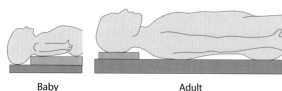

Baby                          Adult

**Fig. 8.1.** Spinal alignment. Reprinted with permission from Hadley (2002) [26]

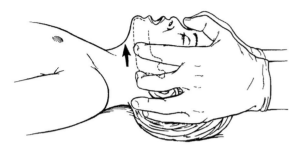

**Fig. 8.2.** Jaw thrust method, airway management. Reprinted with permission from Dziurzynski et al. (2005) [20]

technique will place the patient's head in the recommended position for simultaneous airway opening (Fig. 8.2) [6]. Another consideration is intubation versus bag-mask ventilation. Although intubation is the preferred method of airway management, not all providers are skilled in this area [6]. Children can be ventilated easily and for extended periods of time with a bag-mask, especially if a skilled provider in intubation is not readily available [53]. The decision to continue ventilating with a bag-mask versus intubation becomes a real issue with C-spine injuries where movement of the spine could have devastating results. A small randomized study by Turkstra et al. in 2005 demonstrated, with the aid of fluoroscopy, that normal patients who were positioned in C-spine stabilization demonstrated less C-spine motion during bag-mask ventilation than during intubation. This study also showed that with bag-mask ventilation there was a small amount of flexion compared with extension during intubation. Turkstra concluded "although flexion versus extension movement could be important for some types of injuries, the clinical relevance of this small flexion during ventilation is questionable compared with the magnitude of movement during laryngoscopy" [62]. These findings help support pediatric life support teaching that only providers experienced in intubation of pediatric trauma victims should perform this procedure in the field [6].

Removal of C-spine stabilization upon arrival to the trauma room or to the pediatric intensive care unit should be preceded by a thorough neurological assessment. The patient should be log-rolled off the back board utilizing a team approach. The team member at the top of the bed maintains C-spine precautions during the log-rolling procedures. The rigid collar remains in place until it is determined that a C-spine injury does not exist. According to the National Emergency X-radiography Utilization Study, there are five criteria that are useful when determining that a C-spine injury does not exist. These criteria are midline cervical tenderness, evidence of intoxication, altered level of alertness, focal neurological deficit, and a painful distracting injury. Children who exhibited none of the five of the criteria were considered at low risk for cervical injury. C-spine precautions should be removed upon a written order by the provider when a cervical injury has been ruled out. If one of the criteria was present, the child was a high risk for C-spine injury. These patients should have appropriate radiographs performed [28]. The exceptions to this are patients who have a SCIWORA.

When the radiographic examinations are negative, the patient denies pain on clinical exam and is able to rotate, flex, and extend the neck without pain, then the precautions should be removed [23]. However, if the patient continues to complain of pain or is unable to complete the exam, the precautions should remain in place and a MRI of the C-spine should be done to rule out ligamentous injury. Palpation of the bony structures should not produce pain. Patients who are unable to participate with the clinical exam should remain in precautions until they are either able to cooperate, or a CT scan and/or MRI of the C-spine should be done. It is recommended that C-spine immobilization be removed at the earliest possible time to minimize complications attributed to the hard spinal board (e.g., pressure sores). Children may be very frightened by being restrained, and allowing them to move freely when it is appropriate to do so may ease their anxiety. Ensuring appropriate stabilization of the injured C-spine, or clearing a normal C-spine, will help reduce further SCIs and comorbidities; thus shortening hospital length of stay and overall cost following a traumatic injury [23].

## Cervical Vertebrae-1 injuries

Fractures at C-l account for approximately 3–13% of all C-spine fractures [25]. There are three types of C-1 fractures, rotary subluxation, Jefferson/Atlas fracture and atlanto-occipital dislocation.

## Atlanto-Axial Rotary Subluxation

This is the most common C-spine injury found in children. This type of "fracture" usually occurs spontaneously after a minor trauma, may be associated with an upper airway infection, with rheumatoid arthritis, or without an identifiable causative event. Fielding and Hawkins (1977) identified four types based on radiological attributes (Fig. 8.3) [22]:

**Type I:** unilateral anterior rotation of the atlas pivoting around the dens with a competent transverse ligament. This is the most common type of fracture.

**Type II:** unilateral anterior rotation of the atlas pivoting around the contralateral C-1-C-2 facet. The atlanto dens interval is increased to no more than 9 mm.

**Type III:** anterior subluxation of both C-1 facets with an incompetent transverse ligament.

**Type IV:** posterior displacement of C-1 relative to C-2 with an absent or hypoplastic odontoid process.

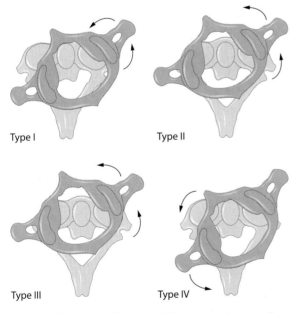

Type I        Type II

Type III        Type IV

**Fig. 8.3.** Four types of atlanto-axial rotary subluxation. Type I: unilateral anterior rotation of the atlas pivoting around the dens with a competent transverse ligament. This is the most common type of fracture. Type II: unilateral anterior rotation of the atlas pivoting around the contralateral C1–C2 facet. The atlantodens interval is increased to no more than 5 mm. Type III: anterior subluxation of both C1 facets with an incompetent transverse ligament. Type IV: posterior displacement of C1 relative to C2 with an absent or hypoplastic odontoid process. Reprinted with permission from Cleary and Wraithe (1995) [15]

## Symptoms

The patient's head is rotated to one side and tilted to the other side; this causes the "cock robin appearance." The patient cannot turn his/her head past midline and any attempts to do so are painful. The child's neurological status is almost always normal [26].

## Radiographs

Cervical spine x-rays (lateral view) may reveal a lateral mass with C-1 rotated anteriorly to the odontoid. An anteroposterior (AP) view may show a rotation of the spinous processes towards the ipsilateral side. A dynamic CT scan is far superior to a static CT scan, as rotary subluxation can be easily seen.

## Treatment

The earlier the patient presents after onset of symptoms, the easier it is to treat the symptoms. Medical treatment rather than surgical treatment is the norm if the symptoms are treated within the first 4 weeks of onset, are easily reducible, or are nonrecurrent. Many subluxations will spontaneously reduce within the 1st week; therefore, no treatment is necessary. If the patient presents late, a halo brace or Minerva cast may be used for up to 4 months. The length of immobilization should be proportionate to the length of time the symptoms were present prior to treatment (Fig. 8.4).

Surgical treatment may be used for those nonreducible or recurrent subluxations. The longer the subluxation exists before treatment, the less likely that medical treatment will be successful or maintained, as these late reductions are more likely to recur. A posterior approach atlanto-axial fusion has been used successfully to reduce recurrent or nonreducible subluxations that present for more than 3 weeks [26].

## Jefferson or Atlas fracture

A four-part burst fracture of the atlas with combined anterior and posterior arch fractures of the ring of C-1 usually resulting from a heavy object falling vertically onto the child's head (Fig. 8.5).

## Symptoms

Presenting symptoms consist of complaints of upper neck pain, although patients are usually neurologically intact. In cases of vertebral artery injury, neurologic injury can occur. This neurologic injury may manifest as Wallenberg's syndrome with ipsilateral loss of cranial nerves, Horner's syndrome (meiosis,

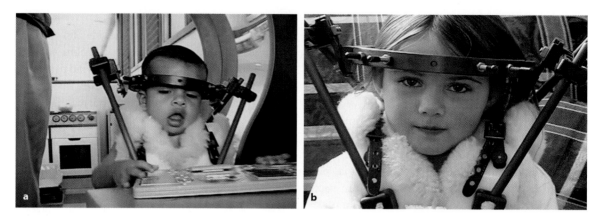

**Fig. 8.4 a, b.** Halo brace use with children (Halo Brace with compliments from PMT Corp./USA 2006)

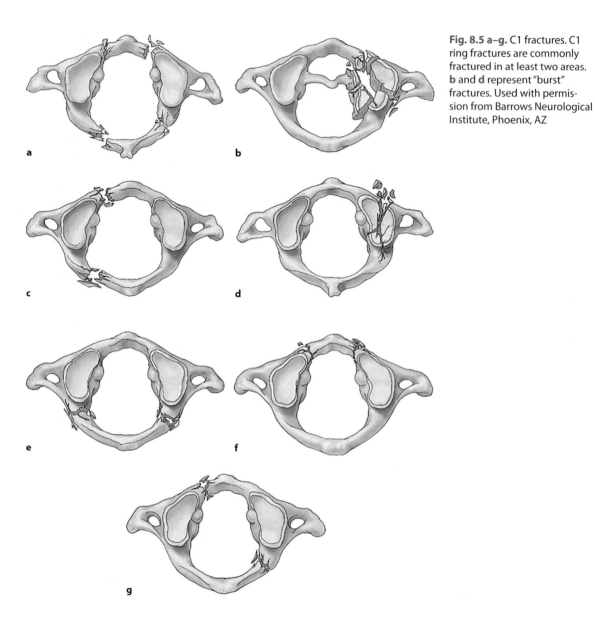

**Fig. 8.5 a–g.** C1 fractures. C1 ring fractures are commonly fractured in at least two areas. **b** and **d** represent "burst" fractures. Used with permission from Barrows Neurological Institute, Phoenix, AZ

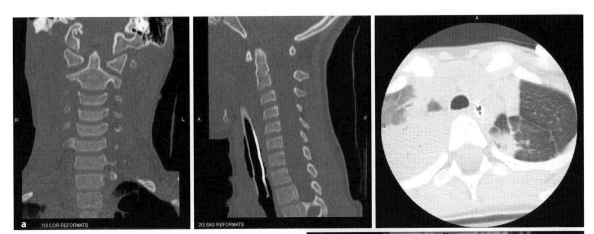

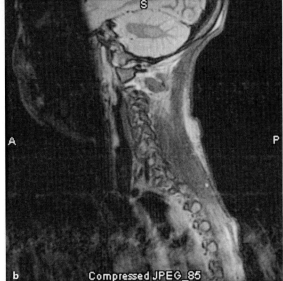

**Fig. 8.6 a, b.** Posterior atlanto-occipital dislocation fractures. Used with permission from Barrows Neurological Institute, Phoenix, AZ

anhydrosis, and ptosis), ataxia, and loss of contralateral pain and temperature sensation.

### Radiographs

An odontoid view shows overlapping of C-1 facets on C-2 facets. The lateral view shows prevertebral soft-tissue widening. Flexion and extension views are usually required to determine transverse ligament disruption. A CT scan is often helpful in delineating the exact displacement of fragments and to help diagnose transverse ligament disruption if the odontoid views are not conclusive.

### Treatment

Stable fractures with an intact transverse ligament and nondisplaced or minimally displaced fractures are usually treated in a rigid neck brace for a period of 3 months. Unstable fractures with a ruptured transverse ligament require prolonged cranial traction (up to 3 months) to reduce the lateral mass displacement. Halo braces may be applied after reduction, but care should be taken to recognize late atlantoaxial instability. Unstable fractures with a greater than 5-mm subluxation of C-1 to C-2 may require a C-1 to C-3 fusion [19].

### Atlanto-Occipital Dislocation

Atlanto-occipital dislocation (AOD) was first reported in 1908 when a 19-year-old man fell to his death. In 1948, a six-year-old child was struck by a car sustaining an AOD injury, but survived this accident with no neurological deficits. Since 1979, AOD represents 1%

of all patients with C-spine injuries who were alive at arrival to the emergency room; however, autopsy studies seem to indicate that this percentage should be 6–8% [35].

### Pathophysiology

The axial strength of the craniovertebral junction is provided by an intricate system of ligaments at the level of the superior facets of the atlas. This system is comprised of the anterior and posterior atlanto-occipital membranes and two lateral atlanto-occipital ligaments. The atlanto-occipital ligamentous structure supplies the majority of the strength at the craniocervical junction. The atlas ring is seated within a ligamentous complex joining the occiput to the axis. This complex consists of the tectorial membrane, the anterior longitudinal ligament, and the uncial ligament. Stability is also supported by the apical dental ligament and the paired alar ligament [31]. A combination of hyperextension with disruption of the tectorial membrane, and a lateral fracture or hyperflexion with disruption of the alar ligaments and posterior atlanto-occipital ligaments are thought to happen simultaneously and cause AOD to occur [65].

This dislocation of the skull from the spine was once thought to be rare and fatal; however, with the improvement in emergency field management, better initial cervical spine immobilization, rapid transport, and increased recognition, more children are surviving. It is important to consider this dislocation with any child who has suffered a head or spinal trauma. Misdiagnosis may impair neurological outcomes [25, 31, 35]. This dislocation may be more common in children due to the less stable craniovertebral junction. This is thought to occur because "the occipital condyles are relatively smaller and the articulation between the cranium and the atlas is more horizontal. This articulation becomes more deeply seated in the superior facets of the atlas as the child grows, and therefore more stable" [31]. In addition, weaker muscles and a relatively large head size, make the ligaments more prone to disruption [65].

The mechanism of this dislocation remains poorly understood. Investigators have suggested that an extreme hyperextension of the cranium on the spine leads to a rupture of the tectorial membrane, or a component of lateral flexion is necessary to disrupt the alar ligaments, or that all of the ligamentous structures must be completely disrupted between the atlantoaxial articulation for an AOD to occur. All agree that a high-energy impact with extreme deceleration is responsible for this dislocation [31].

### Classifications

Three types of AOD have been described and account for 85% of the cases. The remaining 15% consists of other types of nonclassified, rotational dislocations [65].

**Type I:** anterior dislocation with the occiput displaced ventrally to the atlas (40% of cases).

**Type II:** longitudinal dislocation (40% of cases); most unstable.

**Type III:** posterior dislocation of the occiput (5% of cases; Fig. 8.6).

### Symptoms

The initial symptoms of an AOD may be masked by other coexisting injuries. They may have a head injury, facial injuries, multiple organ injuries, or a concurrent SCI, and all will have neck pain. Cranial nerve dysfunction is commonly seen. It is often difficult to diagnosis AOD due to symptoms that often occur in patients with severe brain injuries alone. Because AOD may not always be associated with severe injuries, a high index of suspicion must be held when examining victims of a high-energy impact [31]. Any one or all of the following symptoms may be present: neck pain, loss of consciousness, cervical muscle spasms, diffuse tingling, spasticity, cognitive impairment, dermatomal sensory loss, bradycardia, hypotension, apnea, respiratory distress, spinal shock, muscle flaccidity, facial injuries, nerve palsies, hematomas, vasospasms, and neurogenic shock.

### Radiographs

Recently, there has been much discussion about which radiographic test and which cervical angle measurement techniques should be used to determine AOD. In 1999, Berne et al. demonstrated that complete cervical helical CT scans in addition to routine radiographs should be used when a C-spine injury is suspected in a patient with multiple severe injuries [7]. This study also concluded that complete cervical helical (spiral) CT scans are superior to plain radiographs. In a blinded study done by Dziurzynski et al. in 2005, five methods commonly used to diagnose AOD were compared using plain x-rays and CT scans of the C-spine [20]. The objective of the study was to determine the best method to diagnosis AOD. The conclusion of the study was that the sensitivity, specificity, positive and negative predictive values of all the methods improved when applied to CT scan because of better visualization of anatomic landmarks. Thus, CT scans of the C-spine may be warranted in all trauma patients thought to have cervical spine injuries.

AP and lateral cervical spine films can reveal fractures of the spine and possibly identify AOD, although misinterpretation of plain radiographs is common among physicians who are not used to reading films in young children. Odontoid (open mouth) views are often not efficacious in children under the age of 9 years due to the child's inability to follow instructions and hold their mouths open for an extended period of time. CT scans offer better visualization of the anatomic landmarks thus making identification of

AOD easier. MRI is sensitive in detecting ligamentous disruption and instability not readily seen on radiographs [53].

## Treatment

Treatment should be directed to airway management, adequacy of respiratory and cardiac function, stabilization of a well-aligned neck, nutritional support, skin care, and vigorous physical therapy after stabilization. C-spine stabilization is of immense importance, first by rigid collar then by the application of the halo brace. The halo brace has been found to provide the most secure method of early immobilization, but should not be used to reduce the dislocation. In some cases, redisplacement has occurred in the halo brace before osseous fusion could be attained [35, 65]. Approximately 27% of all patients treated with external stabilization alone showed neurologic worsening [65].

Urgent surgical fusion should be considered with unstable Type I and Type II dislocations [65]. Internal fixation is performed by fusing the posterior C-spine to the occiput. This fixation may result in at least a 50% reduction of flexion, extension, and rotation of the cervical spine [35].

## SCIs Other Than C-spine

SCIs consist of several classifications: spinal cord contusions, Brown Sequard syndrome, central cord syndrome, anterior cord syndrome, incomplete SCI, and complete SCI. Spinal cord contusion is the complete or incomplete transient spinal cord dysfunction which resolves in 1–2 days. A contusion results from the stretching and compression of the spinal cord, which disrupts the gray matter in the spinal cord while preserving the white matter tracks [1].

Brown Sequard Syndrome is an injury to the right or left side of the spinal cord such that movements are lost below the level of the injury on the injured side, but pain and temperature sensation are lost on the opposite side of the injury.

Incomplete SCIs often fall into one of several patterns; the most common of these are the anterior and central syndromes. Anterior cord syndrome is an injury to the motor and sensory pathways in the anterior parts of the spine. Patients are able to feel crude sensation, but movement and detailed sensation are lost in the posterior part of the spinal cord. Central cord syndrome is an injury to the center of the cervical spinal cord, producing weakness, paralysis, and sensory deficits in the arms but not the legs.

Complete SCI will produce total motor and sensory loss below the level of the injury.

## Assessment

A thorough initial neurological assessment is essential to delineate the level of injury and to obtain a baseline with which to compare subsequent assessments. These subsequent assessments will be used to determine improvement or deterioration. Assessments should include basic vital signs, Glasgow Coma Scale, motor function of all muscle groups, sensation levels, and reflexes including checking the anal sphincter for contracture. In addition, diaphragmatic function is assessed to delineate respiratory effort and efficacy. The dermatome chart should be used to assess the level of sensation. Any deterioration noted on subsequent examinations should be reported to the care provider and the appropriate treatment should begin to insure that any secondary injury is minimal [41].

## Treatment

Treatment begins at the scene of the accident with resuscitation, immobilization, and transport. The main consideration of treatment should be to maintain the patient's airway, breathing, and circulation, while decompressing the neural elements and stabilizing the spine to prevent further injury. Basic anatomical and developmental considerations such as future growth, recuperative powers of children, and difficulty in achieving adequate internal or external fixation in the young child must be a part of the treatment plan.

## External Fixation

Halo immobilization has been used successfully in patients <1 year of age and older. The halo ring has more pins (8–10) than the adult version, to distribute the pin pressure around the thinner pediatric skull. The pressure applied by the pins range from finger tight to 2 lb (where 1 lb=0.45 kg). Most of the orthoses or vests are custom made using thermoplastic compounds molded to the child and attached with straps. The neurosurgeon, orthotist, or other trained individual will most likely be the ones who tighten pins. Pin site care is carried out per institutional policy [12].

## Role of Steroids

Several studies are currently looking at the efficacy of high-dose steroids in the initial treatment of SCI. Despite early enthusiasm, much controversy exists concerning their effectiveness. It should also be noted that there were no pediatric patients included in the National Acute Spinal Cord Injury Study data and that no recommendations were made regarding pediatric patients [53]. However, to be complete, current recommendations will be included. An initial bolus of methylprednisolone 30 mg/kg followed by an infusion of 5.4 mg/kg/h should be started within 3 h of the SCI and continued for 24 h. If the treatment is begun 3–8 h after the injury, the treatment should be continued for 48 h. The Congress of Neurologic Surgeons and the American Association of Neurologic Surgeons state that "methylprednisolone for either 24 or 48 hours is recommended as an option in the treatment of patients with acute spinal cord injuries that should be undertaken only with the knowledge that the evidence suggesting harmful side effects (vital sign changes, glucose tolerance changes, and possible harm to the developing nervous system) is more consistent than any suggestion of clinical benefit" [53].

## Surgical Treatment

Injury that requires surgical treatment in the adult patient may only need immobilization in the pediatric patient. Bone and tissue thickness may have a major impact on what orthosis may be applied and what internal constructs may be possible. The vertebrae are partially cartilaginous in the young child, and it may not be possible to apply the same kind of screws or plates that would easily fit a larger patient. Spinal fusion may have a major impact on the developing spine. The spine may not grow normally and scoliosis could result. Therefore, it is important to limit the number of levels fused and to consider the effects of an isolated anterior or posterior fusion on subsequent development of excessive lordosis or kyphosis [53].

## Nursing Care

### Developmental Considerations

Nursing care of the pediatric SCI patient requires a thorough knowledge of pediatric growth and development, the complications of SCI, and implications related to the level of injury. This will alleviate unre-alistic expectations related to the child's ability to participate in the examination that may cause frustration for all. The pediatric neurosurgery nurse is mindful that small children may not be able to describe their pain or other symptoms very well depending on age, the injury, and cognitive function. A thorough history, when it is appropriate to obtain one, will describe the child's social and cognitive level. Some families may not use English as their primary language. A multidisciplinary team including the patient and family should provide comprehensive care and management. Included in this, management of SCI should be anticipatory guidance. The patient and family need to be given information about issues relating to future stages of development.

Children develop along a predictable pattern of physical, intellectual, and emotional growth; therefore, the care of children and adolescents with SCI must be dynamic, developmentally sensitive, and appropriate for each age group. Family-centered care is essential, encouraging family members to take control of the patient's care as appropriate, but also teaching parents to relinquish control of care as the patient becomes an adult. SCI patients require long-term care and an essential part of rehabilitation is appropriate patient and family education. This education must be individualized to the child's and family's needs. The SCI patient's rehabilitation plan should also include return to school.

## Secondary Medical Conditions

The secondary medical conditions that often occur with SCI may be as devastating as the underlying injury if not properly cared for. These complications include: pneumonia, neurogenic bladder or bowel, pressure ulcers, autonomic dysreflexia, spasticity, latex allergy, or deep vein thrombosis. The nurse needs to be able to care for the patient with the following conditions as well as teach the patient and family how to care for themselves.

### Neurogenic Bladder

Neurogenic bladder presents as the loss of sensation of fullness, the inability to voluntarily initiate urination, and inability to completely empty the bladder. This results in urinary retention and/or incontinence. The treatment for this is clean intermittent catheterization, which results in predictable complete emptying of the bladder and reduces the risk of urinary tract infection. Emptying the bladder is important for protecting the kidneys from refluxing of the urine upward from the full bladder. Patients should be taught how to self-catheterize as soon as they are developmentally ready. They must be able to tell the time, recognize the equipment, follow step-by-step instructions, and understand the purpose of equipment. This program can be started at 3 years of age by the parents and then taught to the patient around age 5–7 years. Because managing incontinence in a continent world is very important to children and adolescents, they should be very motivated to manage this aspect of their care themselves. Parental or parental designee supervision is necessary for school-age children, whereas adolescents may need help with problem solving. Continence is an expectation for school age children and adolescents, as dealing with the consequences of diapers can be devastating to the child and to the self-esteem of the adolescent. Continence must be achieved for the adolescent to move on to a productive and satisfying adult life, including issues of sexuality and good self-esteem.

### Neurogenic Bowel

Patients with neurogenic bowel syndrome do not feel the urge to have a bowel movement and are often unable to control them. To manage neurogenic bowel, a regular program of bowel care must be instituted. The goal of this program should be to prevent constipation, provide adequate elimination, and preserve bowel function while providing a convenient, regular, and complete emptying of the bowel. This may be as simple as placing the child on the commode at the same time every day and instructing them to bear down. However, more detailed programs are often necessary. Stool softeners, laxatives, suppositories, enemas, and digital stimulation may be needed to expedite the process. Privacy, consistency, proper seating, and regularity mixed with patience help ensure success. This program can begin at age 3 years, be supervised during the school-age period, and be proficiently performed by adolescents.

### Pressure Ulcers

Pressure ulcers add tremendous cost to already expensive medical care by causing increased hospital stays, surgical repair, and loss of school or work. If left untreated or undertreated, pressure ulcers may lead to an untimely death due to sepsis from the wound.

Good skin care is essential and begins on day one of hospitalization. Prevention is key. A person without SCI will change their position every few minutes by adjusting their weight from one side to the other; this is often done unconsciously. The patient with SCI may not be able to detect the need to shift their weight or have the ability to do so. Children and adolescents should have their positions changed every 2 h while in bed and every hour while sitting in a chair. Their skin needs to remain clean and dry, as moisture leads to skin breakdown. Good nutrition is essential to prevention of pressure ulcers. Parents and patients should be taught the signs of skin breakdown and how to treat them if they should occur.

### Autonomic Dysreflexia

This life-threatening complication of SCI is most often seen in pediatric patients with T6 or higher injuries. Autonomic dysreflexia is caused by an exaggerated response of the sympathetic nervous system to a noxious stimulus below the level of the injury. The inhibitory responses are blocked, resulting in elevation of blood pressure by 15–40 mmHg above baseline (depending on the age of the patient), pounding headache, age-defined bradycardia or tachycardia in young children, profuse sweating, piloerection, cardiac arrhythmias, flushing, blurred vision, nasal congestion, or anxiety. Infants and very young children may exhibit sleepiness or irritability [11].

The most common trigger is bladder distention; however, becoming overheated, kidney stones, urinary tract infections, bowel distention or impaction, pressure ulcers, tight clothing, burns, ingrown toe nails, deep vein thrombosis, menses, pregnancy, labor, fractures, trauma, heterotopic ossification, surgery or invasive procedures, hyperthermia, or any painful stimulus may also trigger autonomic dysreflexia. Recognition of symptoms is paramount to treating this life-threatening process. Assessing and alleviating the triggers is essential. Heart rate and blood pressure measurements should be taken every 2–5 min and antihypertensive medications should be instituted as needed. Caregiver education is essential with children and adolescents prone to this complication. A medical alert bracelet or identification card should be worn or carried at all times.

### Spasticity

Fifty percent of all children with SCI are affected by spasticity. The goals of spasticity management include: improved function, prevention of complications, and alleviation of discomfort and embarrassment. Decreased muscle atrophy and facilitation of standing are potential benefits of the child having some spasticity, and should be considered when determining the plan of care for the child or adolescent. A comprehensive program of range of motion, stretching, and positioning is essential in the management of spasticity. Relief of triggers is also an important part of the management plan. Unique to the pediatric population is hip dislocation, which may occur with spasticity. Any noxious stimulus may exacerbate spasticity.

Baclofen is the drug of choice to manage spasticity that interferes with functioning and is refractory to conservative treatment. Other drugs such as diazepam, clonidine, and tizanidine may be beneficial in spasticity management. A baclofen pump (intrathecal) is an option when other methods of management are not effective.

### Sexuality and Fertility

One of the most socially important topics to cover with SCI patients is the ability to enjoy sexual intimacy and bear children. Males may experience difficulties with erections, ejaculation, and fertility and these topics must be discussed. Why those problems occur and how they may be treated should be covered. Females usually have fewer issues; however, menstruation, lubrication, pregnancy, labor, and delivery should all be discussed. Personal hygiene surrounding incontinence is an issue for both sexes. This information should also be presented to the parent of a child with SCI, as a part of the long-term treatment plan. This will help the parents come to terms with the reality of the injury implications and help them see that there is a future for their child in terms of love, dating, marriage, and children.

### Summary

Pediatric traumatic SCIs are often difficult to diagnose due to the differences in the development of the pediatric spine, inconsistent radiographic quality, and because SCIs are relatively rare. Despite the fact that the pediatric spine offers some natural protection from SCI due to its bony and ligamentous structure compliance, SCI are often severe.

These severe injuries are likely to be due to the high magnitude of force that is necessary to disrupt the tolerance of the pediatric spine. As a result, children often have concomitant neurological injuries that complicate the recovery. Treatment does not stop when the patient leaves the hospital or the rehabilitation facility; it requires a life-long commitment from the family and patient. The cost to the family and patient is astronomical in terms of support, time, effort, and money. Because these injuries are permanent and devastating, injury prevention is paramount.

### Congenital Spinal Cord Disorders

### Spinal Manifestations of Achondroplasia

Achondroplasia is an autosomal dominant genetic disorder affecting endochondral bone formation. It is the most common form of short-limbed dwarfism. The prevalence rate is approximately 1 in 26,000 live births [67]. Achondroplasia occurs as a result of a mutation of the fibroblast growth factor receptor 7 (*FGFR7*) gene, which is involved in the growth and development of bone [5, 59]. Mutation of this gene results in abnormal chondrocyte maturation, causing stunting of bone formation at the epiphyseal plates. The bones in the face, skull base, spine, hands, feet, and proximal long bones, such as the humerus and femur, are especially affected resulting in characteristic features involving these structures [5, 52]. Hydrocephalus, upper cervical spinal cord compression, and spinal stenosis are three neurological problems seen in achondroplasts [50]. The spinal manifestations of achondroplasia will be the primary focus of this section.

### Cervicomedullary Compression

Abnormal development of the bones of the skull base results in abnormalities of the foramen magnum, posterior fossa, and brainstem. These abnormalities contribute to compression at the cervicomedullary junction. The diameter of the foramen magnum is significantly decreased in achondroplasia, leading to compression of the upper cervical spinal cord and distal medulla [54]. The foramen magnum is also displaced anteriorly, resulting in a shallow posterior fossa. As a result, the brainstem is displaced upward and posteriorly, simulating hyperextension of the neck. The compression on the upper cervical spinal cord is exacerbated further because it is often stretched over the edge of the occipital bone [29, 30].

Cervicomedullary compression resulting from foramen magnum insufficiency is usually identified in young achondroplastic patients and is a common cause of early morbidity and mortality in this patient population. It is also thought to be a contributing factor in the hypotonicity and motor developmental delay that is common among achondroplastic infants. The manifestations of this chronic neurological compression can be wide ranging. Patients may be asymptomatic initially but may develop signs and symptoms of upper spinal cord compression, including parasthesias and paresis, which can be progressive, even leading to quadriplegia. Signs of myelopathy, including hyperreflexia and clonus, may be evident even in the patient who is apparently asymptomatic. Symptoms such as spastic quadriparesis may not manifest until adulthood in patients with mild, chronic compression. Respiratory manifestations such as hypoventilation and apnea may also occur because of medullary compression. Simple extension of the neck can cause acute compression of the spinal cord at the cervicomedullary junction, which could lead to sudden death of the achondroplastic infant [29, 30, 42, 54]. The foramen magnum eventually increases in size as the child grows, easing the compression at the cervicomedullary junction [55].

Radiographic evaluation should be undertaken if there is any question of cervicomedullary compromise. A CT scan can provide detailed imaging of the bony architecture of the skull base, foramen magnum, and upper cervical spinal column. Measurements of the foramen magnum can be taken from these scans to determine the degree of stenosis. The diameter of the foramen magnum in achondroplastic infants often measures at least 3–5 standard deviations below the mean diameter for nonachondroplastic infants [30]. MRI provides information on the soft tissue structures including the brainstem and upper cervical spinal cord. Compression of these structures is evident with this study and changes within the upper cervical spinal cord can be identified, including atrophy and abnormal signal within the spinal cord itself [30]. Any patient who exhibits respiratory abnormalities should undergo a thorough evaluation to determine whether there is a neurologic component to their respiratory dysfunction. Additional studies that may be helpful in evaluation of these patients include somatosensory evoked potentials to evaluate brainstem and spinal cord dysfunction, and sleep apnea studies to rule out central versus obstructive apnea [30, 54].

Caution should be exercised in positioning the achondroplastic infant until better control of the head and neck muscles develops. Any position or activity that results in hyperextension of the neck could cause additional impingement of the spinal cord and distal medulla at the craniocervical juncture. Sitting or standing postures without adequate support of the neck and head should be avoided, as well as the use of bouncing-type seats [30]. Surgical intervention may eventually be required, especially if the child develops progressive neurological decline including respiratory compromise, progressive paresis, or evidence of myelopathy. Surgical intervention would involve decompression of the craniocervical juncture, with partial craniectomy and laminectomy of the upper cervical spine [29, 30, 42].

## Thoracolumbar Kyphosis and Lumbosacral Hyperlordosis

Abnormal alignment of the spine, including kyphosis in the thoracolumbar junction and hyperlordosis at the lumbosacral junction, is also frequently seen in this patient population and contributes to the congenital spinal stenosis common in achondroplasia. Kyphosis is very common in the achondroplastic child, with more than 90% of achondroplastic infants under 1 year of age exhibiting a kyphotic deformity [51]. Truncal hypotonicity, ligamentous laxity, the large size of the infant's head, flat chest, and protuberant abdomen are thought to be contributing factors to the development of this deformity. Abnormalities of the vertebral body, such as wedging at the apex of the kyphotic deformity, may be evident in some, but not all, of these patients [2, 37]. Many children will have spontaneous improvement in this deformity once they begin to sit upright and walk; however, up to one-third of these patients will develop a progressive kyphosis into adulthood [2, 37, 51].

Hyperlordosis of the lumbosacral juncture, present in children with achondroplasia, becomes evident as the achondroplastic child begins to walk. The incidence of this deformity increases as these children reach adulthood. This deformity is not thought to be a primary disorder of the spine, but rather occurs as a result of abnormal forward flexion of the pelvis and a horizontally oriented sacrum [24, 33].

Patients with thoracolumbar kyphosis and hyperlordosis of the lumbosacral spine have a very distinct posture. The kyphotic deformity is most notable while patients are in the seated position. The spine assumes a "C" shape and the patient appears to sit with a slumped posture [51]. In the standing position, the kyphotic deformity becomes much less noticeable, but exaggeration of the lordotic curve becomes evident. Plain, lateral view x-rays illustrate these abnormalities well. With these x-rays, the degree of curvature of these deformities can be measured in order to determine the severity. In infants, the thoracolumbar kyphosis generally measures about 15–25º in a neutral position. This curvature will increase to 60–70º in the seated position. The measurement of the lumbosacral lordosis is determined by the sacrohorizontal angle. This is a measurement of the angle comprised of a horizontal line and a line drawn from the first sacral vertebra to the third sacral vertebra. In normal individuals, this measures 25–50º. In achondroplastic patients, this will measure 45–80º in the child, and up to 90º in the adult [33]. Plain, lateral-view x-rays will also demonstrate the presence of remodeling or wedging of the anterior aspect of the vertebral bodies at the apex of the kyphosis. Lateral upright and supine views are helpful in determining the flexibility of these spinal deformities. The presence of anterior vertebral body wedging and immobility of the spinal curvatures increase the possibility that the deformity will progressively worsen over time [33, 51].

The use of positioning restrictions and early bracing techniques has proven beneficial in treating early thoracolumbar kyphosis. These techniques were found to be the most effective if utilized in children under the age of 3 years, while the kyphotic deformity remains flexible and reducible. Parents of achondroplastic children should be instructed to avoid having the child sit in an unsupported position until truncal hypotonia improves. The back should be supported utilizing counter pressure with the hand when the child is held and only hard-backed seating devices should be used. Periodic radiographic follow-up is important during this time to assess for continued progression of the kyphosis. If the kyphosis is determined to progress or if vertebral body wedging is evident, then bracing utilizing a firm brace such as a thoracolumbosacral orthosis can be instituted [33, 51]. In many patients, improvement in the kyphotic deformity will improve with these measures; however, approximately 11% of these patients will develop persistent and progressive kyphosis [4, 33]. In these cases, surgical intervention involving stabilization with fusion and instrumentation is often necessary. Surgery of this nature in the achondroplastic patient carries a significant risk of neurologic injury [2, 4].

Correction of the lumbosacral hyperlordosis has proven difficult. Methods such as bracing, stretching of the pelvic girdle musculature, and release of hip flexor contractures have not proven successful. Surgical treatment involving lengthening of the femur has shown some improvement of the appearance of the hyperlordosis but did not necessarily change the angle of the sacrum [24, 50].

## Spinal Stenosis

The overall diameter of the spinal canal in achondroplastic patients is diminished as a result of abnormalities in the development of the bone of the spinal column. The spinal canal is formed by the posterior aspect of the vertebral body, which acts as the anterior border of the spinal canal, the pedicles that form the lateral borders of the canal, and the lamina which forms the posterior border of the canal [58]. Achondroplastic spines have shortened pedicles, which causes narrowing of the anterior-posterior diameter of the canal. Additional narrowing of the canal also occurs because the distance between the pedicles is decreased in the achondroplastic spine. Normally, this distance between the pedicles increases as the spine progresses caudally; however, in achondroplasia this distance progressively narrows in the lower spinal segments. The result is a progressively stenotic canal in the distal spine [3, 50]. Because achondroplastic patients already have a narrowed spinal canal, they are more susceptible to the stenotic effect caused by aging from ligamentous hypertrophy, disc degeneration, and osteoarthritic changes. Thoracolumbar kyphosis and lumbosacral hyperlordosis can also cause additional narrowing of the canal, placing added stress on the dura and nerve roots exacerbating the stenosis [5, 29, 30].

Symptoms related to spinal stenosis below the cervicomedullary juncture usually do not become problematic until the late teens. In most cases, symptomatic spinal stenosis does not occur until later in adulthood, with the average age of symptom onset occurring late in the third decade of life [3, 29, 30]. Low back pain is a very common complaint in patients with achondroplasia. Neurogenic claudicatorytype symptoms are typical in patients with symptomatic spinal stenosis. These symptoms include pain, parasthesias, and weakness involving the lower extremities with walking. The symptoms are often relieved by rest, bending forward, or squatting. A typical scenario is the patient who must lean on a shopping cart in order to complete the task of grocery shopping. The symptoms usually affect both lower extremities and can progress to the point where they are present even at rest. If the stenosis is severe and ongoing, neurologic changes including weakness, abnormal reflexes, spasticity, alterations in sensation and proprioception below the level of the stenosis, and bladder dysfunction may be present [30].

Radiographic evaluation is warranted in any patient experiencing symptoms of spinal stenosis. Plain x-rays are often the first line of evaluation. These x-rays can determine if abnormalities of spinal alignment, degenerative changes such as the presence of osteophytes, degenerative disc disease, and abnormalities of the shape and configuration of the vertebral body complex are present. CT will provide a detailed evaluation of the bony structure of the spine. Myelogram is very useful for evaluating the spinal canal; however, performing the lumbar puncture necessary for a myelogram may prove difficult because of the anatomical changes of the spine in achondroplasia. MRI provides very detailed information about the soft tissue structures including the spinal cord, ligaments, and intervertebral discs [42].

The treatment of spinal stenosis in achondroplasia is dependant on the severity of the stenosis. Mild symptoms can be managed initially with medications and steroid injections. If the stenosis is severe, symptoms are progressive and limiting, or if neurological symptoms including bowel and bladder dysfunction are present, surgical intervention would be necessary. Surgery involves decompression of the involved neural structures. Surgery of this nature in this patient population carries a high risk for complication including neurologic injury. Special care must be taken during the operative procedure due to the limited spinal canal space. Patients are also at a higher risk for the development of spinal instability and restenosis requiring additional surgery [3, 44, 64].

## Conclusion

Achondroplasia is a complex genetic disorder involving bone formation. The manifestations of this disorder result in abnormalities of the craniocervical juncture and the spine. These abnormalities can become problematic at any time throughout the achondroplast's lifespan; however, cervicomedullary insufficiency and abnormalities of spinal alignment, including thoracolumbar kyphosis and lumbosacral hyperlordosis, are most common in early childhood. Stenosis below the cervicomedullary juncture often does not become symptomatic until later into adulthood, but can begin to manifest in the teenage years. Early recognition and treatment of these disorders is important to promote normal growth and development of the achondroplastic child.

## Klippel-Feil Syndrome

Klippel-Feil Syndrome (KFS) was first described in 1912 by Maurice Klippel and Andre Feil [60]. This syndrome is a rare, congenital disorder that affects the spine as well as many other body systems. This disorder is characterized by "the congenital fusion of any two of the seven cervical vertebrae" [60]. The resulting fusion is caused by a failure of the normal division of the cervical somites vertebrae during early fetal development [60]. Patients with KFS present with a triad of symptoms; short neck, low hairline at the back of the head, and restricted mobility of the upper spine.

### Diagnosis

Diagnosis is based on clinical presentation and radiographic exam. The clinical presentation varies because of the number of associated syndromes and anomalies that can occur. Associated abnormalities may include scoliosis, spina bifida, anomalies of the kidneys and the ribs, cleft palate, respiratory problems, and heart malformations. The disorder may also be associated with abnormalities of the head and face, skeleton, sex organs, muscles, brain and spinal cord, arms, legs, and fingers [16]. Careful evaluation is essential as some associated anomalies may be fatal if not recognized and treated.

### Radiographs

AP and lateral views of the cervical spine are made to determine the presence of anomalies. Flexion-extension radiographs should be obtained if instability or anomalies are suspected or if two fused segments are separated by an open segment. AP and lateral chest radiographs may be obtained to rule out rib fusions and cardiac involvement. CT scans of the entire spine are useful to determine associated abnormalities. MRI scans are indicated in patients with neurological deficits. These scans may reveal cord compression, spinal stenosis, and central nervous system anomalies such as syringomyelia. Renal ultrasound scans are used to determine renal involvement, and an intravenous pyelography is performed to delineate any abnormality found on ultrasound.

## Classification

KFS patients may be placed in three categories when they are determined to be high-risk patients:

**Group 1:** C2–C3 fusion with occipitalization of the atlas. Flexion and extension occurs at C1–C2, which thereby becomes unstable.

**Group 2:** Long fusion below C2 with an abnormal occipitocervical junction

**Group 3:** Single open space between two fused segments [16]

## Treatment

The treatment for KFS is focused on relieving associated symptoms. Medical treatment may involve a wide variety of specialists depending on which anomalies are present. A patient with KFS may be seen by a cardiologist, audiologist, or urologist, among others; physical therapy may be useful. Because the spinal anomalies are often progressive in nature, surgical intervention is often necessary to relieve cervical or craniocervical instability, constriction of the spinal cord, and to correct scoliosis. Depending on the type of surgery needed, neurosurgery, orthopedic surgery, or both, may be necessary to correct the anomalies.

## Outcomes

Careful diagnosis, consistent follow-up, and multidisciplinary care are essential to achieve positive outcomes. Minimally complex patients may lead normal lives with few restrictions. The more associated anomalies, the poorer the outcome and the more restrictions on activities of daily living.

### Patient and Parental Education

KFS, a syndrome that may be progressive and involve other specialties, may be found at any stage of life. Parents should be informed of the possible related anomalies and the symptoms associated with those anomalies.

## Summary

KFS is a rare congenital anomaly with no known etiology. It is diagnosed based on clinical findings with radiographic confirmation. There may be any number of associated anomalies and syndromes occurring with KFS. Treatment should be initiated soon after diagnosis, especially with those patients who are considered high risk or who have progressive disease processes. Patient outcomes vary and are dependent on the extent and number of associated syndromes and anomalies. Careful evaluation, consistent follow-up, and coordination of providers are essential to positive patient outcomes.

## Mucopolysaccharide Disorders

Mucopolysaccharide disorders (MPS), also referred to as lysosomal storage disorder (LSD) were first identified in 1917 [61]. These inherited disorders are errors of metabolism that are progressive in nature. The lysosomal enzyme, normally found in each cell, is needed to degrade and recycle glycosaminoglycans, a long-chain sugar carbohydrate. The acid, mucopolysaccharide, is found intercellularly. The glycosaminoglycans are polysaccharide chains that contain amino sugars, which are located intracellularly, on the surface of the cell, as part of the extracellular matrix, in the basement membrane, and in the structure of proteoglycans [61, 63]. Proteoglycans act as a "shock-absorber," retaining water and forming a sponge-like structure. The proteoglycan is degraded by glycosaminoglycan-chain-specific enzymes. If these enzymes are not degraded and recycled, they accumulate within the cells causing the disease process, with consequent progressive damage to the body [63]. People affected with these disorders either do not produce enough of any one of the 11 identified enzymes that normally degrade and recycle the sugar chains into proteins, or the enzymes do not work correctly to produce the enzyme necessary for degradation.

Mucolipidoses (ML II) disorders are called I-Cell, from their characteristic appearance when viewed through the microscope. This family of disorders was first discovered in 1960 by Dr. Jules Lerory in Belgium [61]. ML III was first identified by Dr. Maroteaux and

Dr. Lamy in France. The mucopolysaccharide enzymes are present in the ML disorders; however, these enzymes are constantly leaking from the cell. Therefore the enzyme is not completely broken down. This group lacks a phosphate that is essential for sending the enzymes into the lysosomes, thus allowing the mucopolysaccharide and lipids material to accumulate in the tissues and cells. The characteristics of the ML disorders are the same as those for the MPS disorders [61].

### Inheritance

The disease relies on autosomal recessive inheritance, an abnormal gene must therefore be inherited from each parent for the disease to manifest. The odds of receiving the disorder if both parents are affected are one out of every four pregnancies. The unaffected child of parents with the gene has a two in three risk of being a carrier, and a one in three chance of being a noncarrier of the disorder. The sole exception is MPS type II (Hunter syndrome), as this is X-linked and recessive inheritance. The Hunter gene is carried by a normal female and there is a 50/50 chance of transmission to each of the male offspring. Estimates have the occurrence in population at 1 birth in 25,000 (Table 8.2) [47, 61].

### Characteristics

Children with MPS may appear normal at birth and develop normally for the 1st year or so of life. The symptoms that prompt further clinical investigation are usually repeated upper respiratory infections, colds, runny noses, and ear infections [61]. Clinical features may produce neurological complications through impaired signals as damage occurs to neurons affecting motor function and pain receptors. Children with MPS are often mentally retarded, hyperactive, suffer from depression, in pain, and their growth and development may be stunted. All children with MPS have coarse facial features and skeletal involvement, as in skeletal dysplasia [15, 39, 46, 57]. Some may have an absence of the odontoid process or odontoideum. They may have a thoracic gibbus deformity, a form of structural kyphosis. The curvature is not smooth, as the posterior curve is angled sharply, and results in a humpback that is more prominent when bending forward.

In Morquio's syndrome, MPS type IV, death commonly occurs by age 7 years from hypoxia secondary to a cervical myelopathy and the effect upon the respiratory system [15, 40]. Other characteristics of MPS may include: general ligamentous laxity thought to contribute to atlantoaxial subluxation [39], corneal clouding, speech or hearing impairment, chronic runny nose, hernias, heart disease, development of congenital hydrocephalus, stiff joints, splenomegaly, liver enlargement, diarrhea, and shortened life expectancy. Symptoms appear as the storage of the enzymes increase. The projected life expectancy of children with MPS is 10–20 years [15, 46, 57, 61].

**Table 8.2.** Types of syndromes associated with mucopolysaccharide disorders (MPS)

| Type/syndrome | Disease name | Deficiency |
|---|---|---|
| MPS I | Hurler/Hurler-Scheie syndrome | $\alpha$-L-Iduronidase |
| MPS II | Hunter Syndrome | Iduronate sulfatase |
| MPS III A | Sanfilippo syndrome | Heparan-$N$-sulfatase |
| MPS III B | Sanfilippo syndrome | $\alpha$-$N$-Acetylglucosaminidase |
| MPS III C | Sanfilippo syndrome | Acetyl CoA: $\alpha$-glycosaminide |
| MPS III D | Sanfilippo syndrome | $N$-Acetylglucosamine-6-sulfatase |
| MPS IV A | Morquio syndrome | Glactose-6-sulfatase |
| MPS IV B | Morquio syndrome | Glactosidase |
| MPS VI | Maroteaux-Lamy syndrome | N-Acetylgalactosamine-4-sulfatase |
| MPS VII | Sly syndrome | Glucuronidase |
| MPS IX | | Hyaluronidase |
| ML II | I-Cell | $N$-acetylglucosamine-1-phosphotransferase |
| ML III | Pseudo-Hurler polydystrophy | $N$-acetylglucosamine-1-phosphotransferase |

## Diagnosis

The diagnosis of MPS may be made through clinical examination, urine, and tissue testing. Genetic counseling and reviewing family history for at least three generations may assist couples to determine if they are carrying the mutated gene responsible for the development of the disorders [14]. Prenatal diagnosis utilizing amniocentesis and chorionic villus sampling at 14–17 weeks gestation should be done to determine if the fetus has the defective gene or is affected by the disorder. Clinical signs and symptoms such as chronic otitis media, chronic rhinitis, macrocephaly, chronic respiratory infections, developmental delay, coarse facial features, inguinal or umbilical hernias, or corneal clouding alone do not demonstrate a diagnosis. Further definitive testing such as enzyme-specific assays for alpha-L-iduronidase, peripheral blood leukocytes, and plasma or cultured fibroblasts should be ordered [27, 45, 46]. For an infant suspected of having an inborn error of metabolism, laboratory studies should include complete blood counts, urinalysis, capillary blood gases, electrolytes, glucose, ammonia, urine-reducing substances, urine ketones, plasma and urine amino acids (quantitative), urine organic acids, and plasma lactate [10].

## Treatment

Currently there is no cure for MPS. Treatment is therefore focused on relieving and treating symptoms as they arise. The Food and Drug Administration approved aldurazyme (laronidase) in 2003 and naglazyme in 2005. These are enzyme replacement therapies for MPS type I and IV, and are proving to be useful in the reduction of the pain and nonneurological symptoms of MPS. They replace the deficient enzymes and are given intravenously once a week for life. Bone marrow transplant, to replace lost enzymes, has been utilized; however, some of the children have heart disease due to the disease process and cannot withstand the chemotherapy required for the transplantation of bone marrow. Bone marrow transplantation, along with umbilical cord blood transplants, is showing limited success with improved survival.

## Summary

Pediatric patients may suffer from congenital anomalies or injuries from trauma. These spinal problems are often difficult to diagnose due to the differences in the development of the pediatric spine compared to the adult spine. Congenital spinal anomalies may not be diagnosed until the child is older, often resulting in irreversible neurological damage. SCIs are often severe. Children may have concomitant neurological injuries from the anomalies, the injury, or the required surgical intervention that complicate the recovery. Because of these concomitant injuries, treatment does not stop when the patient leaves the hospital or the rehabilitation facility; it requires a life-long commitment from the family and patient.

> ### Pediatric Practice Pearls
>
> 1. Smaller children are more prone to injuries of the cervical spine with flexion-extension forces because of the large size of their head in relation to the rest of their body.
> 2. Children require appropriate head support when on a back board because the size and shape of the head could cause extreme flexion. This could lead to worsening of the injury or obstruction of the airway.
> 3. Appropriate immobilization is imperative after a spinal injury to prevent worsening of the injury.
> 4. Frequent neurological assessments must be performed on the newly diagnosed spinal-cord-injured child. Neurological deterioration must reported immediately.
> 5. Autonomic dysreflexia is an exaggerated and possibly life-threatening autonomic response to normal innocuous stimuli seen in injuries of the spinal cord at T6 or above. The offending stimulus must be sought and reversed as soon as possible.

## References

1. Adelson PD, Resnick DK, (1999) Spinal cord injury in children. In: Albright AL, Pollack IF, Adelson PD (eds) Principles and Practice of Pediatric Neurosurgery. Theime, New York, pp 955–972
2. Ain MC, Browne JA (2004) Spinal arthrodesis with instrumentation for thoracolumbar kyphosis in pediatric achondroplasia. Spine 29:2075–2080
3. Ain MC, Elmaci I, Hurko O, Clatterbuck RE, Lee RR, Rigamonti D (2000) Reoperation for spinal restenosis in achondroplasia. J Spinal Disord 13:168–173

4. Ain C, Shirley E (2004) Spinal fusion for kyphosis in achondroplasia. J Pediatr Orthop 24:541–545

5. Alman BA (2002) A classification of genetic disorders of interest to orthopaedists. Clin l Orthop Rel Res 401:17–26

6. American Heart Association (2000) Trauma resuscitation and spinal immobilization. In: Hazinski MF, Zaritsky AL, Nadkarni VM, Hickey RW, Schexnayder SM, Berg RA (eds) PALS Provider Manual. American Heart Association, Dallas, Texas, pp 253–283

7. Berne JD, Velmahos GC, El-Tawil Q, Demetriades D, Asensio JA, Murray JA, et al (1999) Value of complete cervical helical computed tomographic scanning in identifying cervical spine injury in the unevaluable blunt trauma patient with multiple injuries: a prospective study. J Trauma Injury Infect Crit Care 47:896–903

8. Bosch PP, Vogt MT, Ward WT (2002) Pediatric spinal cord injury without radiographic abnormality (SCIWORA): the absence of occult instability and lack of indication for bracing. Spine 32:2788–2800

9. Brown RL, Brunn MA, Garcia VF, (2001) Cervical spine injuries in children: a review of 103 patients treated consecutively at a level 5 pediatric trauma center. J Pediatr Surg 37:1107–1114

10. Burton BK (1998) Inborn errors of metabolism in infancy: a guide to diagnosis. Pediatrics 102:69–73

11. Campanolo DI (2005) Autonomic dysreflexia in spinal cord injury. Accessed on e-medicine, http://www.emedicine.com

12. Carreon LY, Glassman SD, Campbell MJ (2004) Pediatric spine fractures: a review of 137 hospital admissions. J Spinal Disord Tech 22:477–482

13. Cirak B, Ziegfeld S, Knight VM, Chang D, Avellino AM, Paidas CN (2004) Spinal injuries in children. J Pediatr Surg 39:607–612

14. Clarke JTR (2005) A Clinical Guide to Inherited Metabolic Diseases (3rd edn). Cambridge University Press, New York

15. Cleary MA, Wraith JE (1995) The presenting features of mucopolysaccharidosis type IH (Hurler syndrome). Acta Paediatr Int J Paediatr 84:337–339

16. Curcione PJ, Mackenzie W (1995) Klipper-Feil a Clinical Case Presentation at The Alfred I. Dupont Institute in Wilmington, Delaware

17. Dibsie GL (1998) Clearing cervical spine injuries: a discussion of the process and the problems. Crit Care Nurs Q 2:26–41

18. Dickman CA, Zabramski JM, Hadley MN, Rekate HL, Sonntag VK (1991) Pediatric spinal cord injury without radiographic abnormalities: report of 26 cases and review of the literature. J Spinal Disord 4:296–305

19. Duke Orthopaedics (2005) Atlas fracture/Jefferson fracture. Wheeless' Textbook of Orthopaedics. Retrieved December 4, 2005, from http://www.wheelessonline.com

20. Dziurzynski K, Anderson PA, Bean DB, Choi J, Leverson GE, Marin RL, et al (2005) A blinded assessment of radiographic criteria for atlanto-occipital dislocation. Spine 30:1427–1432

21. Ergun A, Oder W (2003) Pediatric care report of spinal cord injury without radiographic abnormality (SCIWORA): case report and literature review. Spinal Cord 41:249–253

22. Fielding JW, Hawkins RJ (1977) Atlanto-axial rotary fixation: fixed rotatory subluxation of the atanto-axial joint. J Bone Joint Surg Am 59A:45–55

23. Freeborn K (2005) The importance of maintaining spinal precautions. Crit Care Nurs Q 28:195–199

24. Giglio GC, Passariello R, Pagnotta G, Crostelli M, Ascani E (1988) Anatomy of the lumbar spine in achondroplasia. In: Nicoletti B, Kopits SE, Ascani E, Mckusick VA (eds) Human Achondroplasia: A Multidisciplinary Approach. Plenum, New York, pp 227–239

25. Greenberg MS (2001) Spine injuries. In: Greenberg MS, Handbook of Neurosurgery (5th edn). Thieme, Stuttgart, pp 686–735

26. Hadley MN (2002) Management of pediatric cervical spine and spinal cord injuries. Neurosurgery 50:S85–S99

27. Hall CW, Liebaers I, Di Natale P, Neufeld EF (1978) Enzymatic diagnosis of the genetic mucopolysaccharide storage disorders. Methods Enzymol 50:439–456

28. Hendey GW, Wolfson AB, Mower WR, Hoffman JR, National Emergency X-Radiography Utilization Study Group (2002) Spinal cord injury without radiographic abnormality: results of the National Emergency X-Radiography Utilization Study in blunt cervical trauma. J Trauma 53:5–8

29. Hunter A, Bankier A, Rogers J, Sillence D, Scott C (1998) Medical complications of achondroplasia: a multicentre patient review. J Med Genet 35:705–712

30. Hurko O, Pyeritx R, Uematsu S (1988) Neurological considerations in achondroplasia. In: Nicoletti B, Kopits SE, Ascani E, Mckusick VA (eds) Human Achondroplasia: A Multidisciplinary Approach. Plenum, New York, pp 153–162

31. Kenter K, Worley G, Griffin T, Fitch RD (2001) Pediatric traumatic atlanto-occipital dislocation: five cases and a review. J Pediatr Orthop 21:585–589

32. Kokoska ER, Keller MS, Rallo MC, Weber TR (2001) Characteristics of pediatric cervical spine injuries. J Pediatr Surg 37:100–105

33. Kopits SE (1988) Thoracolumbar kyphosis and lumbosacral hyperlordosis in achondroplastic children. In: Nicoletti B, Kopits SE, Ascani E, Mckusick VA (eds) Human Achondroplasia: A Multidisciplinary Approach. Plenum, New York, pp 241–255

34. Kriss VM, Kriss TC (1996) SCIWORA (spinal cord injury without radiographic abnormality) in infants and children. Clin Pediatr 35:119–124

35. Labbe JL, Leclair O, Bernard B (2001) Traumatic atlanto-occipital dislocation with survival in children. J Pediatr Orthop 10:319–327

36. Lang SM, Bernardo LM (1993) SCIWORA syndrome: nursing assessment. Dimens Crit Care Nurs 12:247–254

37. Lonstein JE (1988) Anatomy of the lumbar spinal canal. In: Nicoletti B, Kopits SE, Ascani E, Mckusick VA (eds) Human Achondroplasia: A Multidisciplinary Approach. Plenum, New York, pp 219–226

38. Mattera C (1998) Spinal trauma, new guidelines of assessment management in the out hospital environment. J Emerg Nurs 24:523–538

39. Menezes AH, Ryken TC, Brockmeyer DL (2001) Abnormalities of the craniocervical junction. In: McLone DG, Marlin AE, Scott RM, Steinbok P, Reigel DH, Walker LM (eds) Pediatric Neurosurgery – Surgery of the Developing Nervous System (4th edn). WB Saunders, Philadelphia, pp 400–422

40. Menezes AH (1999) Craniovertebral anomalies and syringomyelia. In: Choux M, DiRocco C, Hockley AD, Walker ML (eds) Pediatric Neurosurgery. Churchill Livingstone, New York, pp 151–183

41. Moloney-Harmon PA, Adams P (2001) Trauma. In: Curley MAQ, Moloney-Harmon PA (eds) Critical Care Nursing of Infants and Children (2nd edn). Saunders, Philadelphia, pp 947–980

42. Morgan DF, Young BF (1980) Spinal neurological complications of achondroplasia: results of surgical treatment. J Neurosurg 52:463–472

43. Morris CG, McCoy E (2004) Clearing the cervical spine in unconscious polytrauma victims, balancing risks and effective screening. Anesthesia 59:464–482

44. Nelson MA (1988) Kyphosis and lumbar stenosis in achondroplasia. In: Nicoletti B, Kopits SE, Ascani E, Mckusick VA (eds) Human Achondroplasia: A Multidisciplinary Approach. Plenum, New York, pp 305–312

45. Neufeld EF, Muenzer J (1995) The mucopolysaccharidoses. In: Scriver CR, Beaudet AL, Sly WS, Valle D (eds) The Metabolic and Molecular Bases of Inherited Disease, 7th edn. McGraw-Hill, New York, p 2465–2487

46. Neufeld EF, Muenzer J (2001) The mucopolysaccharidoses. In: Scriver CR, Beaudet AL, Sly WS, Valle D (eds) The Metabolic and Molecular Bases of Inherited Disease, 7th edn. McGraw-Hill, New York, p 3421–3465

47. Online Mendelian Inheritance in Man (OMIM), http://www.ncbi.nlm.nih.gov/Omim/ Hunter's syndrome

48. Pang D, Wilberger JE (1982) Spinal cord injuries without radiographic abnormalities in children. J Neurosurg 57:114–129

49. Pang D, Pollack IF (1989) Spinal cord injury without radiographic abnormality in children – the SCIWORA syndrome. J Trauma 29:654–664

50. Park H, Kim H, Hahn S, Yang K, Choi C, Park J, Jung S (2003) Correction of lumbosacral hyperlordosis in achondroplasia. Clin Orthop Rel Res 414:242–249

51.. Pauli RM, Breed A, Horton VK, Glinski LP, Reiser CA (1997) Prevention of fixed angular kyphosis in achondroplasia. J Pediatr Orthop 17:726–733

52. Poseti IV (1988) Bone formation in achondroplasia. In: Nicoletti B, Kopits SE, Ascani E, Mckusick VA (eds) Human Achondroplasia: A Multidisciplinary Approach. Plenum, New York, pp 109–122

53. Proctor MR (2002) Spinal cord injury. Crit Care Med 53: S489–S499

54. Reid CS, Pyeritz RE, Kopitz SE, Maria BL, Wang H, McPherson RW, Hurko O, Phillips JA (1988) Cervicomedullary cord compression in young children with achondroplasia: value of comprehensive neurologic and respiratory function. In: Nicoletti B, Kopits SE, Ascani E, Mckusick VA (eds) Human Achondroplasia: A Multidisciplinary Approach. Plenum, New York, pp 199–206

55. Rimoin DL (1988) Clinical variability in achondroplasia. In: Nicoletti B, Kopits SE, Ascani E, Mckusick VA (eds) Human Achondroplasia: A Multidisciplinary Approach. Plenum, New York, pp 123–127

56. Ruge JR, Sinson GP, McLone DG, Cerullo .J (1988) Pediatric spinal injury: the very young. J Neurosurg 68:33–53

57.. Scheie HG, Hambrick GW, Barness LA (1962) A newly recognized form of Hurler's disease (Gargoylism). Am J Ophthalmol 67:753–769

58. Schnuerer AP, Gallego J, Manuel C (2001) Basic Anatomy and Pathology of the Spine: Core Curriculum for Basic Spinal Training. Medtronic Sofamor, Daneck

59. Shiang R, Thompson LM, Zhu Y, Church DM, Fielder TJ, Bocian M, Winokur ST, Wasmuth JJ (1994) Mutations in the transmembrane domain of FGFR3 cause the most common genetic form of dwarfism, achondroplasia. Cell 78:335–342

60. Sullivan JA, O'Dononghue DH (2005) Klippel-Feil Syndrome. Accessed on e-medicine, http://www.emedicine.com/orthoped/topic408.htm on May 18, 2006

61. Symptoms and effects of mucopolysaccharide syndrome (April 2006) Retrieved April 22, 2006, from http://www.mpssociety.ca/about/faq.html

62. Turkstra TP, Craen RA, Pelz DM, Gelb AW (2005) Cervical spine motion: a fluoroscopic comparison during intubation with lighted stylet, GlideScope, and Macintosh laryngoscope. Anesth Analg 101:910–915

63. Tuschl K, Gal A, Paschke E, et al (2005) Mucopolysaccharidosis type II in females: case report and review of literature. Pediatr Neurol 32:270–272

64. Uematsu S, Wang H, Hurko O, Kopitx SE (1988) The subarachnoid fluid space in achondroplastic spinal stenosis: the surgical intervention. In: Nicoletti B, Kopits SE, Ascani E, Mckusick VA (eds) Human Achondroplasia: A Multidisciplinary Approach. Plenum, New York, pp 275–281

65. Van de Pol GJ, Hanlo PW, Oner FC, Catelein R (2005) Redislocation in a halo vest of an atlanto-occipital dislocation in a child: recommendations for treatment. Spine 30: E424–428

66. Vogel LC, Hickey KJ, Klass SJ, Anderson CJ (2004) Unique issues in pediatric spinal cord injury. Orthop Nurs 23:300–308

67. Wright MJ, Ain MC, Clough MV, Bellus GA, Hurko O, McIntosh I (2000) Achondroplasia and nail-patella syndrome: the common phenotype. J Med Genet 37:E25

# Neurovascular Disease

9

*Patti Batchelder, Tina Popov, Arbelle Manicat-Emo,*
*Patricia Rowe, Maria Zak, and Amy Kolwaite*

## Contents

## Introduction

Neurovascular malformations are generally congenital lesions that have the potential to produce symptoms at any time. Vascular malformations are a rare occurrence in children but can be quite complex in this population [47]. The vast majority of pediatric malformations fall into one of the following groups: aneurysms, arteriovenous malformations (AVM), cavernous malformations, vein of Galen malformations, venous angiomas, and moyamoya. Vessels within the vascular blood supply are composed of arteries, veins, and capillaries. Table 9.1 describes the characteristics of these three types of vessel.

## Cerebral Blood Supply

The cerebral circulation, as elsewhere in the body, has an arterial system and a venous system, separated by capillary beds. The two systems work in balance to maintain appropriate pressure and perfusion within the brain. There are many physiologic and pathologic factors that can affect blood flow in the arteries and veins of the brain, including acid–base balance, oxygen saturation, and systemic blood pressure. Autoregulation is the ability of cerebral arteries to constrict or dilate to maintain a constant flow in response to such factors. Under normal conditions of autonomic regulation, the mean arterial pressure is maintained at 0–10 cm $H_2O$ [44]. This ensures adequate perfusion of the cerebral capillary beds despite changes in systemic blood pressure.

**Table 9.1.** Description of arteries, capillaries, and veins

| | |
|---|---|
| Arteries | Artery walls are composed of three layers: tunica intima, tunica media, and tunica adventitia. There are three types of arteries: elastic arteries, muscular arteries, and arterioles. Thickness of wall layers and differences in make up of these layers – particularly the tunica media - are elements that further distinguish the different artery types from one another [47].<br><br>**Elastic Arteries**<br>Elastic arteries are the largest type of artery. They expand synchronously with heart contractions and resume their normal shape between contractions [47].<br><br>**Muscular Arteries**<br>These arteries distribute blood to various parts of the body, and for this they are often referred to as *distributing arteries*. Muscular artery walls consist of circularly disposed smooth muscle fibers. The smooth muscle fibers constrict their lumina upon contraction [47].<br><br>**Arterioles**<br>Arterioles are the smallest of the arteries. They have a narrow lumina and thick muscular walls. The degree of tonus of the smooth muscle in arteriole walls is primarily responsible for arterial pressure [47]. |
| Capillaries | Capillaries connect arteries to veins. They are made of endothelial tubes and are arranged in a network known as a capillary bed [47]. The make-up of a capillary wall consists of a single layer of endothelial cells that are surrounded by a thin basement membrane of the tunica intima. Some capillary walls consist of a single endothelial cell with no tunica media or tunica externa. Other capillaries contain oval windows known as fenestrations within the endothelial cells. A thin diaphragm covers the fenestrations [44]. |
| Veins | Vein walls are thinner than artery walls because of the lower blood pressure in the venous system. They are also fibrous, and have a larger diameter. The tunica externa of veins has less elastic tissue than arteries, and as a result, veins do not possess the capacity to recoil as seen in arteries [44]. Valves work to permit blood to flow toward the heart and prevent blood from flowing in the opposite direction. There are three types of veins: small, medium, and large. The adventitia of large veins is composed of wide bundles of longitudinal smooth muscle. Venules are the smallest type of vein [47]. The smallest venules that are closest to capillaries have an inner lining made up of the endothelium of the tunica intima and surrounded by fibrous tissue. The largest venules that are furthest from the capillaries are made of a thin tunica media that consists of a few smooth muscle fibers [47]. |

## Arterial Supply

Arterial blood enters the cranial cavity by way of four large vessels, the paired left and right internal carotid arteries (ICAs) and left and right vertebral arteries. They branch to provide blood flow to the brain and contribute to an anastomotic ring of vessels called the circle of Willis (Fig. 9.1). The arterial supply to the brain can be divided into the anterior circulation and the posterior circulation. The posterior circulation, also referred to as the vertebral basilar system, is fed by the vertebral arteries. It supplies the brainstem, cerebellum, occipital lobe, and parts of the thalamus. The anterior circulation, which is fed by the ICAs, supplies the remainder of the forebrain.

The two vertebral arteries form the basilar artery after passing through the foramen magnum. The pos-terior and anterior inferior cerebellar arteries and the superior cerebellar arteries arise from the vertebral and basilar arteries (Fig. 9.1). The carotid arteries divide in the neck, with the ICA entering the skull. The ICA gives off several main branches including the ophthalmic artery, posterior communicating artery, and anterior choroidal artery. The ICA then terminates by dividing into the anterior cerebral artery and middle cerebral artery. The cortical areas are supplied by the anterior and middle cerebral arteries, and the deep structures of the brain by perforating vessels and the anterior choroidal arteries (Table 9.2). Occlusion of a specific artery often leads to a characteristic clinical picture (Fig. 9.2). Each major artery supplies a certain territory that is separated from other territories by watershed areas (the border of two vascular territories lying adjacent to each other). The two ante-

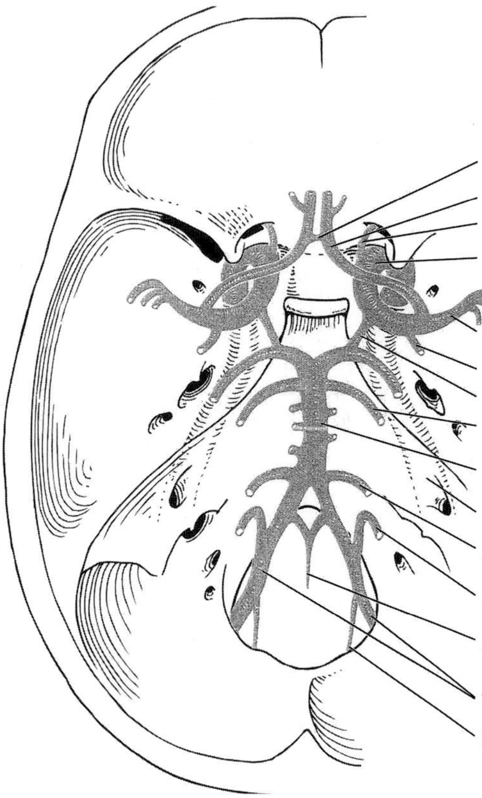

**Fig. 9.1.** Circle of Willis. Principal arteries on the floor of the cranial cavity. From Waxman (2003) [74]

- Anterior communicating artery
- Anterior cerebral artery
- Ophthalmic artery
- Internal carotid artery
- Middle cerebral artery
- Anterior choroidal artery
- Posterior communicating artery
- Superior cerebellar artery
- Basilar artery with pontine branches
- Internal carotid artery in skull base
- Anterior inferior cerebellar artery
- Posterior inferior cerebellar artery
- Anterior spinal artery
- Vertebral arteries
- Posterior spinal artery

**Table 9.2.** The cortical areas supplied by the major cerebral arteries

| | |
|---|---|
| Middle cerebral artery | Supplies many deep structures and lateral aspect of the cerebrum |
| Anterior cerebral artery | Supplies the anterior frontal lobe and the medial aspects of the hemisphere |
| Posterior cerebral artery | Supplies the occipital lobe and choroid plexus of the third and lateral ventricles and the lower surface of the temporal lobe |
| Anterior choroidal artery | Supplies the choroid plexus of the lateral ventricles and the adjacent brain structures |

rior cerebral arteries are joined together by the anterior communicating artery, a part of the circle of Willis. This allows for compensation of blood flow in the event of occlusion of one of the carotid arteries.

## Venous Supply

The blood supply from the brain drains into the dural venous sinuses and subsequently into the internal jugular veins. The dural venous sinuses are lined with endothelial cells, and are found between the endosteal and meningeal layers of the dura mater [44]. The cerebral veins comprise the superficial cerebral veins and the deep cerebral veins. The superficial cerebral veins, also known as the cortical veins, drain blood from the outer surface of the brain into the large dural venous channels, the superior and inferior sagittal sinuses, the great cerebral vein of Galen, and the straight sinus. Blood from the cerebellar surface is drained by way of the cerebellar veins into the superior vermian vein, and then into the great cerebral vein, straight sinus, and transverse sinuses. Blood from the inner regions of the brain is drained by the deep cerebral veins (or central veins). The inner regions include the hemispheric white matter, basal ganglia, corpus callosum, and choroid plexus. The deep cerebral veins also drain blood from several cortical areas [47].

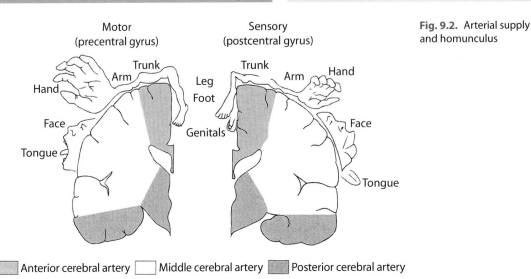

**Fig. 9.2.** Arterial supply and homunculus

Motor (precentral gyrus)  Sensory (postcentral gyrus)

Anterior cerebral artery  Middle cerebral artery  Posterior cerebral artery

## Vein of Galen Aneurysmal Malformations

### Pathophysiology

The vein of Galen, or great cerebral vein, lies under the cerebral hemispheres in the subarachnoid space dorsal to the midbrain and drains the anterior and central regions of the brain into the sinuses of the posterior cerebral fossa [64]. A vein of Galen aneurysmal malformation (VGAM) is a rare intracranial vascular anomaly that is typically found in neonates and infants, but can also present in older children and adults. It accounts for approximately 1% of all cerebrovascular lesions [24]. VGAM is a developmental anomaly of the deep venous structures, thought to arise between the 8th and 11th weeks of gestation [24]. In the VGAM, there is a persistent embryonic channel that forms the aneurysmal or dilated component [57]. Most of the arterial supply of a VGAM comes from the choroidal arteries, or feeders, which include the anterior and posterior choroidal arteries, the pericallosal artery, transmesencephalic branches from the basilar tip, and the proximal posterior cerebral arteries [17]. The VGAM results from multiple fistulous connections or arteriovenous shunts that drain into the central vein, which becomes progressively dilated from the high-pressure flow from the choroidal feeders. It is still not known how these arteriovenous shunts actually form [17].

VGAMs can be classified in two ways, according to their angioarchitecture or their clinical presentation. Based on angioarchitecture, they can be divided into choroidal and mural types [36]. The simplest, or cho-roidal type, receives its arterial contribution from the choroidal arteries, and an interposed network is present before opening into the large venous pouch. The second, or mural type, represents direct arteriovenous fistulas (AVFs) within the wall of the vein of Galen, and it can either be single or multiple. Table 9.3 presents VGAM classification based on clinical presentation, assigning a clinical "score" based on severity of symptoms. Poorer lower clinical scores tend to be found with choroidal-type malformations and higher scores tend to be associated with the mural type. This grading system can be used to help determine treatment. A score of between 8 and 12 entails emergency endovascular management [36].

### Presenting Symptoms

The clinical features of VGAM differ characteristically with the age of presentation [18]. The larger the arteriovenous shunt, the earlier the anomaly will manifest itself clinically. Symptomatic neonates often present with cardiomegaly and congestive heart failure as a result of the high-flow, high-volume arteriovenous shunt caused by the VGAM [18,61]. Severe pulmonary hypertension can also be a complication. Infants may present with an increasing head circumference secondary to hydrocephalus, seizures, and/or hemorrhage, albeit rare [18]. A cerebral "steal" phenomenon, or the siphoning of blood flow away from adjacent brain tissue, can result in cerebral atrophy and periventricular leukomalacia [51]. Intracranial bruits caused by the turbulent blood flow, dilated or

**Table 9.3.** Vein of Galen aneurysmal malformation: neonatal evaluation scoring system. *EEG* Electroencephalogram

| Score function | Cardiac function | Cerebral function | Hepatic function | Respiratory function | Renal |
|---|---|---|---|---|---|
| 5 | Normal | Normal | Normal | Normal | Normal |
| 4 | Untreated overload | Subclinical EEG abnormalities | Normal | Tachypnea but finishes bottle feed | Normal |
| 3 | Stable treated failure | Intermittent neurological signs | No hepatomegaly, normal function | Tachypnea, does not normally finish bottle feed | |
| 2 | Unstable treated failure | Isolated seizure | Hepatomegaly, normal function | Ventilated, normal saturations <25% added O2 | Transient anuria |
| 1 | Ventilated treated failure | Continuing seizures, neurological signs | Abnormal function | Ventilated, normal | Unstable |
| 0 | Resistant to treatment | | Coagulopathy, raised enzymes | Ventilated, desaturated | Anuric |

prominent scalp veins secondary to hydrocephalus, proptosis, and recurrent epistaxis can also present in infants with a VGAM [17]. In older children and adults, headaches tend to be the presenting symptom, which may be attributed to a subarachnoid hemorrhage (SAH) [18]. Older children may also present with seizures, progressive developmental delays, and hydrocephalus.

Noncommunicating hydrocephalus results from aqueductal obstruction or compression of the posterior third ventricle by the VGAM itself. Communicating hydrocephalus can develop secondary to impaired cerebrospinal fluid (CSF) absorption caused by a SAH [27]. Intracranial venous hypertension induced by the VGAM has also been postulated to contribute to the development of communicating hydrocephalus [79].

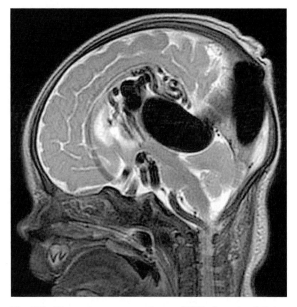

**Fig. 9.3.** Magnetic resonance image (MRI) of a vein of Galen malformation

### Diagnostic Tests

Transcranial ultrasound will help to localize or identify the lesion and color Doppler studies can help to delineate the hemodynamics of the lesion [7,61]. A typical Doppler finding is that of a large, midline, cystic structure with arterialized flow, and visualization of the feeding arteries [3]. Cranial magnetic resonance image (MRI) and/or computed tomography (CT) scan, with and without contrast administration, will help to establish the venous and arterial vascular anatomy of the lesion, as well as to confirm the diagnosis and define the degree of involvement (Fig. 9.3) [3,17,24].

Imaging studies in infants will also demonstrate whether the patient has accompanying hydrocephalus. Magnetic resonance angiography (MRA) may be able to delineate feeding arteries, nidus, and draining veins, as well as distinguish the high-flow feeding vessels from the low-flow venous lesions [3,65]. In patients being considered for surgery or for endovascular therapy, cerebral angiography may be required to define the extent of aneurysmal dilatation and details for arterial feeders [24]. Angiography findings typically show anterior and posterior circulation fistulas supplying a markedly dilated vein of Galen [3]. However, cerebral angiography should only be undertaken as a prelude to therapeutic intervention and is not required purely for diagnosis, as the nature of the condition can be confirmed by MRI [56]. Cardiac ultrasound may be indicated to assess left ventricular function [6].

## Treatment Options

### Endovascular Treatment

VGAMs have proven to be very difficult to treat using standard surgical procedures. Fortunately, this condition can now be treated with endovascular embolization. This involves the injection of embolic agents, such as synthetic cyanoacrylate glue N-butylcyanoacrylate the (NBCA), or a variety of platinum coils. Embolic agents encourage blood clotting and closure of the VGAM [37]. While initial attempts used a transvenous approach, transarterial approaches are the preferred approach, as the literature clearly indicates an improved outcome and fewer complications associated with the arterial approach. Impairing normal deep venous pathways may lead to hemorrhage, and are therefore less favored [39,70,71]. Using x-ray guidance, this procedure involves the insertion of a microcatheter through the femoral artery that is threaded through the arteries until the tip reaches the site of the arterial feeder. The embolic agent is injected through a catheter. Several staged endovascular embolizations are often required to help avoid the occurrence of parenchymal bleeds, the so-called "perfusion breakthrough phenomenon," or massive venous thrombosis potentially endangering the normal venous supply [17]. "Perfusion breakthrough" refers to a hemorrhage or swelling developing from abnormal perfusion from the vessels surrounding the recently embolized lesion. Perfusion breakthrough is more prevalent in patients who are hypertensive. Given that most of these hemorrhages occur within the 1st week after treatment, strict management of the blood pressure in the days immediately postprocedure is imperative.

Nonneurological complications related to embolization are rare [36]. Asymptomatic occlusion of the internal iliac artery, and the microcatheter becoming glued in place have both been reported. Repeated puncture of the femoral artery does not seem to cause significant problems except in the newborn.

In general, the therapeutic window for optimal endovascular management is between 4 and 6 months of age, as long as the infant is hemodynamically stable [17,70]. Neonatal intervention is reserved for the most ill, unstable patients and is associated with a worse outcome. However, excessive delay may lead to intractable hydrocephalus [36]. There is a minority of patients who experience spontaneous thrombosis of the malformation [5,36,37].

### Surgical Treatment

As a result of advances in endovascular management, open surgical obliteration of a VGAM is now only very rarely considered in case of failure of, or as an adjunct to, embolization [17,24]. Surgical interventions are indicated for the evacuation of intracranial hematomas and for the management of hydrocephalus. This can be treated either by endoscopic third ventriculostomy or insertion of a ventriculoperitoneal shunt [17]. Shunt placement has been associated with mortality and morbidity, such as increased risk of mental retardation [70,79]. A diversionary procedure should be considered only after the treatment of the VGAM is unsuccessful in reversing or relieving the hydrocephalus.

### Nursing Care

One of the primary goals of the nursing care for the neonate with a VGAM is maintaining optimal neurologic function. Head circumference measurements should be obtained regularly and monitored carefully to detect hydrocephalus. Patients should be monitored for seizures and managed with antiepileptic medications. Neonates are usually given phenobarbital and phenytoin. Respiratory interventions should include chest physiotherapy and suctioning to maintain the airway. Cardiac management of high-output heart failure is essential. Management includes monitoring of physical activity, oxygen requirements, adequate caloric intake, and strict input and output records. Pharmacological management can include inotropic agents (digoxin, dopamine, dobutamine), diuretics (loop diuretics such as furosemide), and afterload-reducing agents (angiotensin converting enzyme inhibitors such as captopril and enalapril). Other important nursing interventions include maintaining skin integrity, preventing infection and early recognition of sepsis, and providing comfort measures of frequent repositioning and pain medications as needed. In addition, facilitating normal parent–infant bonding, normal grieving and coping, and open communication are other means of providing holistic nursing care [70].

## Family Education

Parents must face the ethically and morally difficult decision of whether or not to treat the child's lesion, particularly for parents of children whose available medical information does not clearly indicate the benefit of one choice over the other [17]. Parents may not fully understand the potentially devastating outcome of a child who is unresponsive to treatment, yet survives, and are therefore ill prepared to adapt to life with a severely debilitated child. Problems include obtaining medical equipment, financial assistance, and certain support services. It is of utmost importance that therapeutic decision-making is a shared process between the clinician and parents, and all elements of defining the child's best interests are considered and discussed [17].

## Outcomes

Before the advent of endovascular embolization, the prognosis for patients presenting as neonates with congestive heart failure was poor. An earlier review reported mortality rates of 100% (9/9) for neonates, 68% (13/19) for infants, and 45% (5/11) for older children and adults [18]. Modifications in the application of newer microcatheters, improved coils, acrylic polymer NBCA, and neonatal care, such as modern imaging and intensive care environments, have improved the outlook for these patients [13]. In a series of 11 patients, no mortality had occurred, and 6 out of the 11 patients were functionally normal up to 30 months follow-up. In a series of 78 neonates, infants, and children who were treated and followed, 7 died; however, 66% of the 71 remaining patients were neurologically normal, 14% had transient neurological symptoms, 11.5% had mild permanent deficits, and 8.5% had severe permanent deficits [37]. In a more recent series of 27 children undergoing endovascular treatment, 4 of whom died in hospital, 61% of the 23 surviving patients had no or minor developmental delay, and 64% had no or mild abnormalities on neurological examination [16].

Resolution of cardiac failure has also been achieved favorably with embolization. In a series of five symptomatic neonates, one died of intractable cardiac failure (20%), whereas control of cardiac failure was achieved by embolization without neurological symptoms in the surviving four patients. One of the patients (20%) demonstrated moderate developmental delay in follow-up [46]. In a larger series of nine symptomatic neonates who underwent endovascular treatment, six (66%) obtained control of cardiac failure and normal neurological functioning, one died from intractable cardiac failure, and two (33%) died later as a result of severe hypoxic-ischemic neurological injury. At 6 months–4 years follow-up, five infants had no evidence of either neurological or cardiac deficits, and one (11%) child had mild developmental delay [12]. Larger series are obviously needed to further reflect the benefits of modern endovascular techniques.

## Cerebral Arteriovenous Malformation in Children

### Etiology

AVMs are a relatively uncommon vascular lesion. Within the general population, the prevalence is estimated to be between 0.5 and 1% [22]. Approximately 10–20% of AVMs are diagnosed in children and adolescents, with a prevalence of between 0.014 and 0.028% in children [21,22,78]. Although AVMs are considered to be congenital in origin, few are diagnosed in the first two decades of life [32,78]. The mean age at diagnosis is 30 years. Approximately 20% of AVMs become symptomatic before the age of 15 years [22,78]. The majority of cerebral AVMs occur sporadically, with no predilection for race or gender. Familial cases have been reported but are very rare [76]. AVMs are known to be associated with a few syndromes, specifically hereditary hemorrhagic telangiectasia (HHT), or Osler-Web-Rendu disease. About 7.9% of children with HHT have an AVM, and HHT should be considered in children diagnosed with multiple AVMs [19,22,60]. Wyburn-Mason syndrome (Bonnet-Dechaume-Blanc) is a rare congenital, nonhereditary disorder that is characterized by multiple cutaneous nevi, and brain and retinal AVMs [60].

## Pathophysiology

AVMs can be very complex neurovascular lesions. They are defined as a tangle of arteries and veins in the brain, or on its surface, which directly shunt arterial blood to the venous system. AVMs have a fairly well circumscribed center known as the nidus, and have been predominantly described as congenital abnormalities arising from persistent embryonic patterns of blood vessels. The embryonic vascular plexus fails to fully differentiate and develop a mature capillary bed in the affected area [66]. Some theories postulate that AVMs are a consequence of stimulation of vascular growth by blood shunting, genetic errors, and mutations in the genes controlling angiogenesis [78].

AVMs are distinguished from other types of cerebral vascular malformations by their direct anastomosis between arterial and venous channels, without any intervening capillary involvement [2,33,60]. There is no brain parenchyma contained within the nidus. The tangled nidus of the AVM receives direct, high-flow arterial blood from multiple feeding arteries. Blood is then shunted straight into the venous drainage system, which is subserved by veins that vary considerably in number, size, and configuration. The blood vessels become progressively dilated, thereby increasing the risk of rupture and subsequent spontaneous intracranial hemorrhage (ICH).

AVMs have a propensity for hemorrhage. The annual incidence of AVM rupture in children is 1 per 100,000 [22]. Tissues adjacent to the AVM may also be mildly hypoxic as the malformation may be shunting blood from the bordering healthy tissue causing chronic ischemia [60,66]; this is known as the "steal phenomenon." Approximately 70–90% of AVMs are located in the supratentorial compartment [19,22]. They occur most frequently in the cerebral hemispheres and in the middle cerebral artery territory. In children, 10–20% of AVMs are located infratentorially [22].

Secondary pathological changes can include cerebral aneurysms; approximately 7% of patients with an AVM develop an aneurysm [66]. Most commonly, aneurysms are found on the artery feeding the AVM and are prenidal. Aneurysms may also occur nidally or postnidally.

## Presenting Symptoms

Clinical symptoms of AVMs at the time of presentation can be varied. Approximately 70–80% of childhood cerebral AVMs present with spontaneous ICH [ 19,22,25,32,33,49,42,45,56,78]. Spontaneous ICH is more commonly reported in pediatric AVMs than in AVMs in the adult population [78]. As the majority of AVMs lie within the cerebral parenchyma, hemorrhages usually present as subarachnoid or intraparenchymal bleeds. Clinical symptoms of an ICH include: sudden and severe headache that is often described as the "worst headache ever," nausea and vomiting, neck stiffness, progressive neurological decline, and rapidly progressing coma [56].

Some patients with AVMs may have intermittent or progressive symptoms, rather than a single catastrophic event [60]. Occasionally, the evolution may be more gradual and characterized by episodes of moderate headache, followed by focal neurological features, such as hemiparesis, hemianopia, and focal seizures over a number of hours. This presentation may lead clinicians to believe that the child has sustained a characteristic occlusive episode, rather than a hemorrhagic one [56]. It may in fact be that periodic small hemorrhages, or thromboses, of a portion of the AVM, causing an infarct in the surrounding brain parenchyma, have occurred [60]. Some patients develop progressive neurological deficits over time without evidence of hemorrhage. This presentation has been attributed to the steal phenomenon.

Seizures without features of spontaneous ICH or fixed neurological deficit are seen in 14–20% of patients [25,33,56]. The seizures are presumably a result of gliosis of the brain due to chronic ischemia adjacent to the AVM [33,56]. Very large AVMs may produce audible cranial bruits [10]. AVMs with large arteriovenous shunts can also present with heart failure in the infant population [10,40,56]. AVMs in the basal ganglia may produce movement disorders [56]. Macrocephaly and prominent scalp veins may also be evident.

## Diagnostic Imaging

In the case of presentation with suspected hemorrhage, a CT scan should be the first radiological study completed. A CT scan will demonstrate the hemorrhage and evidence of subsequent hydrocephalus. A

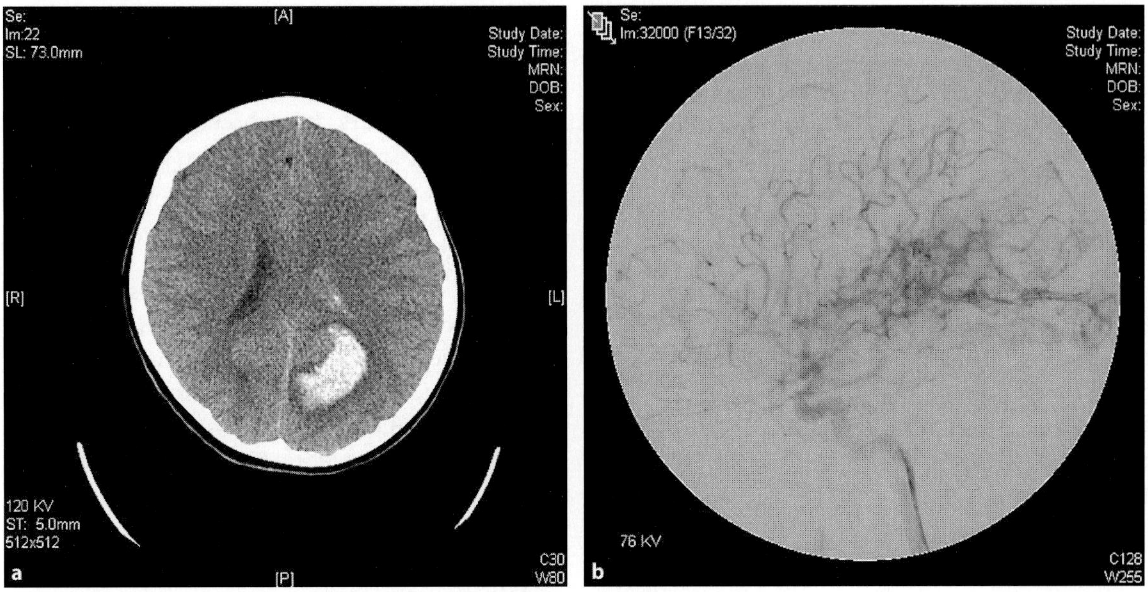

Fig. 9.4 a, b.  a Computed tomography scan and b angiogram of an AVM

noncontrast CT scan may suggest the presence of an AVM by showing calcifications or dilated vessels. Contrast CT will often demonstrate the nidus, the abnormal conglomeration of arteries and veins [22,33,45]. Angiography remains the best diagnostic tool for the study of AVMs (Fig. 9.4) [33]. Angiography of an AVM will show abnormally dilated feeding arteries and the tangle of nidus and draining veins [22]. It is ideal to delay the angiogram until hematomas have resolved, as the presence of a hematoma may lead to failure to visualize all of the malformation and its feeding vessels [56].

MRI is more specific and sensitive compared to CT, and it is essential for surgical planning and functional mapping. In addition to imaging and clinical assessment, a thorough review of all systems, a cardiovascular examination, a full coagulation profile, electrolytes, and complete blood count should be completed on every child in order to establish a diagnosis [2,56].

### ■ Treatment

The primary goals of treatment of AVMS are to eliminate the risk of future hemorrhage, control seizures, and relieve symptoms related to vascular steal [22]. Treatment options of AVMs include conservative management (observation alone), surgical excision, radiosurgery, embolization, or a combination of treatment modalities. Surgical excision is considered by many to be the treatment of choice for parenchymal AVMs in children [2,22,33,78].

Children who present with an acute ICH and associated progressive neurological deficit and/or brainstem compression require immediate surgery [22,32]. The main goal of the surgery in acute presentation is to relieve the immediate increased intracranial pressure (ICP) by evacuating the hematoma. Patients often require a CSF diversionary procedure, such as insertion of an external ventricular drain.

Resection of the AVM is delayed for 2–4 weeks posthemorrhage if a child is clinically stable [22]. This allows for resolution of the hematoma and the opportunity for a complete diagnostic evaluation. The Spetzler-Martin Grading system is often used to determine the surgical candidacy of a patient (Table 9.4). This grading system assigns points to three features of an AVM: the size, area of the brain (eloquent and noneloquent), and the pattern of venous drainage; the sum of the points determines the grading. Surgery is usually recommended for grade I and II lesions. Grade III lesions are dealt with on a case-by-case basis; however, most children undergo surgery. Of patients who receive a score of IV and V, only those with a significant repetitive hemorrhage will require surgery.

Surgery eliminates the risk of immediate bleeding and improves seizure control [2,21,22,66]. Intraoper-

Table 9.4. Spetzler and Martin grading system. *AVM* Arteriovenous malformation

| Graded feature | Points assigned |
|---|---|
| Size of AVM | |
| Small (<3 cm) | 1 |
| Medium (3–6 cm) | 2 |
| Large (>6 cm) | 3 |
| Eloquence of adjacent brain | |
| Noneloquent | 0 |
| Eloquent[a] | 1 |
| Pattern of venous drainage | |
| Superficial | 0 |
| Deep[b] | 1 |

[a] Eloquent brain: brainstem, cerebellar peduncles, deep cerebellar nuclei, internal capsule, basal ganglia/thalamus, motor strips, speech area, visual cortex
[b] Deep drainage is internal cerebral veins, basal vein of Rosenthal and pre-central cerebellar veins

ative complications include hemorrhage, parenchymal injury due to sacrificing of vessels, retraction, and incomplete resection. Immediate complications related to surgical excision of an AVM are hemorrhage, seizures, vasospasm, and retrograde vascular occlusion, with either an arterial or venous thrombosis [22]. Significant postoperative hemorrhages are most likely to occur within the first 12–24 h after surgery. These children will require postoperative management in the pediatric intensive care setting. Postoperative hemorrhage may be due to residual malformation, or insufficient occlusion of the major arterial inputs and normal perfusion breakthrough phenomenon [22,66]. Normal perfusion breakthrough can occur after AVM resection, when blood flow that was directed through the AVM is now redistributed. If the perfusion pressure is greater than the autoregulatory capacity of the surrounding brain, swelling or hemorrhage may occur [22]. Intraoperative angiography should always be considered, if available, to assess for residual AVM during the procedure.

Conventional radiation, while effective in approximately 20% of children, is not often used. Stereotactic radiation or gamma-knife radiosurgery are treatment modalities that are more commonly utilized. These treatments entail the use of high-energy radiation aimed directly on the nidus of the AVM. The radiation induces sclerosis of the blood vessels, and ultimately obliterates the AVM by proliferation and thrombosis [60]. Obliteration of the malformation occurs over 1–3 years. During this period of time, the

child continues to be at risk for recurrent hemorrhage [21,40,56,66,67]. Stereotactic radiosurgery such as gamma knife is noninvasive and can be done as an outpatient procedure. It has been proven to be most efficacious in smaller lesions (less than 2.5–3 cm deep) and those that are surgically inaccessible [66]. Complete obliteration of the AVM has been reported in 50–80% of cases that had an AVM of less than 3 mm [22,40,56,67]. Radiosurgery is seldom performed in children under 2 years of age [40]. The side effects associated with radiation are often transient and due to cerebral edema, and are a result of the AVM size, radiation dose, and AVM location [40]. After radiosurgery has been performed, patients may present with headache, nausea, vomiting, new onset of seizure activity, increase in seizure activity, and new neurological deficits. Treatment with corticosteroids in the postprocedure phase may help with symptom management.

Embolization is rarely a solitary treatment option for children with AVMs [66]. It is usually an adjunct therapy prior to a surgical resection [60,70]. It is helpful in removing the deep vessels that feed the malformation by inducing partial thrombosis, making the operation less bloody and therefore safer. By occluding the flow through the malformation, embolization helps to avoid normal perfusion pressure breakthrough postoperatively [22,78]. In large AVMs, complete embolization in one session carries a higher risk of embolization-related hemorrhage. As a result, a staged treatment approach is recommended [60,78]. During embolization, a catheter is placed inside the blood vessel and blocks off the abnormal vessels supplying the AVM. Various materials can be used for this procedure, including liquid tissue adhesives, microcoils, and particles. The chance of cure of the AVM with embolization alone is 20%. When this treatment is used alone, it has been reported that AVMs can recanalize and reestablish arteriovenous shunting [60]. It is also important to keep in mind that the risk of hemorrhage in a partially treated AVM may be reduced but not eliminated.

Conservative management (observation alone) is used in cases where the AVM is not treatable due to size or location, and is generally associated with poor outcome [78]. Patients and families should be counseled to have the child avoid activities that elevate blood pressure excessively, avoid medications or alternative therapies that may have blood-thinning properties, and have regular medical monitoring and follow-up. Infants with congestive heart failure from shunting through the low-resistance AVM should be stabilized. Seizures should be treated with anticonvulsant medication. All treatment modalities require angiographic follow-up at appropriate intervals to confirm successful and complete obliteration [2,56].

## Outcomes

In the general population, untreated lesions carry a 10–15% mortality rate and 30–50% morbidity rate [22,70]. The risk of hemorrhage from an unruptured AVM is 2–4% per year, which translates into a 30–40% risk of serious morbidity and a 10–15% risk of mortality per decade [22,40,42,60,66]. The greatest risk to a child with an AVM is hemorrhage. Without treatment, the risk for rehemorrhage is nearly 6% in the 1st year after the initial hemorrhage, with a return to 1.5–3% per year thereafter. Hemorrhage results in damage to normal brain tissue, which can lead to loss of normal functional abilities that may be temporary or permanent. The impact of a hemorrhage depends on the location and the extent of associated brain injury. Successful management depends on many factors, including presentation, clinical condition, the age of the child, and neuroanatomical features (size, location, and angioarchitecture) of the lesion [22]. Complete surgical excision of the AVM eliminates the risk of bleeding almost immediately. Nearly 50% of patients with preoperative seizures are eventually seizure-free and off anticonvulsants after resection of the AVM [22].

Excellent or good outcomes can now be achieved in 95% of children with AVMs, with complete angiographic obliteration achieved in over 90% [22]. It is imperative that radiological evaluation in the postoperative period is completed, as there is a risk of incomplete resection or recurrence. Severe complications are reported in approximately 10% of children and operative mortality is between 0 and 8% [22,60]. Despite the treatment options and recent advances, limited options for therapy still exist for approximately 10% of cases [22]. The prognosis for these children continues to be poor [22].

## Cerebral Arteriovenous Fistulas (AVFs) in Children

## Etiology

Cerebral AVFs, excluding VGAMs, are extremely rare [22]. Among all intracranial arteriovenous lesions in children, AVFs account for approximately 10% [22,78]. AVFs can be acquired or congenital in origin [21,22]. The exact etiology is unknown, but most AVFs are thought to be multifactorial. Conditions associated with dural AVFs include intracranial venous hypertension, previous sinus thrombosis, thrombophlebitis, tumor, previous neurosurgical intervention, and cranial trauma.

Much like AVMs, AVFs have a relationship to some childhood syndromes, including HHT (Osler-Weber-Rendu disease), Wyburn-Mason syndrome (Bonnet-Dechaume-Blanc), and Kippel-Trénaunay-Weber syndrome [21,22].

## Pathophysiology

AVFs are abnormal connections between a dural arterial supply and a dural venous channel. There is no intervening capillary channel between the arterial and venous supply [21,22,32]. Unlike the AVM, which has a well-circumscribed discrete nidus, AVFs are composed of a diffuse network of numerous arteriovenous microfistulas [32,78]. AVFs are commonly found in the sigmoid-transverse sinus, cavernous sinus, and superior sagittal sinus [22,32]. Approximately 50% of all dural AVFs are found in the occipital-suboccipital region [32].

In children, AVFs are often solitary entities, but they may also be multiple entities with multiple feeding arteries [22,32]. Arterial supply and venous drainage patterns vary depending on the location of the fistula [78]. Transverse sigmoid dural AVFs are usually supplied by the ipsilateral occipital artery, with additional supply from the anterior and posterior division of middle meningeal arteries, posterior auricular artery, neuromeningeal trunk of the ascending pharyngeal artery, posterior meningeal branches of the ipsilateral vertebral artery, and possibly the meningohypophyseal trunk from the ICA [78]. Venous drainage is variable and can involve the ipsilateral sinus, depending on the degree of sinus obstruction into the contralateral transverse sigmoid sinus or cortical veins [78]. The arterial supply from the coronal segments of either or both middle meningeal arteries, or superficial temporal artery, primarily supplies fistulas that are found in the superior sagittal sinus. Additional supply may be from the anterior falcine artery of the ophthalmic artery and the posterior meningeal branch of the vertebral artery.

Ethmoidal dural AVFs are those found along the anterior cranial fossa floor. They are fed primarily by anterior and posterior ethmoidal branches of the ophthalmic artery and receive a secondary supply from the internal maxillary artery. Venous drainage is usually via a pial vein, commonly associated with a venous varix that is directed towards the superior sagittal sinus [22]. Cavernous dural AVFs are rarely found in the pediatric population. These fistulas receive their arterial supply from dural branches of the cavernous segment of the ICA and from distal internal maxillary artery branches, middle/accessory meningeal arteries, and distal branches of the ascending pharyngeal artery. Venous drainage is via the superior ophthalmic vein, cavernous sinus, or cortical veins.

AVFs can be associated with other vascular lesions such as AVMs and aneurysms [22]. Neonates and children with dural AVFs can develop cerebellar tonsillar prolapse as a result of hydrovenous dysfunction of the posterior fossa, and is reversible after therapy [22,32].

## Presenting Symptoms

Clinical presentation in children with AVFs is variable and specific to age, location, size of the fistula, and the presence of other vascular lesions [21,22,32]. The location and pattern of drainage are key components of the clinical presentation. Cardiac involvement is absent in the adult population, but in children it is often seen and may be the sole presenting feature [78]. Neonates typically present with symptoms of heart failure, cyanosis, and cranial bruits, whereas children outside of the neonatal period present with neurological symptoms [21,22,32]. Children between 1 and 15 months of age (largest group of patients) typically present with hydrocephalus, macrocrania, developmental delay, seizures, and SAH [22]. If a child is 2–15 years of age at the time of presentation their clinical symptoms would often include headaches, fo-

cal neurological deficits, syncope, seizures, and SAH [22].

Hemorrhage from an AVF is relatively uncommon [21,32]. Anterior cranial fossa and tentorial dural AVFs almost always drain into a cortical vein and are associated with a higher degree of intracranial hemorrhage [78]. A dural AVF occurring in the cavernous sinus usually presents with proptosis, cranial bruit, increased intraocular pressure, diplopia, or diminished visual acuity [32,78].

AVFs can be classified into three types:

**Type 1:** (low risk) draining via the ipsilateral sinus, usually present with headaches and bruits, but rarely with neurological deficits or hemorrhage.

**Type 2:** (higher risk) draining toward the contralateral sinus, present with more severe symptoms mostly related to increased ICP or papilledema.

**Type 3:** (highest risk) drain via cortical veins, are at greatest risk of ICH or venous infarction.

Some dural AVFs can spontaneously progress from type 1 to either type 2 or 3 [78].

## Diagnostic Imaging

Conventional cerebral angiography remains the preferred diagnostic test for AVFs. A complete evaluation of head and neck vasculature is required [78]. Plain chest x-rays are utilized to screen for signs of congestive heart failure (i.e., cardiomegaly, pulmonary vascular congestion, and edema).

CT features that may suggest AVFs include: prominent enlargement of arteries or veins, a large varix (tortuous vein), and lack of an obvious nidus [22]. A CT scan is valuable for assessing ventricular size or the presence of ischemic infarctions, and is also used to rule out parenchymal edema related to venous hypertension, SAH, subdural hematoma, and intraparenchymal hemorrhage [22]. Pediatric dural AVFs can have rather large draining sinuses or veins. Sometimes the draining sinus may be so massive on imaging that it can be misinterpreted as an extra-axial mass [78].

MRI in combination with ultrasound can expose abnormally enlarged dural arteries, normal pial arteries, thrombosis of the dural sinus, and multiple parenchymal serpentine vessels without a vascular nidus [78]. MRI is effective in delineating cerebellar tonsillar prolapse. MRA may demonstrate flow-related enhancement of serpentine vessels, and MRV is used to evaluate for the presence of a thrombosis in the recipient sinus [78].

## Treatment

Therapy for dural AVFs in the pediatric population must be performed with the understanding that they are potentially life-threatening lesions. The goal of treatment is to interrupt all the feeding arteries as closely as possible to the fistula while leaving the venous drainage intact, thereby obliterating the fistula [21]. Medical management with inotropic agents and diuretics is often vital at the onset of cardiac manifestations [32].

Treatment options for the AVF include surgical resection, endovascular treatment, or a combination of treatment modalities. Surgery has traditionally been the treatment approach, but endovascular embolization is now commonly used and currently considered the treatment option of choice [32]. Endovascular embolization is often a staged approach, in that it requires more than one intervention [21]. Complications that may occur include arterial collateral recruitment from too proximal an occlusion, or decreased venous out-flow and venous hypertension from an occlusion too distal. Other complications include cerebral edema and hemorrhage. Radiation has been utilized in adults with localized slow flow dural lesions but is not an appropriate treatment in infants or children with extensive dural AVFs [32]. Depending on the complexity of the fistula, treatment may be either palliative for symptom relief or curative.

## Outcomes

Irreversible brain injury was found in cases where dural AVFs were undiagnosed and in cases where cerebral venous hypertension went unchecked for a long period of time [32]. In cases of early presentation in neonates, no presence of lasting radiological or clinical deficits were seen [32].

## Intracranial Aneurysms

### Incidence

The incidence of intracranial aneurysms in children has been estimated at 1 per 1,000,000 per year. There is a bimodal age pattern, with a peak occurring in the first 2 years of life and the second peak occurring in the second decade. Intracranial aneurysms occur predominantly in males, with a male to female ratio of 1.2–2.8:1 [56]. A recent review of the literature has found that pediatric aneurysms account for less than 2% of all aneurysms. Cerebral aneurysms are very rare in patients 18 years old or younger, but are even rarer in the youngest age groups [23].

Features of childhood aneurysms which are different than those of adults include: (1) a predominant incidence in males versus females; (2) a higher incidence of unusual sites, specifically the posterior circulation, and especially the carotid bifurcation location; (3) a predominance of giant aneurysms that account for 20% of the aneurysm types seen in children; (4) a lower incidence of multiple aneurysms; (5) a higher incidence of posttraumatic and infectious causes; and (6) a tendency toward a higher frequency of spontaneous thrombosis aneurysms [70].

### Aneurysm Subtypes

There are five different subtypes of aneurysms that are defined by their shape and form: saccular aneurysms (berry aneurysms), fusiform aneurysms, giant aneurysms, mycotic aneurysms, and traumatic aneurysms.

### Saccular Aneurysms

Saccular aneurysms (berry aneurysms) may be round with a narrow stalk that connects to a parent artery, broad-based with no stalk, or cylindrical. Thought likely to be a result of congenital abnormalities in the media of the arterial wall, saccular aneurysms occur in approximately 25% of the general population. They are rare in childhood [44].

### Fusiform Aneurysms

Fusiform aneurysms are circumferential dilatations of an artery with abnormalities of the arterial wall. They can occur in the cerebral arteries and arteries elsewhere in the body. They are slightly more common in children, particularly occurring with connective tissue disorders. They are also well described after radiation therapy to the pituitary region and following resection of craniopharyngiomas.

### Giant aneurysms

Giant aneurysms are greater than 25 mm in diameter. Approximately 5–8% of intracranial aneurysms are giant aneurysms. Giant aneurysms are commonly found in the basilar arteries or terminal portions of the ICAs. Although uncommon, giant aneurysms do occur more frequently in children than adults. These aneurysms act like space-occupying lesions, and are often mistaken for a tumor on imaging [44].

### Mycotic Aneurysms

Mycotic aneurysms are very rare and result from arteritis caused by bacterial emboli [44]. They typically occur more distally in the cerebral circulation than saccular aneurysms.

### Traumatic Aneurysms

Traumatic aneurysms occur as a result of sustained trauma to the arterial wall, causing a fracture that weakens the wall [44]. They are relatively rare intracranially, occur more commonly at the skull base, and are associated with fractures or cervical spine trauma.

### Etiology

Pediatric aneurysms differ from those of adults in that they are not caused by the classic risk factors associated with adult aneurysms, namely hypertension, flow direction, atheromatosis, shear stress, high fat and high cholesterol diets, oral contraceptive use, vascular disease, and alcohol and tobacco use [29,38]. There are multiple causes of intracranial aneurysms in children, including vascular anomalies, cardiac lesions, connective tissue abnormalities, hematological disorders, infections, and phakomatoses. Miscellaneous causes are surgical complications, penetrating head injuries, and radiation therapy [23,29]. Others feel that intracerebral aneurysms in children are due to a combination of genetic and acquired factors (Table 9.5) [29].

**Table 9.5.** Causes and associated pathologies of intracranial aneurysms in child [56]

| Causes and associated pathologies of intracranial aneurysms |
| --- |
| Vascular anomalies<br>– Cerebral AVM<br>– Moyamoya |
| Cardiac lesions<br>– Coarctation of the aorta<br>– Bacterial endocarditis<br>– Atrial myxoma |
| Connective tissue abnormalities<br>– Marfan's syndrome<br>– Ehlers-Danlos type IV syndrome (rarely in types I and VI)<br>– Fibromuscular dysplasia<br>– Pseudoxanthoma elasticum |
| Hematological disorders<br>– Sickle cell disease<br>– Glucose-6-phosphate dehydrogenase deficiency<br>– Thalassemia |
| Infections<br>– Human immunodeficiency virus<br>– Syphilis |
| Phakomatoses<br>– Neurofibromatosis-1 (especially after radiation therapy)<br>– Tuberous sclerosis |
| Miscellaneous<br>– Surgery for craniopharyngioma<br>– Radiation therapy<br>– Polycystic kidneys<br>– Penetrating or blunt head injury |

### Pathophysiology

Numerous theories exist regarding the pathophysiological mechanisms of childhood aneurysm formation. Some state that childhood aneurysms are not congenital in nature but rather are thought to be related to a weakening process of the vessel wall matrix [70]. Yet other theories purpose that aneurysms form because of an internal elastic membrane defect that is attributed to a congenital anomaly, infectious process, or head injury including birth trauma.

The ICA bifurcation is the most common site for pediatric aneurysms and accounts for 29–54% of all pediatric aneurysms [41]. Some researchers feel that this may be due to the large bifurcation angle. Hemodynamic stress with subsequent impingement of an axial stream of blood causes high shear forces and fenestration of the internal elastic lumina at the apex of the bifurcation. Another theory implicates the augmented blood flow in the vessel wall due to associated vascular anomalies, such as AVMs or coarctation of the aorta, to be causes of aneurysms in younger age groups [34]. The concept of aneurysmal vasculopathies, and a redirection of focus to understanding the biology of the type of arterial wall disease that is associated with an aneurysm, have been entertained in recent years [38]. Aneurysmal subtypes add to the complexity of etiologic theories of aneurysm formation, as most case series that examine specific aneurysm subtypes are too small to arrive at a definitive conclusion [38].

## Presenting Symptoms

It is important to note that most intracranial aneurysms in children are not found incidentally [56]. The most common presenting symptom in children with an aneurysm is sudden massive ICH. Severe and sudden onset of headache, vomiting, meningeal irritation, and increased ICP occur as a result of the blood from the ruptured aneurysm entering the subarachnoid space. Further symptoms such as focal neurologic deficits, deterioration in consciousness, seizures, coma, and retinal hemorrhages occur as a result of progressive bleeding, expansion of the aneurysm, or, in the case of large lesions, mass effect. Retinal hemorrhages are found near blood vessels and may appear flamed shaped, or they may be ovoid and located close to the optic disc. Subhyaloid hemorrhage may occur if the retinal hemorrhages dissect between retinal layers. A sudden increase in ICP caused by an intracerebral hematoma occurs in approximately one-fourth to one-half of all children [29,64].

## Diagnostic Tests

Children who do not have any presenting symptoms, but are at risk of developing an intracranial aneurysm, require diagnostic evaluation by means of MRI/MRA. Children who have a strong family history of aneurysms, risk factors, or comorbidities such as Ehlers-Danlos syndrome or polycystic kidney disease, should have a screening MRA. MRI/MRA can visualize larger lesions of the circle of Willis [29]. To date, cerebral angiography remains the gold standard for preoperative diagnosis of intracranial aneurysms [29,55]. Bruits are rarely heard in children with an unruptured aneurysm.

In the case of ruptured aneurysms, lumbar puncture and cranial CT are used for initial evaluation [29,55]. Lumbar puncture (LP) is used to detect blood in the CSF. Performing an LP is contraindicated if a child has signs and symptoms of increased ICP. MRI/MRA is capable of visualizing aneurysms that are greater than 5 mm. MRI is much better for demonstrating the aneurysm and for delineation of complications in the case of an aneurysmal bleed, such as intraventricular hemorrhage, subdural hemorrhage, intracerebral hematoma, or acute hydrocephalus. In the case of an inconclusive MRI/MRA study, digital subtraction CT angiography is the diagnostic procedure that will allow for the most definitive diagnosis [64].

## Treatment Options

### Medical Management

Today, expectant medical management is not indicated as a definitive therapy [23]. The goal of medical management of children with intracranial aneurysms or suspected aneurysms is to provide prompt stabilization in order to prevent secondary complications of hemorrhage. This includes aggressive control of systolic and mean arterial blood pressure to prevent rebleeding. Strict fluid control and monitoring is required with the aid of indwelling arterial catheters, central venous lines, or Swan-Ganz catheters, and an indwelling urinary catheter. Provision of adequate sedation or analgesia to minimize anxiety and headache must be considered against the need for frequent neurologic assessment. Antihypertensive agents, including calcium channel blockers, beta-blockers, and vasodilators may be required to manage marked hypertension. Anticonvulsant therapy to prevent seizures is often routinely administered. In the postoperative phase, anticonvulsant therapy is often continued for a period of 6 months, or indefinitely, in situations where extensive cortical destruction has occurred after SAH. High-dose glucocorticoids are given in situations of acute aneurysmal SAH. Minimization of fluctuations in ICP as a result of straining, coughing, and vomiting is controlled with stool softeners, breathing treatments, and antiemetic medications [29]. A fibrinolytic inhibitor is administered to delay lysis of blood clots and minimize the overall risk of rebleeding. Bed rest may be indicated in children who are unable to have immediate surgery.

In cases of subarachnoid hemorrhage, vasospasm is of great concern. Vasospasm, or constriction of the arteries, can be a significant source for further morbidity and mortality. The exact mechanism by which vasospasm occurs continues to be a subject of debate; however, it is felt to be related to the release of oxyhemoglobin, a product of blood breakdown. Vasospasm compromises blood flow to the brain, resulting in neurologic deterioration, which can lead to permanent deficits if not treated. The peak incidence for vasospasm is 7–10 days postrupture, but can occur anytime between 3 and 14 days postrupture. A typical presentation is insidious onset of confusion and decreasing level of consciousness followed by focal neurologic deficits [29]. The best treatment for vasospasm is prevention. Volume expansion and the use of cerebroselective calcium channel blockers can help to prevent or minimize vasospasm. When vasospasm does occur, early detection and treatment are critical to prevent permanent deficits. Transcranial Doppler scanning can be used to monitor for increasing velocities and should be performed daily during the period of peak incidence. Suspected acute vasospasm often necessitates emergent angiography and possible balloon angioplasty. Children who have had an SAH should be monitored in the intensive care unit during the period of peak vasospasm risk.

## Surgical Management

The primary goal in surgical treatment of aneurysms is to exclude the aneurysm from the circulation but at the same time preserve the normal vasculature, including the perforating arteries [41]. The conventional surgical approach to treating intracranial aneurysms in children is clipping of the aneurysm neck through an open craniotomy. Increasingly used methods, however, are interventional angiography and endovascular occlusion; these are associated with less morbidity [56]. Vascular reconstruction is considered in cases where clipping of the aneurysm is not possible [41].

In recent years, significant developments have been made in the treatment of cerebral aneurysms. Endovascular balloon occlusion has enabled neurointerventionalists and surgeons to assess for adequate collateral flow by testing for occlusion. Multiple treatment modalities have been widely adopted as standard treatment of intracranial aneurysms, and this in turn has led to significant improvements in patient outcomes [23].

## Assessment of Intracranial Aneurysms

Vigilant assessment of children with ruptured intracranial aneurysms is critical in attaining the best possible outcomes as rapidly as possible. The use of grading scales to assess the severity of a ruptured intracranial aneurysm is valuable. Two outcome predication scales commonly used to assess clinical outcomes are the Hunt and Hess (HH) Grading Scheme and the World Federation of Neurological Surgeons Scale [4].

## Hunt and Hess Scale

The HH scale is the most commonly used tool to assess SAH. The grades of the scale correspond to the neurological deficits with the level consciousness and focal deficits [4]. The HH scale is used to predict prognosis and timing of surgical or endovascular intervention (Table 9.6) [9].

## Outcomes

A good or excellent outcome can be expected in 70–80% of all children who have intracerebral aneurysms [29]. In a recent study, favorable outcomes were seen in 95% of the children followed. These children had better clinical outcomes, lower rates of death, including the greater proportion of children followed in the series that had surgical treatment. Before 1986, good outcomes were achieved in half of all patients, and one-third of all children died [23].

**Table 9.6.** Hunt and Hess Scale [4]

| Grade | Clinical condition |
|-------|--------------------|
| 0 | Unruptured |
| I | Asymptomatic or minimal headache, nuchal rigidity |
| II | Moderate to severe headache, nuchal rigidity, no neurological deficit other than cranial nerve palsy |
| III | Drowsiness, confusion, mild focal deficit |
| IV | Stupor, moderate to severe hemiparesis, possible early decerebrate rigidity and vegetative disturbances |
| V | Deep coma, decerebrate rigidity, moribund appearance |

## Venous Angiomas (Developmental Venous Anomaly)

### Etiology

Venous angiomas are considered a subset of developmental venous anomalies that occur because of arrested development. The cause of this arrested development is not known. They are the most common form of vascular malformation and are found at autopsy in approximately 3% of cases [44]. The natural history of venous angiomas is unknown, as diagnosis is made only after surgical intervention [1].

### Pathophysiology

A venous angioma is an extreme variation of veins that drain normal brain tissue within its region of distribution [30]. Venous angiomas consist of primitive embryologic veins that form in a radial pattern and feed a central vein or "collector vein" [44]. The collector vein is often located on the surface of the brain, but it may also be found in the deeper regions [30]. The veins of the angioma drain their respective vascular regions [1]. Normal parenchymal tissue is found between the veins that make up the venous angioma. Venous angiomas are often found near the frontal horns of the ventricles or in the cerebellum [30].

### Presenting Symptoms

Unless combined with another type of vascular malformation, venous angiomas alone rarely become symptomatic. When they do, the presenting problems are seizures or hemorrhage. Both are extremely rare in a venous angioma alone.

In the extremely rare case of rupture of a venous angioma, signs and symptoms of a hemorrhage would include sudden onset of headache, which may be associated with nausea, vomiting, somnolence, hemiparesis, or other focal neurological deficit. The formation of a thrombus in one or more veins can cause local venous hypertension, resulting in a headache. Venous angiomas may also cause seizures [30].

### Diagnostic Tests

Cerebral angiography will define a venous angioma well, but is rarely indicated. Angiography shows the caput medusae pattern (a cluster of veins that resemble a "head of snakes") that drain into a collector vein. The caput medusae originate from a main venous trunk [63]. MRI with and without contrast is now the diagnostic modality of choice and shows the venous angioma along with any other vascular abnormality through multiple imaging sequences. Magnetic resonance venography may be able to detect a venous angioma if it is not too small. CT angiography may also be used; however, it is not effective in detecting commonly associated vascular malformations, such as a cavernous hemangioma, if it is too small [30]. Venous angiomas are detected primarily using neuroimaging, as they are usually not problematic

### Treatment Options

#### Medical Management

Venous angiomas on their own are almost always benign and do not require any form of treatment, unless they are associated with seizures. If seizures are present, neuroimaging should be used to ensure there is no other vascular malformation. If none is present, anticonvulsant medications are used to treat the seizures [30].

#### Surgical Management

Surgical resection of venous angiomas alone, without an associated vascular malformation, is only recommended in cases where a patient has suffered a massive or recurrent hemorrhage due to rupture of the angioma, or if the venous malformation is causing debilitating seizures. Resection of venous malformations yields a risk of venous stroke due to venous congestion, as venous malformations are thought to drain normal brain tissue [30]. Venous angiomas are frequently associated with cavernous malformations that tend to be problematic and often require surgical intervention [30].

## Capillary Angiomas and Telangiectasia

Capillary angiomas and telangiectasias are two distinct entities. They are often mistakenly thought to be interchangeable terms [64].

## Capillary Angiomas

In capillary angiomas, the neural tissue is usually gliotic and contains no neurons. The vessels in angiomas tend to be variable in diameter, thin-walled, and they resemble the smaller vessels seen in cavernous angiomas. Capillary angiomas are found in the posterior fossa, primarily in the pons or medulla, and occasionally in the cerebellum. They are also found in the subependymal deep cortical region, where they are solitary. Capillary angiomas, like telangiectasias, are often discovered as an incidental finding at autopsy. Capillary angiomas may lead to catastrophic hemorrhages because of their location in the brainstem or subependymal region [64].

## Telangiectasias

In cerebral telangiectasias, the parenchyma between the vessels in the telangiectasia is normal and there are normal neurons, a normal concentration of glial cells, and normal fibers with variable ratios, depending on the region of the brain involved. Vessels in telangiectasias tend to be more constant in size and are morphologically consistent with capillaries found in telangiectasias. Telangiectasias, unlike capillary angiomas, tend to be asymptomatic in nature. They do not cause intraparenchymal hemorrhage or neurologic deficits. They do not irritate neurons, and nor do they provoke seizures. Telangiectasias are commonly found in the basis pontis. They are usually discovered as an incidental finding at autopsy [64].

## Cavernous Malformations

## Etiology

Cavernous malformations, also known as cavernous angiomas or cavernous hemangiomas, are vascular lesions that can be asymptomatic or present with varying neurological symptoms. Cavernous malfor-

mations make up 5–13% of all vascular lesions [75]. These lesions are found more frequently with the increased use of imaging studies for surveillance imaging for various disease entities. They are most commonly seen in the third and fifth decade of life and are rare in childhood [14,75]. Fortuna et al., in a retrospective review of cavernomas in children, found a bimodal pattern of distribution at 0–2 years of age and 12–14 years of age [11].

The causes of cavernomas are both familial and sporadic. Although the exact cause of cavernomas is unknown, factors associated with sporadic formations of cavernous malformations are previous irradiation, genetics, and hormones [11,35,54]. The genetic predisposition for cavernomas is associated with an autosomal pattern of inheritance and has been found to be more predominant within the Hispanic population [14,75]. This familial tendency to develop cavernomas has been linked to the CCM 1 locus on the long arm of chromosome 7 in Hispanic families and 7q21-22 in non-Hispanic families [14,75].

## Pathophysiology

Cavernous malformations are vascular lesions that are composed of cystic vascular spaces lined by a single layer of endothelial cells. There is a distinct absence of smooth muscle elastic fibers, which signifies the immaturity of the vessels. The sinusoidal vessels form a compact mass with no intervening neural parenchyma between the vascular structures. The immaturity of the blood vessels, no intervening neural parenchyma, and lack of recognizable arteries and veins, differentiates the cavernoma from other vascular lesions.

The appearance of a cavernous malformation is that of a discrete, well-circumscribed, reddish mass with distinct lobulations. It is a low-flow lesion that lacks an arterial supply. It may have both cystic and calcified components, and is often characteristically described as a cluster of mulberries. Several forms have been identified in childhood. They have been classified as solitary, multiple, iatrogenic, and familial lesions. Cavernous malformations most commonly occur in the supratentorial region and less commonly in the spine and posterior fossa [8,11]. In the cerebral hemisphere, cavernomas have been reported in the parietal lobes, periventricular area, temporal lobes, and occipital lobes. They are generally independent lesions, but have been found to occur with associated venous malformations, specifically developmental venous anomalies [28,35].

Most cavernomas show evidence of recent or remote hemorrhage. They often contain clots and blood products of various stages of evolution within the lesion, as well as calcification and gliosis. These lesions have a propensity to hemorrhage because of the fragility of the sinusoidal channels. Microhemorrhages may not manifest clinically; however, overt hemorrhages result in neurological deterioration. The risk of bleeding of a cavernous malformation is 0.6%, but this increases to 4.5% per year for cavernous malformations with a history of hemorrhage [14,75]. There has been some evidence in the literature to suggest that the location of the cavernous hemorrhage influences the rate of hemorrhage, specifically brainstem cavernomas [35,52,53]. However, this may be more related to the eloquence and sensitivity of the surrounding brain to show clinical events, as opposed to other areas of the brain [35].

Cavernomas have a tendency to grow over time. This is one of the characteristics that differentiate them from other vascular lesions [75]. One of the theories regarding the growth of the cavernoma is the hemorrhagic angiogenic proliferation theory, which suggests that recurrent microhemorrhages are followed by fibrosis, reorganization, or calcification, which leads to growth [14,75]. It has also been theorized that cysts occur with clot absorption and rehemorrhage. The cysts enlarge because of osmotic forces favoring movement of fluid into the cyst cavity. Biological factors, such as estrogen, have also been found to play a role in the growth of cavernous malformations [11,14,75].

## Presenting Symptoms

As previously indicated, cavernomas can be asymptomatic. Those that are symptomatic generally present with seizures, hemorrhage, and neurological deficits. Seizures are the most common presenting symptom in children: 45% of patients with a cavernoma present with seizure, followed by 27% with hemorrhagic syndrome, and 16% with focal neurological deficits [11]. Children experience headaches and neurological deficits less often than adults. The seizures have been theorized to be related to cortical irritation, the presence of calcification, and gliosis around the

surrounding parenchyma, or the accumulation of iron-containing substances produced by silent microhemorrhages [11,75]. Further symptoms such as headache, nausea and vomiting, deterioration in the level of consciousness, and irritability are related to hemorrhage-induced increased ICP. Neurological deficits will be dependent on the location of the cavernoma and can be either acute or progressive. The deficit can be a symptom of overt bleeding or gradual enlargement of the lesion causing the brain to become dysfunctional. Although extremely rare in children, patients with spinal cavernomas may present with hydrocephalus and myelopathies secondary to small hemorrhages and a spinal cord compression. Progressive paraparesis and sensory changes are often seen in symptomatic patients with spinal cavernous malformations [33].

## Diagnostic Imaging

Cavernomas are detectable both on CT and on MRI; however, MRI, with its high resolution, is the diagnostic tool of choice for diagnosing cavernous malformations and for their follow-up. Noncontrast CTs show cavernous malformations as focal areas of increased density, representing calcium or blood within the brain without mass effect. On MRI, cavernous malformations are best seen on T2-weighted images, which show high-intensity lobulated lesions surrounded by a low-intensity hemosiderin ring, an appearance that resembles popcorn. Hemorrhages can produce areas of encephalomalacia, cyst, or calcification. The absence of large flow voids, suggestive of feeding arteries or draining veins, suggests strongly the diagnosis of cavernous malformation (Fig. 9.5). MRI gradient echo imaging, which shows hemosiderin more prominently, is performed to reveal other lesions elsewhere in the brain. Cavernous malformations can be classified into four types based on their appearance on MRI (Table 9.7). They are not seen on angiography.

## Treatment

There is no standard treatment for children with cavernous malformations. As each child is an individual, each cavernoma needs to be assessed on an individual basis using a risk–benefit approach. It has been gener-

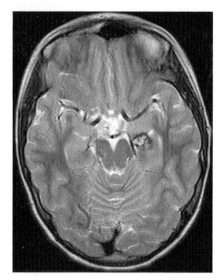

**Fig. 9.5.** MRI of a cavernoma

because the curative rate from seizures with a surgical procedure is between 65 and 100% [11,33]. Surgical management is generally considered for symptomatic lesions, lesions showing growth, and those with large hemorrhages [14,75]. The location of the lesion near eloquent or superficial areas of the brain needs to be taken into consideration when deciding upon surgical management. The location would impact the surgical risk and associated morbidity of the surgical resection.

The use of stereotactic radiosurgery for the treatment of cavernomas remains controversial. There have been studies pertaining to the adult population using radiation for inaccessible lesions [72]. Generally, the role of radiation surgery remains unclear in the pediatric population.

 **Outcomes**

**Table 9.7.** Classification of cavernous malformation based on magnetic resonance imaging

| Type I | Subacute bleed hyperintense on T1-weighted sequences |
|---|---|
| Type II | Popcorn appearance, heterogeneous T1- and T2-weighted sequences |
| Type III | Isointense/hypointense T1- and T2-weighted images, chronic blood products |
| Type IV | Tiny punctuate foci, hypointense T1- and T2-weighted sequences |

ally accepted that cavernomas found incidentally, and that are asymptomatic, do not require treatment. Surveillance for these lesions is recommended with follow-up MRI.

Treatment options for a symptomatic cavernoma can be either medical or surgical. Medical management, or conservative therapy, involves the use of antiepileptic drugs for seizures, treatment for headache, and physiotherapy. Medical management is considered for lesions with medically controlled seizures, lesions in critical areas without severe symptoms, and cases of multiple cavernous malformations for which the actual symptomatic lesion is unidentified [14,75]. When considering medical/conservative management, one needs to take into account the cumulative risk of hemorrhage for the child, the lifetime costs associated with antiepileptics, and the long-term effects of being on antiepileptics. This becomes controversial

Patients who undergo complete surgical resection of their cavernous malformation are relieved of their symptoms [33]. The literature regarding seizure resolution indicated that 65–100% of patients show resolution of their seizures postoperatively [11,33]. In a pediatric series, Fortuna et al. found that 73% of patients were cured from their seizures, 20% had improvement and 3% experienced worsening symptoms [11]. Location of the cavernoma will also affect the outcome. Deep cavernomas, or those involving the brainstem, are associated with significant morbidity and mortality. In a review of 20 pediatric patients with brainstem cavernomas who underwent surgical excision, 6 had excellent results, 10 had good results with neurological improvement, and 2 had worsening of symptoms [8].

Recovery of the neurological deficit is dependent of the number of hemorrhagic events. Tung et al. reported that of patients who had experienced a single hemorrhagic event, 80% experienced a transient deficit [72]. Porter et al. report that one-third of patients experiencing an event will recover fully, one-third will have no significant recovery, and one-third will have partial recovery [52].

For patients with spinal cavernomas that present with hydrocephalus, the hydrocephalus may resolve postresection [9,58]. With regard to functional ability postresection, the more functional the patient is preoperatively, the more likely the patient is to do well after surgical excision of the lesion.

## Moyamoya Syndrome

### Etiology

Moyamoya is a rare vascular disorder that leads to irreversible blockage of the ICAs. It is a chronic occlusive cerebrovascular disorder of unknown etiology that was initially reported and discovered in Japan [69]. The annual incidence of moyamoya is 1 per 1,000,000, with the highest prevalence in Japan [15]. Moyamoya in Japanese means "puff of smoke" and was named this due to the characteristic appearance of abnormally fine collateral vessels on angiography. The disease is found predominantly in children, has a bimodal presentation at the first and fourth decade of life, and has a female preponderance of 1:1.8 (male/female ratio). Although its exact etiology is unknown, the disease has a genetic link carried on chromosomes 1–22 [26]. Other factors associated with moyamoya have been cranial radiation, Down syndrome, neurofibromatosis, sickle cell anemia, congenital cardiac conditions, renal artery stenosis, meningitis , tuberous sclerosis, and being of Asian descent [50].

### Pathophysiology

Moyamoya disease is characterized by progressive intracranial vascular stenoses due to thickening of the intima of the vessel. It is commonly seen in the distal carotid artery, proximal anterior artery, and the middle cerebral arteries [50]. The progressive narrowing leads to a decrease in arterial blood flow, resulting in cerebral ischemia. The brain induces the growth of net-like moyamoya vessels in order to establish collateral blood flow to areas distal to the site of vascular stenosis [20]. Although the exact cause of the thickening of the intima is unclear, it has been suggested that it is related to elevated basic fibroblast growth factor, platelet activation, and systemic alterations in cellular function [50].

### Presenting Symptoms

Children with moyamoya present with ischemic symptoms, whereas adult patients tend to present with cerebral hemorrhage [31]. It manifests itself as monoparesis, hemiparesis, sensory deficits, and dysphasia [77]. Initially children will develop transient ischemic attacks (TIAs) that can progress to cerebral infarction. TIAs can be precipitated by crying, coughing, hyperventilation, or straining, which ultimately reduces cerebral blood flow. In general, 40% of children present with TIAs, 40% present with stroke, and 80% present with extremity weakness [50]. Repeated TIAs are manifested predominantly by seizure (20–30%) and motor hemiparesis (70–80%), as well as headache and speech difficulties, which are strongly indicative, although not pathognomonic, of moyamoya [15].

### Diagnostic Test

Radiologic criteria for moyamoya are: (1) stenosis or occlusion at the terminal portion of the ICA and proximal portion of the anterior cerebral artery and middle cerebral artery; (2) abnormal vascular network near the arterial occlusion, and (3) bilateral involvement [15]. Moyamoya had been traditionally diagnosed with angiography; however, multiple diagnostic techniques can be used to diagnose moyamoya. This disease entity can be well characterized radiologically on either MRI or MRA (Fig. 9.6). CT scans can show cerebral ischemia, but will not visualize the abnormal vessels. MRIs show flow voids and MRAs show stenosis of the cerebral arteries. Positron emission tomography (PET) and single photon emission CT (SPECT) are diagnostic tests used that provide important information regarding the cerebral hemodynamics. The findings are indicative of cerebral perfusion and metabolism, depicting areas of ischemia, which are important when planning surgical intervention. Electroencephalograms can also be useful in moyamoya disease. Characteristic findings are a "rebuild-up" of slow waves after cessation of hyperventilation that relate to decreased perfusion reserve of the ischemic brain [15].

### Treatment Options

Currently there is no curative medical/surgical treatment for moyamoya. Treatment is based on symptom management and begins with medical management. Initially, when the child presents with their first TIA, they may be started on antiplatelet agents, anticoagulants, nonsteroidal anti-inflammatory drugs (NSAIDs), and calcium channel blockers [50]. Treat-

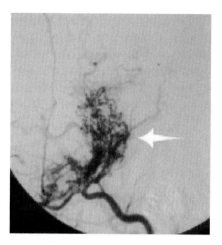

**Fig. 9.6.** Angiogram of a moyamoya "puff of smoke"

ment transitions to surgical as ischemic episodes progress. The goal of surgical therapy is to increase the blood supply to the hypoperfused brain by establishing collateral circulation for the ischemic brain to prevent cerebral infarct. Multiple types of bypass procedures have been effective for moyamoya and can be classified as direct or indirect bypass. Ultimately, bypass procedures bring blood to the brain and bypass areas of blockage.

Direct bypass, namely superficial temporal artery–middle cerebral artery anastomosis is a procedure in which a scalp artery is directly sutured to a brain surface artery and burr holes are place in the skull to allow for regrowth. This procedure is generally not used in children as they often do not have a recipient cerebral artery large enough for anastomosis and are at increased risk for stroke [73].

Indirect bypass involves leptomeningeal anastomosis from the external carotid artery directly onto the ischemic brain. Indirect can be either single or multiple, depending on the number of vessels used. Single procedures, such as encephaluduroarteriosyangiosis and encephalomyoarteriosyangiosis, are limited in their abilities to form collaterals and hence cover the ischemic area. The failure rate for a single procedure is 20–30% [20]. Hence, multiple indirect bypass procedures have been developed to improve the possibility of revascularization and have a success rate of 94% [20]

Postoperatively, success is determined by the change in frequency and clinical presentation of the TIAs in the patient. Postoperative imaging entails angiograms (during the follow-up period), MRA to demonstrate collateral revascularization, and SPECT and PET scans to show improvements in cerebral perfusion.

## Outcomes

Without surgical intervention, the prognosis is poor, with the majority of individuals experiencing mental decline and multiple strokes because of the progressive narrowing of arteries [20]. Without surgical management, the incidence of TIAs may decrease but the intellectual and motor disturbances tend to increase. Outcome is dependent on the individual, as it varies from patient to patient. Patients who have sustained extensive ischemic morbidity preoperatively do not recover their abilities postoperatively. If sufficient collaterals form, TIAs may decrease or disappear within months; however, this is difficult to predict as patient factors influencing collateral formation is unknown.

## Nursing Care

Close monitoring after surgery is vital in these children. After surgery, children should be initially managed in an intensive care unit environment. Patients should be sedated and remain normotensive and well hydrated. In the immediate postoperative period, neurologic status, arterial blood pressure reading, and fluid status should be carefully monitored to prevent serious ischemic complications.

## Patient and Family Education

Family members should be educated on signs and symptoms of cerebral ischemia, cerebrovascular accident, and seizures, as well as the importance of follow-up with the neurosurgeon. Follow-up angiography is done during the 1st year after surgery in order to evaluate the growth of cerebral circulation.

## Nursing Care for Vascular Brain Lesions

### Monitoring of Neurological Status

Careful monitoring of neurological status and vital signs is critical in assessing the child with a vascular anomaly. Nurses should monitor for signs of increased ICP by observing for signs of changes in the child's level of consciousness, abnormal cranial nerve finding, abnormal eye movements, papillary abnormalities, focal motor deficits, and increasing headache. Signs of headache and focal neurological deficits may indicate rebleed or vasospasm. Consistent documentation and communication of the patient's neurological status must exist amongst all caregivers assessing the child so that subtle changes in neurological status can be appreciated. Any changes indicative of worsening neurological function needs to be reported to the neurosurgical team.

### Cerebral Perfusion – Monitoring and Maintenance

Cerebral perfusion requires careful maintenance and monitoring. Specific neurological signs of decreased cerebral perfusion include decreasing level of consciousness, complaints of diplopia, headache, and blurred vision. To increase cerebral perfusion, the administration of hypervolemic and/or hypertensive therapy may be required. In addition to monitoring for signs of decreased cerebral perfusion, children should be monitored for signs and symptoms of vasospasm, including the insidious onset of confusion, disorientation, focal neurologic deficits corresponding to a specific vascular territory, and decreased level of consciousness. It is also important to maintain the child's blood pressure within the parameters indicated as per institutional protocols. Administration of hypertensive medications and vasopressors may be required and, if used, their effect must be carefully monitored.

### Monitoring for Seizures

Children with vascular lesions have a high propensity for seizure activity in both the preoperative and postoperative phase. Surgical intervention may involve stimulation of the parenchyma that in turn can provoke seizure activity in the postoperative stage, therefore necessitating careful observation of the child for seizure activity. If the child is seizing, anticonvulsants are administered with subsequent monitoring of therapeutic drug levels to ensure adequate dosing. It is important to educate the family and child regarding seizures and their management.

### Management of Environmental Stress

To avoid complications related to vascular lesions, precautions should be instituted to decrease the environmental stimulus and minimize stress. Depending on the institution, patients may have an extended stay in the critical care unit during their postoperative period to allow for the child to remain ventilated, sedated, and hemodynamically stable. Further precautions include reducing edema by maintaining the head of the bed at 30°, maintaining the child on bed rest, and minimizing stimuli such as bright light, noise, anxiety, and pain. Precautions should also include limiting activities to avoid elevations in blood pressure and ICP. Administration of stool softeners is important to minimize an increase in ICP as a result of straining. Children who experience extreme agitation may require medication to reduce their level of agitation.

### Management of Pain and Anxiety

Pain management needs to be addressed in the postoperative period. Obtaining a child's pain history is critical in helping to gauge their response to pain. Speak with the child and his/her parents to determine how they have responded to pain in the past and what modes of pain management were successful and unsuccessful. This will help in the assessment and treatment of the child's pain. The use of age-appropriate pain scales (e.g., the Oucher scale, Faces Scale, or numeric rating scale), observation of physical manifestations such as increased blood pressure, increased respiration rate, alteration in mood or behavior, and monitoring of vital signs should be completed on an ongoing basis. Particular attention should be paid to signs of worsening of headache. Pain management is individualized and can vary from acetaminophen to opioids, depending on institution and surgeon preference. NSAID medications can inhibit platelet aggregation and prolong bleeding time. For this reason, they may not be used in patients with vascular anomalies, particularly if they have had a hemorrhage or are in the immediate postoperative period. The nurse should discuss concerns regarding pain management with the neurosurgical team. In addition to the administration of analgesics, techniques should be employed to provide nonpharmacological modes of pain management through methods such as distraction (e.g., engage in therapeutic play with the Child Life specialist, experience a visit with a therapy dog, listen to favorite music, establishment of a quiet, dark environment that is conducive to rest, blowing of bubbles).

Anxiety often accompanies pain and can intensify pain. To reduce anxiety in children, it is important to explain all procedures that will occur, ensure parental presence when possible for comfort, and provide an anxiolytic if clinically indicated. Risks in masking the symptoms of increased ICP must be weighed against the benefits of providing an anxiolytic. Sedatives such as chloral hydrate, pentobarbital, midazolam, diazepam, and lorazepam may be administered to manage anxiety. As for opioid administration, cardiorespiratory equipment must be available at the bedside to manage respiratory distress or oversedation (Table 9.8). Ready access to benzodiazepine antagonists is essential [25].

### Management of Nausea and Vomiting

Children often experience nausea and vomiting postoperatively as well as in nonoperative situations. Administration of antiemetics such as dimenhydrinate, metoclopramide, and ondansetron may be effective. The nurse should not administer these drugs repeatedly if there is suspicion that the child's nausea and vomiting are due to increased ICP. Intravenous fluids may be required if the child is unable to take adequate fluid orally. For some patients in the initial postoperative period their intravenous fluids are run above maintenance to allow for adequate cerebral perfusion.

**Table 9.8.** Bromage sedation scale

| | |
|---|---|
| 0 | Awake |
| 1 | Occasionally drowsy, easily arousable |
| 2 | Frequently drowsy, easily arousable |
| 3 | Somnolent, difficult to arouse |
| S | Normal sleep |

With prolonged intravenous hydration, electrolytes need be closely monitored.

### Monitoring for Signs of Infection

Postoperatively, the child should be observed of signs of infection. These include fever, discharge from the wound, redness or swelling around the incision site, stiff neck, vomiting, irritability, and headache. Parents need to be educated regarding the signs and symptoms of infection.

### General Postoperative Care

Other needs that require attention include an adequate diet, good pulmonary care, mobilization issues, rehabilitation plans, skin care, and adequate rest and emotional care. Referral to other professional services such as social work, occupational therapy, physical therapy, speech pathology, and Child Life therapy should be initiated if clinically indicated.

### Patient and Family Education

Always assess for the level of readiness in the parent of a child when providing teaching regarding neurovascular disease and the treatment. The level of anxiety may prohibit the intake of information and will often require a step-by-step approach to information exchange and teaching. Repeating and re-explaining the child's condition and treatment is often required to ensure adequate understanding by parents and children. Teaching aids in the form of handouts, diagrams, web-based teaching tools, or physical models of the brain are excellent tools to use in helping parents and children understand their condition. Allowing parents and children to view the child's own neuroimaging is often a very effective way to teach about the child's condition.

Parents and children (if age appropriate) should be provided with information on their vascular malformation in both written and verbal forms. In situations where the child is being managed medically by observation, the parents and children (if age appropriate) should be taught to watch for any potential signs and symptoms such as seizure activity, or signs of hemorrhage such as severe headache, and the emergency action they need to take. Thorough instructions regarding activity restrictions need to be reviewed.

Parents and children should be taught emergency management of seizures – particularly prolonged seizures lasting greater than 5 min. Education regarding a prescribed anticonvulsant medication, along with side effects and adverse reactions, should be reviewed. Assessment of the parent's level of understanding should be completed on a daily basis and opportunities for ongoing teaching need to be included in the daily care of the child.

At the time of discharge, it is important to provide written information that indicates the exact name of the child's condition, the type of treatment the child received (including the surgical procedure), the medications required for ongoing management, instructions for dressing and wound care, information on level of activity, follow-up appointments, and contact numbers in case of emergency or questions. In situations where ongoing care will be required in the home, homecare arrangements will need to be made. This includes providing the homecare agency with accurate and detailed instructions on care and the name of a nurse the homecare agency can contact for further advice if required. If a parent or child is to perform ongoing care in the home, teaching of the procedure and opportunities for return demonstrations must be provided during the child's admission.

When providing Web-based information to patents and children, ensure that the information comes for a credible site. Warn parents and children about Web sites that may provide inaccurate information or that lack credibility. Provide families with Web sites that are known to be credible. For a list of Web sites pertaining to neurovascular disease in children see Appendix 9.1

## Spinal Arteriovenous Malformations

Spinal vascular malformations in children are rare. They consist of the same malformations seen in the brain and include cavernous malformations, AVFs, and AVMs. The majority of spinal vascular malformations seen in the pediatric population are AVMs [43,49,59,68].

## Etiology

AVMs in the spine are similar in structure to their cerebral counterparts. They are congenital malformations that result from failure of arteriovenous connections to differentiate properly early in embryogenesis [43,59,68,73]. An AVM is a tangle of arteries and veins without the typical intervening capillaries. The result is a so-called "high-flow" lesion where blood is shunted directly and quickly from the arterial to the venous side [49,59,68,73]. AVMs of the spine can have varying numbers of feeding arteries and draining veins. The number and size of vessels involved can vary considerably. At the core of these vessels is the nidus [48,68,73]. Simply stated, the nidus is where the arterial side meets the venous. A nidus can be small and compact, or large and diffuse. AVMs in children have been shown to increase in size over time secondary to increased flow through poorly differentiated vessels and the ability to recruit collateral vessels or proliferate new ones [73]. Poorly differentiated and dilated vessels in an AVM have a propensity for hemorrhage. The overall risk of hemorrhage is 2–4% per year and the incidence is cumulative with age [73]. Children with spinal AVMs therefore have a high lifetime risk of hemorrhage [73]. In children, hemorrhage tends to occur more often in the second decade of life than in the first.

AVMs of the spine can exist with a familial tendency. They can also be associated with syndromes, as mentioned previously in this chapter [73,49]. Most occurrences, however, are often the first within a family. Like their cerebral counterparts, spinal AVMs can have an associated aneurysm; however, such occurrences are rare [59,68,73].

## Pathophysiology

Spinal AVMs can occur anywhere along the spinal axis and the location of the AVM relative to cord parenchyma can vary. AVMs can arise from vessels on the surface of the cord or within the cord parenchyma itself. AVMs with the nidus involving the cord parenchyma are called intramedullary AVMs and are the most frequently occurring in children (Fig. 9.7) [59]. They derive their arterial blood supply directly from the spinal cord vasculature, either the anterior or posterior spinal arteries, and often involve very high blood flow and high pressure [49,68].

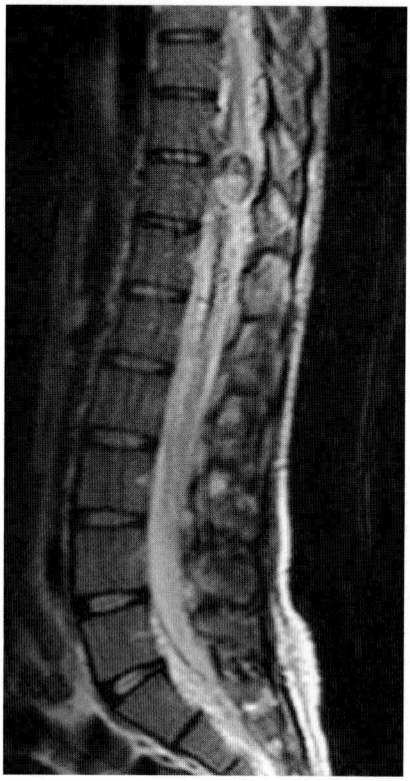

**Fig. 9.7.** Intramedullary arteriovenous malformation

Extradural-intradural AVMs can involve not only the cord itself, but the surrounding tissues including the covering meninges, vertebrae, and surrounding soft tissue [59]. These AVMs can have an intramedullary component to them, but often are on the surface of the cord. Their arterial blood supply typically comes from multiple medullary arteries, which in turn are branches off the spinal arteries [48]. They can be large with a large number of arterial feeders and are associated with very high flow [59,61,68]. When the AVM involves all tissue types, it is referred to as Cobb's syndrome [59,61,68]. These are very rare, but do occur more frequently in the pediatric population than in adults.

AVMs affecting the terminal portion of the spinal cord are called conus arteriovenous malformations. They involve the conus medullaris and the cauda equina. The blood supply tends to be from one or more of the spinal arteries and they are also a high flow lesion [59].

Spinal AVMs can produce symptoms secondary to hemorrhage, compression, vascular steal, and venous congestion [48,68,59,73]. Hemorrhage can occur in one catastrophic event or in repeated smaller ones. Symp-toms produced will vary depending on the location and extent of the hemorrhage. Compression on the cord or nerve roots can result from hemorrhage, the mass of the AVM itself, or from largely dilated vessels. Compression can also result from surrounding edema that may be a result of hemorrhage or cord ischemia. Vascular steal is a result of blood being shunted into the malformation and away from arteries supplying the surrounding healthy tissue. Vascular steal leads to ischemia, which can result in cell death and cord atrophy [48]. Venous congestion leads to venous hypertension, which can impair perfusion pressure to the cord by causing ischemia. It can also progress to venous thrombosis, causing a spinal cord infarct [48].

## Presenting Signs and Symptoms

The presenting clinical picture is dependent on the location, size, and the pathophysiology of the AVM. The majority of children will present with an acute hemorrhage. The hemorrhage may be into the subarachnoid space, into the cord parenchyma, or both. Signs and symptoms of an acute hemorrhage include sudden onset of back or neck pain, extremity weakness or loss of function, sensory changes, and bowel and bladder dysfunction. The pain and neurologic deterioration may be nonspecific and subtle in onset, causing the symptoms to be overlooked [49].

Compression and ischemia can also present with pain and loss of motor and sensory function. Pain from compression or ischemia is more likely to be present in affected limbs. The exact location and nature of pain and neurologic deficit is dependent on the location of the AVM. For example, an AVM in the cervicothoracic area will cause symptoms in the upper extremities, whereas an AVM in the conus will cause lower extremity and bowel and bladder dysfunction. Motor dysfunction can range from weakness to paralysis in the affected extremities. Tone may also be affected and can be increased or decreased. Sensory manifestations can result in diminished or heightened perception of stimuli. Diminished sensation can result in a loss of discrimination to touch, temperature, sharpness, and proprioception. Hypersensitivity can result in pain with minimal stimulation. Paresthesias, such as tingling and numbness, may be present. Because of the fragility of the spinal cord, most patients will present with some degree of neurologic dysfunction. The nature and severity of the dysfunction depends on the location of the AVM, presence of hemorrhage, and damage done to the cord.

## Cavernous Malformations and Arteriovenous Fistulas of the Spine

Cavernous malformations of the spine are rare in children but do occur. They have been described to occur more frequently in children who have received spinal radiation and typically present secondary to signs and symptoms following repeated hemorrhages [59]. Occasionally, they are an incidental finding [59]. Cavernous malformations have a typical appearance on MRI, with a focal area of abnormal signal with surrounding hemorrhage of various ages and hemosiderin (Fig. 9.8) [59]. They are angiographically occult. The only treatment option is surgery and is reserved for cases of an easily accessible lesion or significant neurologic compromise.

AVFs of the spine are similar in physiologic structure to their cerebral counterparts. They can occur anywhere on the spine; however, certain types do occur more frequently in the thoracic region [68]. They tend to occur on the surface of the cord versus within the cord parenchyma [62,68]. They can exist outside, within, or beneath the dura, and can occur on the anterior or posterior surface of the cord [68]. The location and extent of shunting dictates the presenting symptoms [68]. Presentation with acute hemorrhage is less common in AVFs than AVMs. Presentation is usually progressive myelopathy and is the result of cord compression or vascular steal [63]. Treatment of spinal AVFs is most often accomplished with endovascular techniques alone. Surgery is required less often [63].

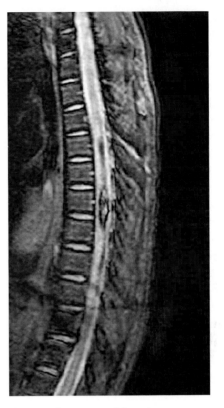

**Fig. 9.8.** Cavernoma of the spine

MRA can be performed at the time of the MRI and may be useful in helping to identify the anatomy of the malformation. However, selective angiography remains the test of choice in defining the vascular architecture of an AVM, and is absolutely necessary for treatment planning [43,48,49,73]. In the case of an acute hemorrhage, angiography may be postponed until after the clot has resolved. The presence of the clot can make defining the structure of the AVM difficult.

### Diagnostic Tests

All patients with a suspected cord lesion will undergo an MRI of the spine. The MRI will often be performed with and without gadolinium to help differentiate an AVM from other vascular abnormalities or tumor. The MRI will define not only the location and nature of the malformation, but also the presence of blood and its location. The MRI can help determine if the blood appears to be acute or subacute. It will also further define any associated pathology such as an intravascular thrombosis, syrinx, associated cord edema, or cord atrophy [43,48,49,59].

### Treatment Options

As with cranial AVMs, the goal of treatment is complete obliteration of the malformation to eliminate the risk of future hemorrhage. However, because of the vulnerability of the spinal cord, this is not always possible. Treatment options include conservative management, surgical excision, and embolization; often, a combination of these options is used.

Surgery in the acute presentation phase is typically reserved for children who are experiencing continued neurologic deterioration, and where a need for decompression of the cord exists. Surgery may be staged, with the first being evacuation of the clot. Then, after further work-up with angiography and stabilization of neurologic function, further surgery may be done in an attempt to resect the residual AVM. Sometimes, especially in the case of small AVMs, the AVM may be removed with the clot at the time of the original surgery. AVMs that sit close to, or on the cord surface, with a compact nidus, are most amenable to surgery. Some AVMs, given their location and relationship with the cord, are not surgically treatable.

The potential risks of surgery include new hemorrhage and injury to the spinal cord or nerve roots. Both of these would result in worsening neurologic function. There is also a risk of infection and postoperative CSF leak.

As with cerebral AVMs, endovascular embolization is an important treatment option. Embolization is rarely solely curative with spinal AVMs, but may be the only treatment option in lesions that are surgically inaccessible [59]. Embolization is often used prior to surgery to decrease the number of vessels in the AVM, thus decreasing the risk of hemorrhage. Embolization in the spine involves the same technique and materials used with cerebral lesions. The same risks of post embolization hemorrhage, venous congestion, and edema exist. All of these could lead to further cord injury and loss of function [43,49].

When a child presents with acute hemorrhage, a conservative approach is often taken initially if they are neurologically stable. During this phase, symptoms are managed and neurologic function is allowed to stabilize. Also during this phase, the clot is allowed to resolve so that a full diagnostic work-up can take place. Angiography and treatment planning can proceed most effectively after the hemorrhage has resolved. All treatments pose a risk of causing new deficits or worsening existing ones. Therefore, careful planning and weighing of the risk:benefit ratio will help to determine an individual treatment course for each patient.

## Nursing Care

The most important aspect of nursing care for children with spinal AVMs is serial neurologic examinations. The frequency of exams will vary dependent on the stage of treatment and should be documented thoroughly. Neurologic examination in children is detailed elsewhere in this book (Chap. 1). The key point of the neurologic exam is to know the child's baseline (or pretreatment) deficits and be able to note changes from that. Following surgery, or embolization, it is critical to note changes in existing deficits and whether the changes are for the better or worse. Good and descriptive communication must exist between all caregivers assessing the child so that subtle changes can be noted. Any sign of worsening neurologic function should be reported to the neurosurgical team.

Pain management is important throughout all stages of the patient's care. Pain is most acute following the initial hemorrhage or surgery. In these instances, a combination of narcotics and NSAIDs are typically used. A muscle relaxant such as diazepam may be added if muscle spasms are problematic.

Radicular pain, or pain originating from the cord or nerves, can be particularly painful and difficult to control. Narcotics often are not completely affective in these situations. Certain neuroepileptic drugs, such as gabapentin (neurontin), can be beneficial in helping to control this type of pain.

Depending on the location of the spinal surgery, the neurosurgeon may request that the patient remain flat for a period of time, typically 24 h. The purpose of this restriction is to help prevent a CSF leak. To operate on the spinal cord, the dura must be opened. It is sewn closed, but CSF can easily leak through until the incision has sealed. Typically, the patient can lie on their side, prone, or supine, as long as they remain flat. Other positioning or activity restrictions may be imposed dependent on the location of the incision and nature of the surgery. These are usually meant to help protect the integrity of the incision and prevent CSF leaks.

The incision must be monitored for signs of drainage, particularly for a CSF leak. Some drainage from the incision in the first 8–12 h following surgery can be normal. Persistent drainage increases the risk of infection. It is important to note the character of the drainage and identify signs of a CSF leak, such as those that appear watery or leave a ring sign. A CSF leak can also present itself as a swelling under the incision. Patients with a CSF leak will often experience a severe headache accompanied by nausea, dizziness, and photophobia. The symptoms are often worse when the patient is upright and improve when lying down. Treating a CSF leak may include resuturing the incision if there is an external leak. A conservative approach of strict bed rest is often tried first. In some cases a lumbar drain may be placed to drain CSF and encourage sealing of the leak. On rare occasions, the leak must be repaired surgically.

Positioning and mobility are essential components of nursing care. Care must be taken to ensure frequent turning and range of motion, especially in children who have paralysis or have positioning and activity restrictions. Children should begin mobilizing as soon as it is cleared by the neurosurgery team.

Children who have undergone angiography with embolization will have a brief period of immobilization. Typically, the child is required to lie flat for 6 h following the procedure to prevent bleeding from the arterial puncture site and decrease the risk of thrombus formation. Postembolization care involves serial neurologic checks to monitor for signs of complications as the hemodynamics in the AVM change. It is important to monitor perfusion in the limb where arterial access was gained. Serial checks of pulses and perfusion distal to the puncture site are necessary to monitor for signs of a clot.

Many children who present with spinal AVMs present with neurologic deficits. These deficits may improve or possibly resolve with treatment. However, a significant number of these children will have neurologic deficits that do not completely resolve and, therefore, will need initiation of therapies and involvement of the rehabilitation team. Physical and occupational therapy should be consulted and involved from the onset of care. Other disciplines, such as urology, may be needed depending on the exact deficits. The sooner a multidisciplinary team is brought together to address each child's specific needs, the sooner discharge planning can become a reality.

Paying attention to the emotional care is an aspect that should not be overlooked. Many of these children will present with new and life-altering deficits. Coping may be difficult due to anxiety and pain. It is important to monitor how the patient and their family are dealing with the situation and offer assistance at an early juncture. Counseling may be helpful. Anger and depression are not uncommon, especially as the treatment course progresses. Providing encouragement to the patient and family is important.

## Outcomes

Complete obliteration of the spinal AVM is not always possible. If a residual AVM is present, so is a continued risk for hemorrhage. Presenting deficits are often permanent due to the fragility of the spinal cord, however, neurologic improvement can continue over several weeks to months.

Family education should focus on not only the disease process and treatments, but also on the deficits the child may have and how life adaptations may be possible. The patient and family will rely on the healthcare team to guide them in addressing such issues as mobility and care at home and at school. There may be a need for adaptive equipment or learning new bowel and bladder management. Good communication between the multidisciplinary team and the family is essential.

## Conclusions

Neurovascular disease in children is generally the result of a congenital lesion, and although each specific type of malformation is uncommon, vascular malformations as a whole are seen regularly in the pediatric neurosurgery population. Lesions can become symptomatic at any time and have the potential to cause lasting, life-altering affects.

It is important for the attending nurse to have an understanding of neurovascular malformations, their treatment, and potential outcomes in order to provide these patients with the best possible care. Treatment of neurovascular diseases in children is changing and improving at a rapid rate, and outcomes for the more severe disorders are strikingly different today compared to a decade ago. Keeping abreast of current information will allow the nurse to provide better care and support to patients and families affected by neurovascular disease.

## Appendix 9.1

### Neurovascular Websites for Parents

www.birthmarks.org/info.asp
(Arkansas Children's Hospital site f)
www.novanews.org
National Organization of Vascular Anomalies
www.brainandspine.org.uk/information/publications/brain_and_spine
www.sickkids.ca/childphysiology/
Excellent site for learning about brain anatomy and physiology
www.cincinnatichildrens.org/health/info/vascular/diagnose
http://neurosurgery.mgh.harvard.edu/neurovascular/

## Pediatric Practice Pearls

- VGAM typically present in neonates with high-output cardiac failure, and during infancy with hydrocephalus, seizures, and (rarely) hemorrhage. Headaches tend to be the presenting symptom in older children and adults. Older children may also present with focal seizures and developmental delay.

- Intracranial aneurysms in children are not an incidental finding

- Increased or new drainage from the incision, accompanied by headache, nausea or vomiting, can signal a CSF leak.

- The Pediatric Glasgow Coma scale should be used when documenting a neurological examination.

- Use appropriate pain scales and include the Child Life team whenever possible.

- Narcotics alone are rarely successful in treating neuropathic pain.

- Siblings are often profoundly affected by the child's illness. They need to be included in teaching sessions (if age appropriate) so that they may gain an understanding of their sibling's condition. They need to be included in the illness experience and their informational needs should be met.

## References

1. Abe M, Hagihara N, Tabuchi K, Uchino A, Miyasaka Y (2003) Histologically classified venous angiomas of the brain: a controversy. Neurol Med Chir (Tokyo) 43:1–11
2. Ali MJ, Bendok B, Rosenblatt S, et al (2003) Recurrence of pediatric cerebral arteriovenous malformations after angiographically documented resection. Pediatr Neurosurg 39:32–38
3. Blaser SI, Illner A, Castillo M, Hedlund GL, Osborn AG (2003) Pocket Radiologist PedsNeuro Top 100 Diagnoses (1st edn). WB Saunders, Utah
4. Cavanagh SJ, Gordon VL (2002) Grading scales used in the management of aneurismal subarachnoid hemorrhage: a critical review. J Neurosci Nurs 34:288–295
5. Cheng A, Williams BA, Sivrahan BV (eds) (2003) The HSC Handbook of Pediatrics (10th edn). Elsevier, Saunders, Toronto, ON
6. Chevret L, Durand P, Alvarez H, Lambert V, Caeymax L, Rodesch G, Devictor D, Lasjaunias P (2002) Prognosis significance of hemodynamic parameters in neonates presenting with severe heart failure owing to vein of Galen arteriovenous malformations. Intens Care Med 28:1126–1130
7. Deeg K, Scarf J (1990) Colour Doppler imaging of arteriovenous malformation of the vein of Galen in a newborn. Neuroradiology 32:60–63
8. DiRocco C, Iannelli A, Tamburrini G (1996) Cavernomas of the central nervous system in children. Acta Neurochir 138:1267–1274
9. Drucker DE (2006) Neurologic disorders. In: Nettina S (ed) Lippincott Manual of Nursing Practice (8th edn). Lippincott Williams Wilkins, Philadelphia, pp 465–557
10. Elixson EM (1992) Intracerebral arteriovenous malformations presenting as neonatal congestive heart failure. Crit Care Nurs Clin North Am 4:537–542
11. Fortuna A, Ferrante L, Acqui L, Mastronardi L, Acqui M, d'Addetta R (1989) Cerebral cavernous angioma in children. Childs Nerv Syst 5:201–207
12. Frawley GP, Dargaville PA, Mitchell PJ, Tress BM, Loughnan P (2002) Clinical course and medical management of neonates with severe cardiac failure related to vein of Galen malformation. Arch Dis Child Fetal Neonatal Ed 87:144–149
13. Friedman DM, Verma R, Madrid M, Wisoff JH, Berenstein A (1993) Recent improvement in outcome using transcatheter embolization techniques for neonatal aneurysmal malformations of the vein of Galen. Pediatrics 91:583–596
14. Frim DM, Gupta N, Scott RM (2001) Cavernous malformations. In: McLone DG (ed) Pediatric Neurosurgery. Surgery of the Developing Nervous System. Saunders, Philadelphia, pp 1097–1104
15. Fukui M (1997) Current state of study on Moyamoya disease in Japan. Surg Neurol 47:138–43
16. Fullerton HJ, Aminoff AR, Ferriero DM, Gupta N, Dowd CF (2003) Neurodevelopmental outcome after endovascular treatment of vein of Galen. Neurology 61:1386–1390
17. Gailloud P, O'Riordan DP, Burger I, Levrier O, Jallo G, Tamargo RJ, Murphy KJ, Lehmann CU, (2005) Diagnosis and management of vein of Galen aneurysmal malformations. J Perinatol 25:542–551
18. Gold AP, Ransohoff J, Carter S (1964) Vein of Galen malformation. Acta Neurol Scand 40:1–31
19. Griffiths PD, Blaser S, Armstrong D, et al (1998) Cerebellar arteriovenous malformations in children. Neuroradiology 40:324–331
20. Hannon K (1996) Pial synangiosis for treatment of Moyamoya syndrome in children. AORN J 64:540–560
21. Hoh B, Ogilvy C, Butler W, et al (2000) Multimodality treatment of nongalenic arteriovenous malformations in pediatric patients. Neurosurgery 47:346–358
22. Horgan M, Florma J, Spetzler RF (2006) Surgical treatment of arteriovenous malformations in children. In: Alexander M, Spetzler RF (eds) Pediatric Neurovascular Disease: Surgical, Endovascular, and Medical Management. Thieme, New York, pp 104–115
23. Huang J, McGirt MJ, Gailloud P, Tamargo RJ (2005) Intracranial aneurysms in the pediatric population: case series and literature review. Surg Neurol 63:424–433

24. Huhn SL, Lee JA, Steinberg GK (2006) Surgical treatment of vein of Galen malformations in children. In: Alexander M, Spetzler RF (eds) Pediatric Neurovascular Disease. Thieme, New York, pp 116–128

25. Humphreys RP, Hoffman H, Drake J, Rutka J (1996) Choices in the 1990s for the management of pediatric cerebral arteriovenous malformation. Pediatr Neurosurg 25:277–285

26. Ipone T, Ikezaki K, Susazuki T (2000) Linkage analysis of Moya Moya disease on chromosome 6. J Child Neurol 15:179–182

27. Jaegar JR, Forbes RP, Dandy WE (1937) Bilateral congenital cerebral arteriovenous communication aneurysm. Trans Am Neurol Assoc 63:173–176

28. Kamezawa T, Hamada J, Niiro M, Kai Y, Ishimaru K, Kuratsu J (2005) Clinical implication of associated venous drainage in patients with cavernous malformations. J Neurosurg 102:24–28

29. Khoo LT, Wallace MJ, McComb JG, Levy ML (1999) Pediatric aneurismal disease. In: Albright AL, Pollack I, Adelson PD (eds) Principles and Practice of Pediatric Neurosurgery. Thieme, New York, pp 1133–1152

30. Khurana VG (2005) Venous angiomas: developmental venous anomaly (DVA). Retrieved from http://www.brain-aneurysm.com/dva.html

31. Kitamura F, Fuku M, Oka K, Masushima T, Kurokawa T, Hasuo K (1998) Moyamoya disease. In: Handbook of Clinical Neurology (vol 2) pp 293–306

32. Kondziolka D, Humphreys RP, Hoffman H, et al (1992) Arteriovenous malformations of the brain in children: a forty year experience. Can J Neurol Sci 19:40–45

33. Kondziolka D, Pollock B, Lunsford LD (1999)Vascular malformations: conservative management, radiosurgery and embolization. In: Albright A, Pollack I, Adelson PD (eds) Principles and Practice of Pediatric Neurosurgery. Thieme, New York, pp 1017–1031

34. Krishna H, Wani AA, Behari S, Banerji D, Chhabra DK, Jain VK (2005) Intracranial aneurysms in patients 18 years of age or under, are they different from aneurysms in adult population? Acta Neurochir 147:469–476

35. Larson J, Ball W, Bove K, Crone K, Tew J Jr (1998) Formation of intracerebral cavernous malformations after radiation treatment for central nervous system neoplasia in children. J Neurosurg 88:51–56

36. Lasjaunias P (1997) Vein of Galen aneurysmal malformation. In: Lasjaunias P (ed) Vascular Diseases in Neonates, Infants and Children Berlin. Springer-Verlag, Germany, pp 67–202

37. Lasjaunias P, Garcia-Monaco R, Rodesch G, TerBrugge K, Zerah M, Tardieu M, de Victor D (1991) Vein of Galen malformation. Endovascular management of 43 cases. Childs Nerv Syst 7:360–367

38. Lasjaunias P, Wuppalapati S, Alvarez H, Rodesch G, Ozanne A (2005) Intracranial aneurysms in children aged less than 15 years: review of 59 consecutive children with 75 aneurysms. Childs Nerv Syst 21:437–450

39. Levrier O, Gailloud P, Souei M, Manera L, Brunel H, Raybaud CA (2004) Normal galenic drainage of the deep cerebral venous system in 2 cases of vein of Galen aneurysmal malformations (VGAM). Childs Nerv Syst 20:91–97

40. Levy E, Niranjan A, Thompson T, et al (2000) Radiosurgery for childhood intracranial arteriovenous malformations. Neurosurgery 47:834–842

41. Maher CO, Meyer FB (2006)Surgical treatment of cerebral aneurysms in children. In: Alexander MJ, Spetzler RF (eds) Pediatric Neurovascular Disease. Thieme, New York, pp 83–89

42. Maity A, Shu H, Tan J, et al (2004) Treatment of pediatric intracranial arteriovenous malformations with linear-accelerator-based stereotactic radiosurgery: The University of Pennsylvania experience. Pediatr Neurosurg 40:207–214

43. Mawad ME (1994) Interventional radiology. In: Cheek WR (ed), Pediatric Neurosurgery: Surgery of the Developing Nervous System. WB Saunders, Philadelphia, pp 539–544

44. McCance KL, Huether SE (2002) Pathophysiology: The Biologic Basis for Disease in Adults Children (4th edn). Mosby, St. Louis, MS

45. Meyer P, Orliaguet G, Zerah M, et al (2000) Emergency management of deeply comatose children with acute rupture of cerebral arteriovenous malformations. Can J Anesth 47:758–766

46. Mitchell PJ, Rosenfeld JV, Dargarville P, Loughnan P, Ditchfield MR, Frawley G, Tress BM (2001) Endovascular management of vein of Galen aneurismal malformations presenting in the neonatal period. AJNR 22:1403–1409

47. Moore KL, Agur AM (1995) Essential Clinical Anatomy. Williams Wilkins, Toronto, ON

48. Murasko K, Oldfield E (1990) Vascular malformations of the spinal cord and dura. Neurosurg Clin North Am 1:631–652

49. Muszynski C, Berenstein A (2001) Interventional radiology. In: McClone D (ed) Pediatric Neurosurgery: Surgery of the Developing Nervous System. WB Saunders, Philadelphia, PA, pp 1155–1171

50. Ohaegbulam C, Magge S, Scott M (1999) Moya Moya disease. In: Albright AL, Pollack I, Adelson PD (eds) Principles and Practice of Pediatric Neurosurgery. Thieme, New York, pp 1077–1089

51. Pasqualin A, Mazza C, Da Pian R, Dala BB (1982) Midline giant arterio-venous malformations in infants. Acta Neurochir 64:259–271

52. Porter P, Willinsky R, Harper W, Wallace C (1997) Cerebral cavernous malformations: natural history and prognosis after clinical deterioration with or without hemorrhage. J Neurosurg 87:190–197

53. Porter R, Detweiler P, Spetzler R, Lawton M, Baskin J, Derksen P, Zabramski J (1999) Cavernous malformations of the brainstem: experience with 100 patients. J Neurosurg 90:50–58

54. Pozzati E, Acciarri N, Tognetti F, Marliani F, Giangaspero F (1996) Growth, subsequent bleeding and de novo appearance of cerebral angiomas. Neurosurgery 38:662–670

55. Proust F, Toussaint P, Garnieri J, Hannequin D, Legars D, Houtieville J, Freger P (2001) Pediatric cerebral aneurysms. J Neurosurg 94:733–739

56. Punt J (2004) Surgical management of paediatric stroke. Pediat Radiol 34:16–23

57. Raybaud CA, Strother CM (1986) Persisting abnormal embryonic vessels in intracranial arteriovenous malformations. Acta Radiol Suppl 369:136–138

58. Rivera P, Willinsky R, Porter P (2003) Intracranial cavernous malformations. Neuroimaging Clin North Am 13:27–40

59. Riina H, Lemole M, Spetzler R (2006). Surgical treatment of spinal vascular malformations in children. In: Alexander MJ, Spetzler RF (eds) Pediatric Neurovascular Disease. Thieme Medical, New York, pp 129–134

60. Roach ES, Riela A (eds) (1995) Pediatric Cerebrovascular Disorders (2nd edn). Futura, New York

61. Rodesch G, Hui F, Alvarez H, Tanaka A, Lasjaunias P (1994) Prognosis of antenatally diagnosed vein of Galen aneurysmal malformations Childs Nerv Syst 10:79–83

62. Rodesch G, Hurth M, Alvarez H, Tadie M, Lasjaunias P (2002) Classification of spinal cord arteriovenous shunts: proposal for a reappraisal – the bicetre experience with 155 consecutive patients treated between 1981 and 1999. Neurosurgery 51:374–380

63. Rodesch G, Hurth M, Alvarez H, Tadie M, Lasjaunias P (2005) Spinal cord intradural arteriovenous fistulae: anatomic, clinical, and therapeutic considerations in a series of 32 consecutive patients seen between 1981 and 2000 with emphasis on endovascular therapy. Neurosurgery 57:973–981

64. Santos CC, Sarnat HB, Roach ES (2005) Cerebrovascular Disorders. In: Menkes JM, Sarnat HB, Maria BL (eds) Child Neurology. Lippincott Williams Wilkins, Philadelphia, pp 1–76

65. Santos CC, Sarnat HB, Roach ES (2006) Cerebrovascular disorders. In: Menkes JM, Sarnat HB, Maria BL (eds) Child Neurology. Philadelphia, Lippincott Williams Wilkins, pp 843–844

66. Smith M, Sinson G (2006) Intracranial arteriovenous malformations. http://www.emedicine.com/med/topic3469.htm. retrieved January 9 2006

67. Smyth M, Sneed P, Ciricillo S, et al (1997) Stereotactic radiosurgery for pediatric intracranial arteriovenous malformations: the University of California at San Francisco experience. J Neurosurg 97:48–55

68. Spetzler RF, Detwiler P, Riina H, Porter RW (2002) Modified classification of spinal cord vascular lesions. J Neurosurg Spine 96:145–156

69. Takeuchi K, Shimuzu K (1957) Hypoplasia of bilateral internal carotid arteries. Brain Nerve 19:37–43

70. TerBrugge K (1999) Neurointerventional procedures in the pediatric age group. Child Nerv Syst 15:751–754

71. TerBrugge K (2006) Endovascular treatment of vein of Galen malformations in children. In: Alexander M, Spetzler RF (eds) (2006) Pediatric Neurovascular Disease: Surgical, Endovascular and Medical Management. Thieme, New York, pp 176–185

72. Tung H, Giannotta SL, Chandarasoma P (1990) Recurrent intraparenchymal hemorrhages from angiographically occult vascular malformations. J Neurosurg 73:174–80

73. Ventureyra E, Vassilyadi M (2001) Arteriovenous malformations. In: McLone D (ed) Pediatric Neurosurgery: Surgery of the Developing Nervous System. WB Saunders, Philadelphia, PA, pp 1105–1111

74. Waxman SG (2003) Clinical Neuroanatomy (25th edn). Lange Medical Books/McGraw Hill, New York, p 171

75. Yeh D, Crone K (2006) Cavernous malformations in children. In: Alexander M, Spetzler RF (eds) Pediatric Neurovascular Disease: Surgical, Endovascular, and Medical Management. Thieme, New York, pp 65–71

76. Yokoyama K, Asano Y, Murakawa T, et al (1991) Familial occurrence of arteriovenous malformations of the brain. J Neurosurg 74:585–589

77. Yonekawa Y, Kahn N (2003) Moya Moya Disease. Adv Neurol 92:113–118

78. Zaidat O, Alexander M (2006) Endovascular treatment of cerebral arteriovenous malformations in children. In: Alexander M, Spetzler RF (eds) Pediatric Neurovascular Disease: Surgical, Endovascular, and Medical Management. Thieme, New York, pp 167–175

79. Zerah M, Garcia-Monaco R, Rodesch G, TerBrugge K, Tardieu M, de Victor D, Lasjaunias P (1992) Hydrodynamics in vein of Galen malformations. Childs Nerv Syst 8:111–117

# Surgical Management of Epilepsy

10

*Mary Smellie-Decker, Jennifer Berlin, Trisha Leonard,*
*Cheri Salazar, and Kristin Wall Strother*

## Contents

## ▪ Introduction

Epilepsy affects approximately 0.5–1% of the world's population, with initial onset most frequently occurring during childhood [1]. Prior to initiating treatment, it is important to determine whether or not the described behaviors are epileptic seizures. A detailed and thorough history will help confirm whether the described behaviors include periods of unresponsiveness, altered awareness, interruption in the child's activity, or a period of postictal depression. Additionally, an electroencephalogram (EEG) is performed to provide further formation about the seizure type.

A system for classification of epilepsy and epileptic syndromes was published in 1989 [12]. This provided a consistent description of the nomenclature used to classify epileptic seizures. The classification system includes both partial and primary generalized seizures. Simple partial seizures originate from a somatosensory region of the brain (aura) and consciousness is usually not altered. They generally last for less than 1 min, but may progress to a generalized seizure. In complex partial seizures, there is a loss of consciousness lasting 1–3 min or longer. The individual is usually confused after the event and does not remember it occurring. These seizures also contain a component of automatism (involuntary repetitive movements such as lip smacking or finger snapping).

Several types of seizures are classified as primary generalized seizures. Myoclonic seizures are composed of quick muscle jerks, which can be unilateral or bilateral. Consciousness is usually not impaired during the episode. Tonic seizures consist of tonic spasms of truncal and facial muscles. There is flexion of the upper extremities and extension of the lower extremities. Clonic seizures, which are common in children, may resemble myoclonus, but the repetition rate is slower; and there is also loss of consciousness. Atonic seizures, also called drop attacks, produce a sudden loss of muscle tone. Individuals having these types of seizures have no prior warning that the event is going to occur. The person witnessing the event will see a drop of the head, loss of posture, or a sudden collapse. These seizures last only a few seconds but are dangerous because an individual could be injured. Generalized tonic clonic seizures, also known as grand mal seizures, are the most common type of seizure. These seizures occur suddenly, without warning, and consist of a tonic contraction of the trunk interrupted by short periods of relaxation. There is an increase in heart rate and blood pressure. Tonic clonic seizures may progress to status epilepticus. Consciousness may not be regained for 10–15 min or longer.

Once the type of seizure is identified, appropriate treatment can be instituted. In the majority of cases drug therapy is the method utilized to manage seizures. Some patients will continue to have persistent seizure activity despite maximal medical treatment, resulting in severe debilitation. Practitioners' opinions vary as to the number, combination, and length of time a child must be on antiepileptic drug (AED) therapy before defining the seizures as medically intractable [4, 11]. "Because intractable seizures in children have a malignant natural history with eventual declines in both intellectual and behavioral functions, surgery has become an acceptable early treatment modality for these patients" [1]. Children whose seizures are bilateral and multifocal are not candidates for seizure surgery. Seizures must originate from one side of the brain in order for the procedure to be successful. If they do not meet this requirement and are unsuccessful with AEDs, then they may be a candidate for the ketogenic diet or vagus nerve stimulation. The ultimate goal of epilepsy surgery is freedom from seizures while trying to prevent negative long-term effects on the child's quality of life [11]. This is best accomplished by the utilization of a team approach. The specialized team may include neuropsychologists, epileptologists, neurologists, neurosurgeons, nurses, and EEG technicians. Parents are also very important members of the team.

## Preoperative Preparation

After it has been determined that a child is a candidate for surgery, an attempt is made to further localize the seizure focus. This is accomplished by combining information from different sources. The child's medical history will provide a description of the behavior at the onset of the seizure, as well as seizure pattern [11]. The EEG can give helpful information by verifying the presence of an epileptogenic focus. Sometimes epileptic spikes may be multifocal and identifying the epileptogenic zone may be difficult, resulting in the need for further evaluation [17]. Video EEG monitoring can provide further information in this ongoing evaluation. The testing is usually done in an inpatient setting for 23 h. When necessary, a child's medication can be safely withheld in order to elicit seizures. The information obtained provides a large sample of ictal and interictal phases. In addition to recording the patient's seizures, it also allows correlation of the EEG findings with the recorded patient activity. This information is recorded by a family member who stays with the patient. The video monitor can capture early clonus, tonic postures, head and eye movements, as well as auras that are indicative of a partial focus that are not able to be visualized in other tests [11]. The data is analyzed by the epileptologist to obtain information about the ictus and interictal activity, as well as information about whether or not the seizures are partial or generalized.

All children who are candidates for surgery require a magnetic resonance imaging (MRI) scan to identify structural abnormalities that may contribute to the epilepsy. MRI can also identify neoplastic lesions, vascular malformations, and heterotopias (normal tissue in an abnormal location). These are areas of grey matter that have infiltrated into white matter, which can become seizure-provoking areas. Although a tumor or other space-occupying lesion may be present, the EEG findings may not be localized to the area of the mass. Specialized MRI techniques can also be used to further study subtle areas of abnormalities [15].

Two other imaging techniques utilized are positron emission tomography (PET) and single-photon-emission computed tomography (SPECT) scan. These tests differ from other diagnostic studies because they provide functional information. PET has become a routine part of preoperative evaluation at centers where it is available. PET can assist by defining metabolically abnormal brain regions correlating with the epileptogenic focus when MRI images are negative or inconclusive [11, 16]. It identifies areas of brain hypometabolism after an infusion of a nuclear reagent. The various reagents used are fluorodeoxyglucose, flumazenil, and alpha methyl-L-tryptophan (AMT). Each reagent provides specific localizing information in surgical candidates. Flumazenil has been useful in studying patients with temporal lobe epilepsy. AMT has been helpful in localizing epileptogenic tubers in patients with tuberous sclerosis [17].

A SPECT scan is a functional imaging technique used to help determine whether there is a localized abnormality corresponding to the region of seizure onset. During a seizure, the regional focus receives greater blood flow because of increased metabolic demands. The SPECT scan has been used to localize epileptogenic zones during the ictal and interictal phases after an injection of tracer. In comparison to the PET scan, the SPECT scan does not need to be performed at a specific time following the injection of tracer. It should be noted, however, that SPECT does not provide the same degree of image resolution as PET [14, 15, 17].

Neuropsychological testing is another essential component of the preoperative evaluation. A psychologist familiar with issues surrounding the epileptic patient and the effects that it can have on neuropsychological function performs the evaluation. The primary goal is to establish the patient's baseline cognitive function and then to compare it with postoperative function [11]. Areas that are measured include intelligence, attention, and motor skills. Of particular concern are memory and language function in relationship to the underlying anatomic lesion. In selective cases, intracarotid sodium amytal testing (the WADA test, named after Juhn Wada) is used to determine lateralization of language and verify that memory will not be affected by the proposed surgery. While the patient is awake, sodium amytal is injected into each carotid artery, one at a time, causing the injected half of the brain to become nonfunctional. The examiner takes the child through a series of tests looking for changes in speech and memory on the opposite side of the brain. This is done to determine whether there is right- or left-side dominance in language and memory [15]. Functional MRI can also be performed to identify eloquent areas. Once testing is completed, a case conference is held to review the data. Recommendations are made and a treatment plan is developed. Some children will proceed to surgical resection while others will require invasive monitoring to further define the seizure focus.

## Invasive Monitoring

Noninvasive testing does not always provide a complete picture of the seizure zone. This results in the need to further define the seizure focus using invasive monitoring as part of a two-stage surgery. Children who require invasive monitoring frequently have extra-temporal-lobe seizures [11]. This technique is also used in children who have seizure onset areas that are hard to localize and are in close proximity to the eloquent cortex. The eloquent cortex can be defined as any part of the brain that has observable function, such as language, sensorimotor, and visual pathways [1, 2, 5, 10].

Invasive monitoring may also be required when a lesion is identified on the MRI but the seizure focus zone extends beyond the lesion or is in a different part of the brain. Some areas of the brain are not identified by routine EEGs, and in other instances the scalp electrodes can interfere with the recording. It can also be difficult to differentiate electrical abnormalities in the brain due to the location of the seizure origination [5].

There are several different invasive monitoring methods that can be utilized. In the awake craniotomy, electrocorticography, cortical mapping, and surgery are performed on a patient while awake. This procedure requires that a patient cooperates and follows instructions during the procedure. This type of intervention has limited utility since it is anxiety producing, involves patient cooperation, and requires the surgeon to resect the focus in a limited period of time. There are also some concerns about anesthesia reducing the seizure threshold and impacting the motor mapping [2].

When subdural grids or strips are used to evaluate children, the information obtained enables the epileptologist to identify and define the entire region of the seizure focus (Fig. 10.1). Information collected from ictal and interictal data are used to map out the seizure focus, adjacent tissue, and eloquent cortex [5, 10]. The implanted electrodes can be used to map out the language and sensorimotor strip. Children who previously were not candidates for seizure surgery due to the location of the lesion, or the seizure focus being in close proximity to the eloquent cortex, are now able to undergo a resection [10, 11].

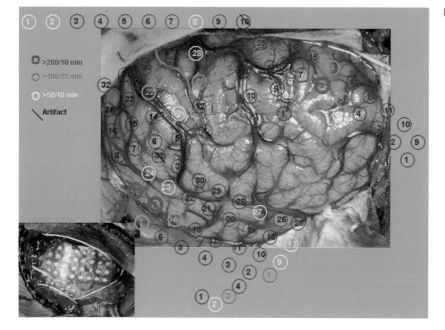

**Fig. 10.1.** Grids/mapping

The importance of removing the entire seizure focus to remain seizure free has been reported in numerous studies [1, 10, 11, 16]. If a lesion has been identified but the seizure zone appears to be larger than the lesion area, then the entire region needs to be resected. In nonlesional epilepsy, the entire seizure focus zone must be resected to become seizure free. Utilizing the subdural grids for monitoring, information can be collected to further define the seizure focus. Depth electrodes are also utilized when the origination of the seizure focus is deep in the brain and unclear.

### Procedure

A craniotomy is performed, the dura is exposed, and the grids are placed over the desired cortical regions (Fig. 10.2). A strip is used when just a small section of the brain needs to be evaluated and it can be placed through a burr hole. Subdural grids are used when a larger area of focus in the brain needs to be evaluated. The grids are placed on the side that previous noninvasive testing indicated may be the seizure focus. If there is a question of both sides of the brain being involved, then a grid can be placed along the falx to provide information about the seizure and its path [11]. Depth electrodes can be utilized if the seizure focus originates deep within the brain. These thin wires are inserted at different depths into the brain parenchyma, usually under stereotactic guidance. Once the grids are placed, then each electrode wire is passed percutaneously and sewn tightly into place to prevent

it from becoming dislodged. A Jackson Pratt (JP) drain and an intracranial pressure (ICP) monitor can also be placed at this time. The intracranial grids are connected to an EEG monitor to verify that they are functional prior to wound closure.

### Mapping

Following the procedure, the patient will be transferred to the intensive care unit for overnight monitoring. The next day the child will be transferred to a monitored unit for video-monitoring EEG (VEEG). It is important that this process begin as soon as possible so that seizure events can be recorded. In many cases, antiepileptic medications need to be withheld to evoke seizures. A family member should be present and documents seizure activity during the VEEG. The information from the VEEG is then correlated with the direct recording from the subdural grids for a better interpretation of the seizure focus. The next step is to map out the eloquent cortex area with regard to the language and motor strips. Stimulation of the electrodes with an electrical current from a generator is performed to help map out the sensorimotor and language strips. The mapping is performed on the unit by the epilepsy team. It is also helpful to have a family member present with the child during the testing to get accurate and repeatable data (Fig. 10.3) [1].

The goal is to obtain data about the child's seizures. If at any time the child's health becomes compromised, however, the seizure should be stopped. A plan

**Fig. 10.2.** Placement of the grids

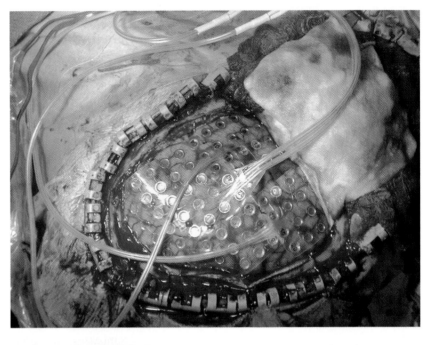

**Fig. 10.3.** Patient being monitored

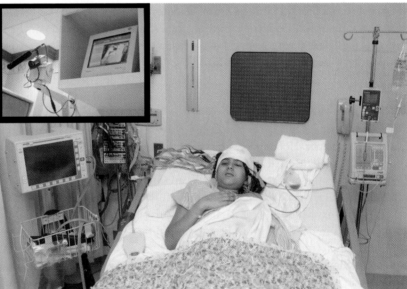

should be established that dictates the management of a seizure that lasts over 3–4 min. For example, if seizure lasts for over 3 min, the nurse may have a standing order to give midazolam. Once the necessary information has been obtained, the AEDs will be restarted. The epilepsy team will meet again and review all of the data to plan for the second stage of surgery. A map is developed by the epileptologist utilizing all of the collected data. The surgeon then uses the map to identify the exact area of resection (Fig. 10.4).

## Seizure Surgery

There are a variety of surgical procedures that are categorized as seizure surgery. The specific procedure utilized is dependent on the location of the seizure origination as well as the results of testing. When compared with adults, children have a more extensive seizure focus. All procedures require a craniotomy with a flap to visualize the affected area. At times, stereotactic surgical navigation systems will be utilized

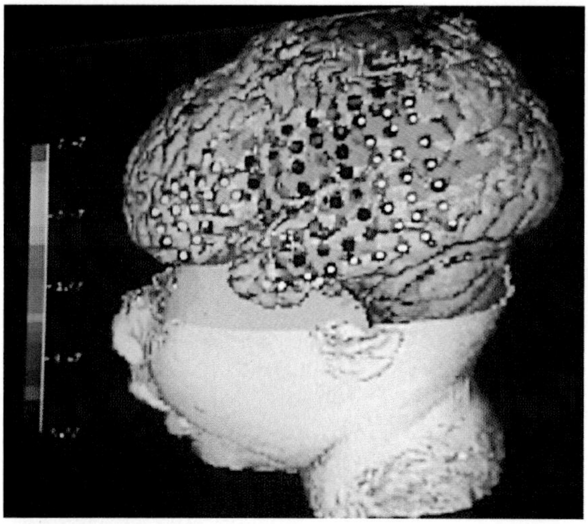

**Fig. 10.4.** Coregistration three-dimensional magnetic resonance imaging, positron emission tomography (PET), and grids. The black areas show the seizure focus, the red areas are the PET scan, and the small circles are the grids

to localize a specific area in the brain. Patients are also monitored with EEG intraoperatively for a short period to verify adequate placement of the brain electrodes prior to beginning the procedure.

## Temporal Lobectomy

Historically, temporal lobe epilepsy has been the most common surgically treated form of epilepsy because of its distinct pathology and accessible location, low morbidity of surgery, and excellent outcomes. It is the origin of approximately 30% of partial complex seizure disorders in children. It has been reported that 78% of children undergoing this procedure are seizure free following the procedure [1, 5, 21, 23]. Seizures are most frequently identified in the anterior temporal lobe. Over-resection of the dominant temporal lobe may injure speech centers that cannot be reliably localized visually; therefore, mapping is used to determine the location of the speech centers [8].

## Frontal Lobectomy

A frontal lobectomy is the second most common surgical procedure for epilepsy. It is used in the treatment of partial seizures. On rare occasions, when there is a structural abnormality identified as the seizure focus, parietal and occipital lobectomies are also performed.

## Lesionectomy

A lesionectomy is undertaken to remove a damaged or abnormally functioning area of the brain identified as the focus of the seizure. This includes scars from brain injury, infection, tumors, or vascular malformations, which can be identified on imaging. In contrast, a cortisectomy is undertaken when there is no identifiable lesion on imaging. Mapping identifies the seizure focus. Once the seizure focus is mapped out the surgeon utilizes the map to resect it. In both incidences the seizures stop once the focus has been removed.

## Hemispherectomy

Another type of procedure that can be utilized is the hemispherectomy. The term hemispherectomy encompasses many procedures. For example, the hemisphere may be completely removed (anatomic hemispherectomy) or the frontal and occipital portions of the hemisphere are preserved but disconnected (functional hemispherectomy) [1, 24]. Walter Dandy first described the hemispherectomy procedure in 1928 to treat malignant brain tumors. Although surgical neuroonclogy containment was not achieved, the patient had acceptable postoperative neurologic function and the foundation for anatomic resection of the cerebral hemisphere was introduced. Numerous modifications to Dandy's surgical technique have been made to reduce the morbidity and long-term complications of hemispherectomy, without reducing long-term seizure control. Hemispherectomy should be considered whenever there is extensive unilateral epileptiform activity, implying that the other hemisphere appears to be functioning normally. The abnormality must involve the majority of the hemisphere so that piecemeal resections are not valid, and the epileptogenic tissue must be confined to a single hemisphere. The child usually develops a contralateral hemiparesis and hemianopsia, since undergoing this procedure will result in loss of function. Candidates for hemispherectomy include children with hemispheric dysplasia, Rasmussen's encephalitis, infantile spasms, hemimegalencephaly, and Sturge-Weber syndrome [17, 20].

## Subpial Resection and Corpus Callosotomy

The final two procedures to be discussed are the subpial resection and the corpus callosotomy. Neither of these procedures is considered curative. Subpial resection is done if the area of seizure focus is a vital area and resection would have a significant negative impact. Shallow cuts (transections) are made into the cerebral cortex. The cuts interrupt fibers that connect functional areas in the brain. The result is a reduction in seizures without eliminating function.

In a corpus callosotomy the nerve fibers that cross between the two cerebral hemispheres are cut, thus interrupting the propagation of epileptic discharges across one side of the brain to the other [1]. This usually involves the anterior two-thirds of the corpus callosum [1, 8, 21]. If this is unsuccessful, then the fibers in the posterior portion of the corpus callosum can be cut in a second procedure. The procedure is generally reserved for severely impaired patients because it can result in a disconnect syndrome: messages from one half of the brain do not cross over to the other half of the brain causing somatosensory, auditory, and visual disorientation

## Complications

The most common complication of seizure surgery appears to be leakage of cerebrospinal fluid (CSF) from the exit site of the electrodes. A CSF leak may resolve spontaneously or require a purse-string suture to stop it. At the time of grid placement, electrode wires can be tunneled to decrease the risk of CSF leak. Wound infection is the other complication reported following subdural electrode grid placement and resection. Studies vary in the rate of infection from 2 to 9%. Antibiotics can be used prophylactically to decrease the risk of infection.

Grid placement may cause cerebral swelling. The grids are very thin and pliable, but may still cause compression on the brain resulting in a subdural hematoma and vascular compression [1, 5]. A JP drain placed at time of grid placement can help reduce swelling around the grids. Some surgeons will remove the bone flap to control the swelling and mass effect seen from the grid placement. The bone flap is then replaced during the second surgery [11]. An ICP monitor can also be used to monitor the pressure following grid placement [11, 18]. Other complications that

may occur include dysphasia, memory deficits, injury to cranial nerves (especially the third cranial nerve), injury to blood vessels leading to ischemic damage, and decrease or loss of motor function [1, 5, 21, 24]. A small group Fever is also seen on occassion it may or may not be signifigant, further workup for fever is required. A small group of patients are also at risk for developing hydrocephalus. There is also the rare complication of death. However, many feel that the lifelong benefits outweigh the possible complications of the seizure surgery procedure.

## Nursing Care

Following resection or grid placement, the child will be admitted to the intensive care unit for close monitoring overnight and then transferred to the monitoring unit. Patients should be watched for changes in ICP, as well as changes in neurological status. This can be done by routinely monitoring vital signs and neurological function, including an assessment of level of consciousness, pupillary response, and changes in motor function. Assessments should be documented and changes reported to the appropriate staff. The staff should be identified at time of admission to the unit. If an ICP-monitoring device is utilized, pressures should be recorded hourly and guidelines should be established with regard to normal ranges. When a patient is having a seizure, ICP will be elevated, but they should return to normal after the seizure is completed.

Children undergoing a craniotomy are at risk for fluid and electrolyte imbalances. Brain swelling can occur during this time, which can cause the patient to develop syndrome of inappropriate antidiuretic hormone (SIADH). Electrolytes should be drawn daily and strict intake and output should be maintained. Specific gravity should be done at least every 8 h to monitor hydration status. If abnormalities are identified, then appropriate interventions should be instituted (e.g., if the serum sodium value becomes abnormal, the amount and type of fluid the patient is receiving will need to be adjusted).

It is also important to monitor closely for CSF leak and wound drainage, as a CSF leak will greatly increase the chance of infection. This can occur following the first or second stage procedure. A JP drain can be placed to help promote drainage from the incision site and reduce pressure on the incision. If a JP is placed, it is usually done at the time the grids are placed. If there is no drainage and the ICP is increasing, then the JP suction may need to be increased. If the ICP is negative and there has been a large amount of drainage, then the JP suction would be decreased. The drain is normally removed at the time of the second procedure. During monitoring, if a patient's dressing becomes saturated it is normally changed by the surgical team. When the dressing is removed, the underlying incision is examined to determine whether further intervention is required. Care is taken not to cut the grid wires. If a child has had a resection, then the dressing can usually be removed 24–48 h after surgery. If a patient is developmentally delayed, an assessment must take place to determine if the patient will scratch at the surgical incision. Steps should be taken to prevent this from occurring. This might include keeping the incision covered, putting mittens on the child's hands, elbow restraints, or continuous monitoring by a parent or sitter.

Pain assessment with age-appropriate pain scales should be done on a regular basis, as these are painful procedures. Narcotic and nonnarcotic analgesics in addition to nonpharmacological interventions should be administered.

Occasionally, a patient with grids attached to a VEEG may need to be taken emergently from the monitoring area for testing. The ground electrode must first be disconnected or the patient could receive an electrical shock. The electrodiagnostic staff should be contacted for assistance.

Some of the children will require long-term inpatient or outpatient therapies due to loss of function. Involving the social services, physical therapy, occupational therapy, and speech therapy early in the treatment will help to facilitate discharge planning. Prior to discharge, a discussion should also take place regarding AEDs and follow-up studies.

Although there are discussions prior to seizure surgery, reassessment should occur throughout the process so that the families' concerns can be addressed. Successful surgery is dependent on a team approach and the child's family is an integral part of the team.

## Vagal Nerve Stimulator

## History

The Food and Drug Administration (FDA) approved the use of the vagal nerve stimulator (VNS) in 1987 as an adjunctive treatment for refractory partial-onset seizures in individuals over 12 years of age [19]. In 1988, Dr. Jacob Zabara trialed the VNS for treatment of refractory partial seizures. Since that time, it has also been used to treat generalized tonic/clonic seizures, Lennox-Gastaut syndrome, and absence seizures [19]. Although it is not clear exactly how the VNS controls seizures, it has been shown that stimulation of the vagal nerve desynchronizes the EEG rhythms of seizures. In most institutions, the VNS placement surgery is done as an outpatient. Candidates for the VNS are those individuals who have refractory seizures despite multiple AED therapies. VNS is an option for those who do not wish to have a lobectomy or hemispherectomy, or whose seizures are not localized enough to have these procedures. Most studies found a 40–60% reduction in seizure activity with the VNS; however, most patients continue to require one or more AEDs [3, 5, 6, 9, 13].

## Surgical Procedure

An incision is made in the left side of the neck to expose the left vagal nerve. The left vagal nerve is chosen because there is less interference in cardiac conduction compared to the right, which innervates the heart. The surgeon must be careful with the dissection in order to avoid the carotid artery and the jugular vein, which lie on either side of the vagal nerve. The VNS electrodes are wrapped around the nerve in two places and an anchor tether is wrapped at the bottom of the exposed nerve. A second incision is made in the chest wall just below the clavicle, allowing the generator to be placed in the subcutaneous cavity. A tunneling tool is used to advance the electrodes from the neck incision to the chest incision. The electrodes are then connected to the generator and both incisions are closed (Fig. 10.5). In some institutions the generator is activated in the operating room; in others it is activated 2 weeks later to allow healing time. Those individuals who have had a prior vagotomy cannot have a VNS placed. Cardiology clearance is necessary for any person who has a known cardiac arrhythmia.

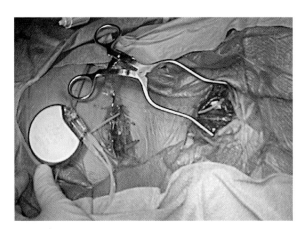

**Fig. 10.5.** Vagal nerve stimulator

## Complications

The most common side effects of VNS therapy are hoarseness, coughing, and gagging. They are more prominent when the vagal nerve is overmanipulated in the procedure. In some patients this complication may be severe, leading to vocal cord paralysis. Fortunately, in most cases the symptoms resolve in a few weeks [5]. There have also been reported cases of cardiac arrhythmias during intraoperative testing of the electrodes, although there have been no reported cases of arrhythmias after implant [6, 19]. Infections, though rare, may develop. If they are superficial, they can be treated with a course of oral antibiotics. If severe infection occurs, the VNS must be explanted and cannot be reimplanted for 6–8 months [7, 22].

## Function

The programming of the generator is carried out after the operative procedure. The programming device (magnet) is placed directly over the generator and communicates with a portable computer. The generators are initially set low and the current is increased at specific intervals based on patient tolerance. There is an on/off cycle to the current, usually 7–60 s on, followed by 7 s–180 min off. In addition, the patient or care provider is given a magnet to take home to permit additional stimulation of the generator if an aura is sensed by the patient.

The lithium battery in the generator has a life of 3–5 years. A patient will usually sense an increase in seizures as the battery wears out. At this time the patient must undergo local or general anesthesia to change the generator. The incision below the clavicle is opened and the electrodes are disconnected from the old generator and discarded. A new generator is connected to the electrodes, placed back in the pocket and the incision is closed. The new device is programmed to the settings of the old generator. Patients initially have follow-up every 2 weeks during the programming phase, and then every 1–3 months thereafter. At every visit the efficacy of the VNS, seizure activity, AEDs, and side effects are evaluated [7, 19].

## Nursing Care

Parents should be taught to look for signs of infection (i.e., redness, swelling, pain, drainage at the site). They should also be given instructions on how the stimulator works and utilization of the wand (or magnet). It is very important that information regarding safety and electromagnetic fields be given to the patient and caregivers. Patient information is available from the company that manufactures the device. It is also readily accessible on the Internet.

## Conclusion

Today, there are options for children who have seizures. Some may no longer need to continue a medication regimen that may or may not provide optimum seizure control. The future of surgical epilepsy management is likely to grow as neuroimaging advances and technology improves. The desired outcome is for a child to be seizure free or significantly reduce the amount of seizures, while preserving the child's development, intellect, and quality of life.

---

**Pediatric Practice Pearls**

- Be careful not to cut wires when changing dressings.
- Have an established plan for a child who is being monitored.
- Identify who should be called with problems and for medications to be used if a child starts to have a seizure.
- Always talk to the parents.

# References

1. Albright AL, Pollack IF, Adelson PD (2001) Operative techniques in pediatric neurosurgery. Thieme, New York, pp 247–274
2. Cohen-Gadol A, et al (2003) Nonlesional central lobule seizures: use of awake cortical mapping and subdural grid monitoring for resection of seizure focus. J Neurosurg 98:1255–1266
3. Crumrine P (2000) Vagal nerve stimulation in children. Semin Pediatr Neurol 7:216–223
4. Duchowny M, Morrison G (2001) Epilepsy classification and evaluation. In: McClone DG (ed) Pediatric Neurosurgery: Surgery of the Developing Nervous System (4th edn). WB Saunders, Philadelphia, pp 1017–1024
5. Foldvary N, Nashold B, Mascha E, Thompson EA, Lee N, McNamara JO, et al (2000) Seizure outcome after temporal lobectomy for temporal lobe epilepsy: a Kaplan-Meier survival analysis. Neurology 54:630–634
6. George R, Kliniek HB (1995) A randomized controlled trial of chronic vagus nerve stimulation for treatment of medically intractable seizures. Neurology 45:224–230
7. George R, Salinsky M, Kuzniecky R (1994) Vagus nerve stimulation for treatment of partial seizures. Epilepsia 35:637–43
8. Greenberg M (2001) Handbook of Neurosurgery (5th edn). Thieme, New York, pp 277–281
9. Handforth A (1998) Vagus nerve stimulation therapy for partial-onset seizures. Neurology 51:48–55
10. Holmes G (2002) Epilepsy surgery in children: when, why, and how. Neurology 58:S13–20
11. Lee J, Adelson PD (2004) Neurosurgical management of pediatric epilepsy. Pediatr Clin North Am 51:441–456
12. Leppik IE (2000) Contemporary Diagnosis and Management of the Patient with Epilepsy (5th edn). Handbook in Health Care, Newton, Pennsylvania
13. Murphy J (1999) Left vagus nerve stimulation in children with medically refractory epilepsy. J Pediatr 134:563–566
14. Murphy M, O'Brien T, Morris K, Cook M (2004) Multimodality image-guided surgery for the treatment of medically refractory epilepsy. J Neurosurg 100:452–462
15. Nordli D Jr, Kelley KR (2001) Selection and evaluation of children for epilepsy surgery. Pediatr Neurosurg 34:1–12
16. Ojemann S. Peacock W (2001) Surgical treatment of epilepsy. In: Mclone DG (ed) Pediatric Neurosurgery: Surgery of the Developing Nervous System (4th edn). WB Saunders, Philadelphia, pp 1025–1034
17. Olson D.M (2001) Evaluation of children for epilepsy surgery. Pediatr Neurosurg 34:159–65
18. Onal C, Otsubo H, Arakitet T, Chitoku S, Weiss S, Elliot I, et al (2003) Complications of invasive subdural grid monitoring in children with epilepsy. J Neurosurg 98:1017–1026
19. Schmidt D, Schacter S (2000) Epilepsy: Problem Solving in Clinical Practice. Martin Dunitz, London
20. Shimizu H (2005) Our experience with pediatric epilepsy surgery focusing on corpus callosotomy and hemisphereotomy. Epilepsia 46:30–31
21. Sinclair DB, Acronym K, Snyder T, McKean J, Wheatley M, Bhargava R, et al (2003) Pediatric temporal lobectomy for epilepsy. Pediatr Neurosurg 38:195–205
22. Smyth M, Tubbs R, Bebin E, Grab P, Blount J (2003) Complications of chronic vagus nerve stimulation for epilepsy in children. J Neurosurg 99:500–503
23. Tellez-Zenteno JF, Dhar R, Wiebe S (2005) Long-term seizure outcomes following epilepsy surgery: a systematic review and meta-analysis. Brain 128: 1188–1198
24. Vining E, Freeman J, Carson B (1994) Hemispherectomy. In: Wyler AR, Hermann BP (eds) The Surgical Management of Epilepsy. Butterworth-Heineman, Boston, pp 146–154

# Surgical Management of Spasticity

*Herta Yu and Mary Szatkowski*

**11**

## Contents

## Pathophysiology of Spasticity

Spasticity is a disorder of motor function that is characterized by tight or spastic muscle activity. The anatomy and pathophysiology of spasticity is not fully understood. Spasticity occurs as a result of any damage or lesion within the central nervous system (CNS) that impairs the mediation of inhibitory inputs down the descending motor pathways and impedes relaxation [12, 13, 25].

Spasticity begins with attempted muscle movement, which originates in the muscle fibers. Within the muscle fibers, there must be a reflex arc for muscle movement to occur (Fig. 11.1). Reflex arcs contain a receptor, an effector muscle, and either two or three neurons that transmit the signal for muscle movement. The afferent (or sensory) neurons arise from the gray matter in the dorsal (or posterior) horn of the spinal cord and transmit impulses from the sensors to the CNS. The efferent (or motor) neurons rise from the ventral (or anterior) horn of the spinal canal and carry impulses from the CNS to the effector muscle. Stimulation of the

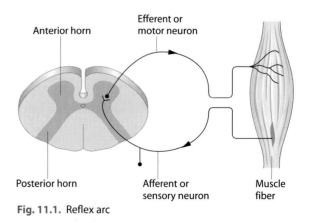

**Fig. 11.1.** Reflex arc

sensory neuron causes the flow of chemical transmitters across the synaptic space to depolarize the next neuron and continue the flow of the impulse to the muscle cell. The muscle cell sends a signal back to the sensory neuron that the action is completed and inhibition occurs, creating relaxation. This completed cycle is a reflex arc. Spasticity occurs when there is an increase in reflex arcs and a lack of inhibition from the sensory neurons to the motor neurons, which creates a loop that continues to stimulate the muscle fibers and can even spread to other muscle groups [18].

Spasticity presents as involuntary, velocity-dependent increase in tonic stretch reflexes, meaning that a sudden rapid stretch would elicit greater resistance to movement than a slow, steady, sustained stretch [23]. Spasticity may have a cerebral or spinal origin, depending upon whether the damage is located in the cerebral cortex, brainstem, or spinal cord. Cerebral causes of spasticity include cerebral palsy, intracranial hemorrhage, hydrocephalus, brain tumor, multiple sclerosis, stroke, or head injury. Spinal causes of spasticity include spinal injury, inflammatory disease, and nontraumatic conditions that result in spinal compression [25, 28].

The clinical presentations of spasticity include increased muscle tone, exaggerated reflexes, flexor and extensor spasms, persistent primitive reflexes, clonus, and decreased coordination. In severe cases, the patient may develop contractures and musculoskeletal deformities resulting in physical disabilities and severe pain [22]. In addition, many patients with spasticity experience fatigue, sleep disturbance, anxiety, depression, immobility, infections, and decreased cognitive development. Spasticity has devastating consequences affecting function, comfort, care delivery, and quality of life [9]. Table 11.1 shows the clinical presentations of spasticity, and the symptomatic and functional problems created.

Managing spasticity requires a multidisciplinary approach involving rehabilitative services, nursing, social work, medical treatments, and possible surgical procedures. The primary goal for treating spasticity is to improve the quality of life for both the patient and family members. Treatment plans will differ according to each patient's conditions and needs, with the following objectives: (1) to relieve symptoms, (2) to enhance comfort, (3) to facilitate personal care, and (4) to promote mobility and function. Nurses play an important role in promoting quality of life by providing superior care, as well as advocating and coordinating the multidisciplinary approach to managing spasticity.

## ■ Baclofen

Baclofen is recognized as a medication that is effective in reducing the tone and symptoms of spasticity. It is structurally similar to gamma-aminobutyric acid (GABA). GABA is a primary inhibitory neurotransmitter in the CNS that promotes relaxation. Spasticity develops when the damage in the CNS impairs the release of GABA from the descending motor neuron that innervates muscle fibers, which would cause them to relax. Baclofen is a GABA agonist and binds to presynaptic GABA receptors to restrict calcium influx at the presynaptic terminal, thereby inhibiting the release of excitatory neurotransmitters across the synaptic junction at the level of the spinal cord to decrease muscle tone [2, 17, 26]. Baclofen can be administered both orally and intrathecally via an implantable pump.

**Table 11.1.** Clinical presentation and complications of spasticity

| Clinical Presentation | Complications | |
|---|---|---|
| | Symptomatic Problems | Functional Problems |
| Increased muscle tone, stiffness | Fatigue | Daily personal care |
| Increased deep tendon reflexes | Sleep disturbance | Difficulty with positioning and mobility |
| Persistent primitive reflexes | Stress | Impaired ambulation |
| Contractures | Bone deformity | Depression and anxiety |
| Clonus | Pain | Psychosocial deficits |
| Clasp-knife rigidity | | |
| Decreased coordination, strength, and endurance | | |

The primary goals of treatment with baclofen are to decrease muscle tone and improve the functional status of the patient. Major adverse effects of baclofen administered orally or intrathecally include sedation, somnolence, seizure activity, muscle weakness, orthostatic hypotension, dizziness, headaches, and ataxia. Cognitive and psychological side effects include confusion, memory deficit, decreased attention span, and depression [7, 17, 19, 27]. Adverse effects are highly dose dependent, with a high dose creating a greater risk of more severe adverse effects. Withdrawal of the medication is another major issue related to baclofen treatment. Baclofen withdrawal may result in rebound severe spasticity, rigidity, tachycardia, hypotension, hyperthermia, and seizures. Table 11.2 shows the characteristics of both oral baclofen and intrathecal baclofen.

## Oral Baclofen

Oral baclofen was introduced in the 1960s as an effective treatment for spasticity [7]. When administered orally, the drug is rapidly absorbed and partially metabolized by the liver. It is excreted by the kidneys largely unchanged. The half-life of oral baclofen is about 3.5 h [17]. Oral baclofen does not readily cross the blood–brain barrier, and requires large doses to reach therapeutic concentrations in the cerebrospinal fluid (CSF). Within the CSF, oral doses are distributed evenly both at supraspinal and spinal levels, resulting in unwanted central side effects [19]. Large oral doses can produce high risks for severe adverse effects. Extremely high doses can result life-threatening overdose symptoms including coma and death [27].

## Intrathecal Baclofen

Intrathecal baclofen (ITB) was first approved in the United States for use to treat spasticity of spinal origin in 1992, and subsequently (1996) to treat spasticity of cerebral origin [7]. ITB infuses directly into the CSF at the targeted spinal level. The half-life of ITB is about 5 h. An implantable pump inserted into the subcutaneous tissue of the abdominal wall delivers ITB. A catheter is connected to the exit port and tunneled through the subcutaneous tissue, inserted into the intrathecal space of the lumbar spine, and threaded up to the appropriate thoracic levels predetermined by the neurosurgeon. For some cases, the catheter may be threaded to higher spinal levels to account for specific patient symptoms and needs. Figures 11.2 and 11.3 illustrate the location of pump implantation and catheter placement.

High drug concentrations of ITB are found in the CSF at only fractions of the oral dose required to achieve therapeutic effects. Some reports indicate that intrathecal doses at only one-hundredth of the oral dose are necessary to reach the same effect [2, 21]. Clearance of ITB occurs via caudalcephalic bulk flow, similar to the flow of CSF in the spine. Cerebral or brainstem drug concentrations are only about one-quarter of the concentration found in the lumbar spine region following ITB administration. The risks of dose-related adverse effects and overdose are greatly minimized. The literature supports the established efficacy of ITB in managing spasticity in conditions of both cerebral and spinal origin, including cerebral palsy, head and/or spinal trauma, multiple sclerosis, and stroke [4, 10, 15, 26].

Withdrawal symptoms are more severe and much more problematic with intrathecal administration of baclofen as compared to oral administration, and may potentially be life-threatening. In addition, abrupt

**Table 11.2.** Overview of baclofen

| Oral Baclofen | Intrathecal Baclofen |
|---|---|
| Lipophilic, rapidly absorbed and partially metabolized in liver, and excreted by kidneys | Delivered directly into the spinal subarachnoid, intrathecal space |
| Barely passes the blood–brain barrier, therefore relatively low concentrations in the spinal cord and cerebrospinal fluid | Allows high levels to diffuse along the spinal cord without cerebral side effects |
| Require large dose to achieve effect | Only fractions of oral dose to achieve effect |
| Withdrawal occurs with symptoms relieved once medication re-established | Withdrawal symptoms are more severe and may become life-threatening if left untreated for greater than 24–48 h |

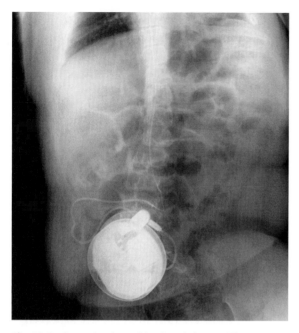

**Fig. 11.2.** Pump implanted in the abdomen. The pump is implanted into the subcutaneous tissue in the abdomen. The catheter is connected to the exit port, threaded around to the back, and inserted in the intrathecal space in the lumbospine (courtesy of Dr. Drake)

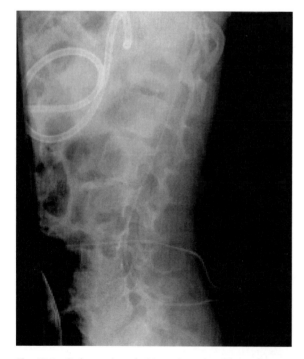

**Fig. 11.3.** Catheter threaded into the spine. The catheter is threaded from the pump to the spine, where it enters the intrathecal space at the lumbar levels and then threaded upward to the appropriate predetermined thoracic or cervical levels (courtesy of Dr. Drake)

disruption of intrathecal administration may result in rhabdomyolysis with elevated plasma creatine kinase level, renal and hepatic failure, disseminated intravascular coagulation, and sometimes death if not treated promptly [7]. When the drug is restarted or replaced with appropriate oral antispasmodic therapy, the symptoms usually resolve within 24–72 h.

## Intrathecal Baclofen Therapy

Management of spasticity with ITB therapy should follow a systematic approach and a multidisciplinary team perspective that involves the rehabilitative services, including occupational therapist, physiotherapist, and social worker. Medical and nursing staff from various services such as orthopedics, neurology, neurosurgery, and pediatric medicine may also be required. The patient requires continuous care from a primary practitioner to assess, monitor, and titrate the medication according to the patient's changing needs. The neurosurgeon not only inserts the pump, but is also required to follow up on possible complications and ensure pump function. Of course, the most important partner in the team will be the primary caregiver(s), who will assume responsibility to care for the patient and ensure that the patient continues with follow-up appointments for assessments, monitoring, and refills.

## Baclofen Pump and Programmer

ITB therapy consists of the administration of continuous ITB via an implanted, programmable pump. The pump contains a reservoir to hold the medication and a catheter access port. Contrast is injected through this port to radiographically assess pump function and catheter integrity when complications are suspected. The pump is a circular device measuring 2.5×3.5 inches (6.25×8.75 cm) and implanted into the subcutaneous space. This is powered by a battery that lasts about 5–7 years. Once the battery runs low, replacement of the battery or the entire pump apparatus is required. An external handheld programmer that includes a computer, printer, and programming head, is used to program and interrogate the pump.

Refills of ITB into the reservoir are required at regular intervals to ensure a continuous supply of medication. It is important to know the maximum capacity of the pump reservoir in order to facilitate appropriate refill schedules. The primary practitioner uses the programmer to easily interrogate and program the pump to deliver prescribed doses of medication according to the needs of the patient. The pump also has built-in alarms set to warn the patient and family members when the reservoir needs to be refilled and when the battery is running low.

Using the Medtronic Synchromed II pump as an example, there are two available sizes with reservoirs having a maximum capacity of 20 ml and 40 ml, respectively, for medications. The batteries of these pumps presently last approximately 7–8 years. The primary practitioner can set the soft, but audible, reminder alarm that beeps intermittently at 2–3 days prior to the reservoir's predicted emptying date. This alarm will alert the patient and caregiver that refilling is needed soon. A more continuous emergent alarm is preset to go off a few months prior to the end of the battery life, and serves to remind family members and primary practitioners to arrange surgery dates to change the battery or reinsert a new pump (Figs. 11.4 and 11.5).

### Patient Selection

ITB therapy is indicated for those patients with spasticity from conditions of cerebral or spinal origin that has been unresponsive to oral antispasmodics. Patients suffering from unacceptable adverse effects from effective doses of oral antispasmodics may also be considered for ITB [7]. The patient needs to be assessed for function and level of spasticity to establish a baseline by which to compare the effectiveness of ITB treatments during a screening trial. The most common scale used to assess spasticity is the Ashworth Scale Scores [3, 19, 25], which is a five-level scale ranging from no increase in tone to rigidity in flexion or extension of affected limbs, as described in Table 11.3. A severity level of 3 on the spasticity score may be a good indication for consideration for ITB

therapy. In addition, assessment should include feedback from the caregiver regarding the patient's quality of life.

### Patient Screening and Test Dosing

Selected patients then need to undergo a screening process or test dosing to ensure that they will respond positively to ITB prior to surgically implanting the

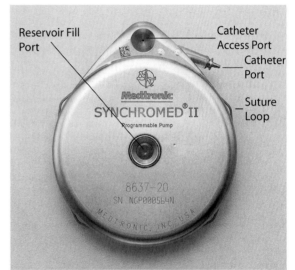

**Fig. 11.4.** Photograph of the Medtronic Synchromed II pump (courtesy of Medtronic)

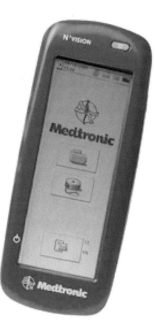

**Fig. 11.5.** Photograph of the Medtronic Synchromed II handheld programmer (picture courtesy of Medtronic)

**Table 11.3.** Spasticity levels

| Score | Description of spasticity level |
|-------|--------------------------------|
| 1 | No increase in tone |
| 2 | Mild increase in tone, giving a catch when affected limb is moved in flexion or extension |
| 3 | More marked increase in tone, but affected limb can be easily flexed |
| 4 | Considerable increase in tone; passive movements difficult with affected limb |
| 5 | Affected limbs rigid in flexion or extension |

pump. The child can undergo testing in one of two ways. The traditional method requires the patient to have a lumbar drain inserted and then receive three consecutive increasing doses of ITB through the drain over 2–3 days. The test doses are usually 50 µg, 75 µg, and 100 µg. The effect of the medication peaks at about 4 hours, and the patient is assessed for any sign of improved spasticity [26]. During this testing period, the child needs to remain on bed rest to prevent possible leakage of CSF from the drain. It is usually difficult for children with severe spasticity to undergo this more extensive testing. These children are at high risk for CSF leak and respiratory complication related to their spasticity and bed-rest protocols. The child must also be monitored closely during the entire testing period for any adverse effects from the medication.

A more recent testing practice involves the instillation of a single test dose of 50 µg or 100 µg into the intrathecal space via a lumbar puncture. The child undergoes evaluation after this dose, similar to the traditional method, but may be discharged home on the same day or the following day. This second testing method helps to minimize the complication risks associated with repeated doses. The neurosurgeon must be confident in his/her assessment of the therapeutic response with the single dose. Another advantage of the single test dose is that the child and family can return home to fully prepare the patient both clinically and physically for the procedure to insert the pump.

When considering ITB, the family should have a team meeting with the primary practitioner, neurosurgery, and the rehabilitation team to discuss the process of pump implantation and possible complications associated with the procedure. In addition, associated issues of ITB therapy need tp be explained, such as the continous follow-up appointments and repeated medication refills for the duration of treatment. The family must be emotionally, physically, and finacially prepared for the issues surrounding lifelong ITB.

## Complications of ITB Therapy

There are many complications associated with intrathecally administered baclofen. Similar to CSF shunts, ITB delivery systems are foreign devices with different parts and few connections. ITB therapy has inherent risks of developing complications that are classified into the following categories: skin or wound, catheter-related, pump apparatus, and infection.

Skin- or wound-related complications are associated with the physical and health condition of the child. Many children with cerebral palsy or other spastic illnesses are malnourished, suffer physical deformities, and are immobilized or bedridden. These physical conditions predispose the child to develop wound complications. Most commonly, inflammation and swelling forms a pocket of fluid or seroma around the pump as part of the natural healing mechanism of the body in response to surgery. The seroma can become excessive and provoke related problems, such as skin breakdown, dehiscence of the incision, CSF leakage, and superficial incisional wound infection. The application of an elastic abdominal binder will help reduce the swelling and prevent seroma development [26]. Skin breakdown over the pump site can result from stretching and continuous compression of the skin by the implanted pump [5]. Poor nutritional status adds to the complications by compromising skin integrity.

Catheter-related complications are by far the most frequently encountered problems. These complications include catheter breakages, microfracture, puncture, or kinking [8, 11]. The catheters may become disconnected at the connection ports or dislodged from the appropriate intrathecal space in the spinal cord, thereby disrupting the adequate administration of the medication [14]. The patient usually presents in the emergency room with increased spasticity, decreased level of consciousness, pain, and other symptoms indicative of ITB withdrawal. X-rays can assess the placement of the catheter and any disconnections or kinks within the catheter system. If no disconnections or possible kinking is noticed, then the integrity of the catheter should be investigated further by injecting contrast medium into the catheter access port to identify breakage or fractures.

Pump-related complications are few but may be serious. There are reports of cases where the pump flips over in the abdominal cavity [14]. The phenomenon is associated with the development of seromas creating a space for the pump, moving it from its implanted space. Other pump-related complications are linked to the electronic mechanism of the pump itself, resulting in pump failure and under- or overdelivery of the medication. Any confirmed catheter or pump complications necessitate surgical intervention to repair, reinsert, and reestablish medication infusion.

### Infection

The most serious complication associated with ITB therapy is infection. Infection can originate from the pump, the catheter, or the wound bed [10]. Possible causes of pump infection can be attributed to the surgical procedure, contamination of the pump apparatus at the time of surgery, and poor sterile technique when accessing the port for medication refill. Untreated, or poorly treated surgical wound site infections may eventually contaminate the pump and catheter.

Pump infections pose the greatest threat to patients, as they may potentially lead to a series of adverse consequences. Bacteria invading the wound and pump may spread along the catheter and enter the spinal canal causing CSF infection or meningitis. Treatment of pump infections involves a process that needs to be initiated promptly to avoid such consequences. When a pump infection is suspected, oral baclofen needs to be restarted, the pump and associated hardware removed, and the patient started on an extensive course of antibiotic therapy. When the infection is resolved, the pump is reinserted and therapy reestablished [5]. This process must be carried out efficiently to avoid inducing withdrawal symptoms and the life-threatening sequela of rhabdomyolysis with acute renal and hepatic failure.

### Nursing Considerations

Nurses can play an important role in the care of patients with spasticity and selection for pump insertion. Nurses are in a unique position to coordinate necessary resources and communicate with members of the multidisciplinary team. During each stage of the ITB therapy process, nurses have distinct and important functions. These stages can be divided into: (1) the planning and screening stage, (2) the preoperative preparation stage, (3) the immediate postoperative hospitalization stage, and (4) the follow up and monitoring stage.

#### Trial Screening Stage

During the planning and trial screening stage of ITB therapy, nurses need to provide appropriate education to patients and their families to help them understand test procedures, as well as the potential benefits and complications. The family needs to have complete disclosure of all possible issues and barriers involved with ITB treatment. The nurse can coordinate the services of a social worker to help facilitate available resources for financial support to the family for long term medication costs. If the trial screening test fails, family members require empathetic emotional support and education about other available resources to the patient for spasticity management.

#### Preoperative Preparation Stage

During this stage, nurses can help to prepare the child to become physically and emotionally ready to undergo surgery and pump implantation. A thorough assessment of the patient's physical condition, nutritional status, clinical presentation, and family readiness can help minimize the risk for potential complications.

The child needs to be in optimum physical condition before surgery. Children with spasticity tend to have poor nutritional intake as a result of their underlying disease. Compounding poor intake, these children are in nutritional catabolic states burning calories at greater rates than intake [24]. The resulting picture presents undernourished children with low body weights, disturbed immune systems, and poor skin integrity. All these conditions predispose the children to infection and seroma development. During this preoperative stage, bringing together a team consisting of a dietician/nutritionist, physical therapists, occupational therapist, social worker, and nurse to work with the family will optimize the physical condition of the patients and address any health problems.

#### Postoperative Stage

The postoperative stage is focused primarily on prevention of both surgical and pump-specific complications. Infection is again the major concern in this stage. The Centers recommends a 24-h course of prophylactic antibiotics postoperatively. Any extended length of antibacterial course would be unwarranted unless actual infection is evident. A firm abdominal binder may prevent seroma development and the associated issues.

The contractures and physical deformity associated with spastic disease predisposes patients to develop the postoperative complications associated with surgery, such as, for example, atelectasis, aspiration pneumonia, ileus, and emodynamic and electrolyte imbalances. Nursing care should rather than encourage mobility, hygiene, and nutrition to facilitate healing. Good skin care, frequent turning and repositioning, and provision of adequate nutrition, will help prevent the skin/wound-related problems and post-operative complications.

Pain associated with the surgical incision may exaggerate spasticity in the immediate postoperative period. Adequate pain management is necessary to promote activities and healing. Postoperative analgesics given at regular intervals to maintain appropriate serum levels are highly recommended to promote comfort. In addition, management of postoperative nausea and vomiting is equally important in this patient population.

### Follow-up and Monitoring Stage

A child with a baclofen pump requires dedication and commitment on the part of the patient and family. It is important that the family keep regularly scheduled follow-up appointments with the entire healthcare team. Missed or delayed appointments may provoke life-threatening and withdrawal conditions. Plassat et al. suggested that dose increases are required up to years following implantation [20]. In many cases drug tolerance and drug sensitivity can become a problem with therapy. Dose change requirements are exaggerated during altered states of health, including fevers and cold. Family members should report any physical and functional changes, possible technical pump problems, or withdrawal symptoms to their care provider. This stage is a complete partnership between patient, family, and medical team. Review and evaluation of the risks and benefits of the therapy occur constantly.

Unlike other surgeries, the insertion of a baclofen pump is similar to that of CNS shunts; once the operative incision is made, an unbreakable bond is established between the family and the healthcare team. Continual support and education from the entire healthcare team help ensure success for ITB therapy and positive outcomes.

## Rhizotomy

## History

The idea of rhizotomy as a method for relieving spasticity was first suggested in 1888 by a New York neurologist by the name of Dr. Charles Dana in a letter to Dr. Robert Abbe. This idea was put into action by Dr. Abbe on a select few patients. He found that indeed, cutting nerves relieved spasticity and the accompanying pain, but also resulted in loss of needed sensation and function. Thereafter, in 1908, a German neurologist by the name of Foerster began to section the posterior lumbar nerve roots, but he also had less than desirable long-term results. It wasn't until the 1970s that an Italian physician by the name of Fasano, along with his colleagues, developed a technique to separate the individual nerve fibers (also called fascicles or rootlets). By using electrical stimulation, he cut the fascicles, relieving the most severe spastic symptoms without losing the desirable sensory function [18].

## Patient Selection

Currently, patients are carefully evaluated and selected for rhizotomy. Ideal candidates are usually children who have walked, have the potential to attain ambulation with rhizotomy, have spasticity that interferes with functions such as sitting, or have hip dislocations caused by spasticity [1]. Review of patient records and examination is performed by a team consisting of a neurologist, physical and occupational therapists, an orthopedist, a developmental specialist, and a neurosurgeon. Patients are screened based on their muscle strength and contractures as well as their ability to cooperate with therapists. Although previous orthopedic procedures may not exclude the child from selection, they will need to have more extensive testing to qualify. Patients are usually between the ages of 4 and 9 years, as they have been found to have the best response. Children younger than 4 years generally are not able to cooperate fully with physical therapy or have the developed muscle strength to get the full benefit of the surgery. Children older than 9 years, and adults, have usually developed contractures and these are not responsive to rhizotomy [18].

## Procedure

A rhizotomy is performed to relieve spasticity in the areas where the reflex arcs are the most pathological. The patient is taken to the operating room and given a short-acting muscle relaxant for intubation and to allow the neurosurgeon to access the area. The paralysis is then reversed to permit electric stimulation and recording. The patient continues under anesthesia and may also be given a narcotic to relieve the pain of the electric stimulation. Electrical stimulation and recording is carried out to identify the specific root level and differentiate between motor and sensory nerve bundles as they exit the foramen. The sensory bundles are separated into rootlets. Then the rootlets are gently separated and stimulated to test the effect on various muscles and to find those creating the spasticity. The rootlets that stimulate an abnormal reflex arc to the muscles and cause tetany are cut [6].

### Postoperative Nursing Care

Pain control is usually the main postoperative nursing consideration. The patient may feel a burning sensation in the back and legs from the severed nerves. It is exacerbated with movement or any change in sensations, such as hot or cold, or movement of clothing or linens. There are several ways to achieve pain control. One is to place an intrathecal catheter and administer several epidural doses of morphine in the first 48 h after surgery. Another is intravenous analgesia, usually morphine or fentanyl, but this produces some undesirable side effects, the most important being respiratory depression at the doses required to achieve patient comfort [18]. The patient should be monitored for muscle spasms. Valium may be used in addition to analgesia to control spasms.

Postoperatively, the patient is positioned on either side or prone for the first 1–2 days. The patient often wants to curl up in a fetal position after surgery. The application of knee splints holds the legs in a natural, extended position. Physical therapy is started on the 3rd day postoperatively and will continue after discharge. Complications in rhizotomy patients include asthma attacks and pneumonia from aspiration of vomit. This usually occurs in children with a history of asthma or recent respiratory infection. There may also be a temporary inability to urinate spontaneously and the patient should be monitored for urinary retention. Once the burning pain subsides, the child may report a "pins and needles" feeling or patchy numbness to the legs and/or feet. This may resolve or be permanent [1, 16].

Long-term results from rhizotomy are as varied as the patients themselves. Approximately 80% of rhizotomy patients have some improvement in spasticity. Some children go on to require further surgeries to correct shortened tendons or hip dislocations [16].

### Pediatric Practice Pearls

■ Rapid withdrawal of intrathecal baclofen, whether from pump removal, pump malfunction, or incorrect dosing, can result in severe withdrawal symptoms and death. Appropriate doses of oral baclofen should be used in the interim.

■ It is imperative that parents of children who are candidates for ITB understand the long-term commitment they must make for follow-up.

■ Videotaping the patient before rhizotomy and at various times after surgery will show the parents how much progress has been made.

■ Explain to parents that after rhizotomy it sometimes takes a while to regain some skills, such as walking, as it is necessary to retrain muscle groups to do these functions.

### References

1. Abbott R (1999) Selective dorsal rhizotomy. Retrieved August 16, 2005, from http://cerebnet. netfirms. com/selective. htm
2. Albright AL (2003) Neurosurgical treatment of spasticity and other pediatric movement disorders. J Child Neurol 18:S67–S78
3. Awaad Y, Tayem H, Munoz S, Ham S, Michon AM, Awaad R (2003) Functional assessment following intrathecal Baclofen therapy in children with spastic cerebral palsy. J Child Neurol 18:26–34
4. Bergenheim AT, Wendelius M, Shahidi S, Larsson E (2003) Spasticity in a child with myelomeningocele treated with continuous intrathecal Baclofen. Pediatr Neurosurg 39:218–221
5. Boviatsis EJ, Kouyialis AT, Boutsikakis I, Korfas S, Sakas DE (2004) Infected CNS infusion pumps: is there a chance for treatment without removal? Acta Neurochir 146:463–467
6. Cheek WR (1996) Atlas of Pediatric Neurosurgery. WB Saunders, Philadelphia
7. Dario A, Tomei G (2004) A benefit–risk assessment of Baclofen in severe spinal spasticity. Drug Safety 27:799–818
8. Dawes WJ, Drake JM, Fehlings D (2003) Microfracture of a Baclofen pump catheter with intermittent under- and overdose. Pediatr Neurosurg 39:144–148
9. Dietz V (2000) Spastic movement disorder. Spinal Cord 38:389–393
10. Fitzgerald JJ, Tsegaye M, Vloeberghs MH (2004) Treatment of childhood spasticity of cerebral origin with intrathecal Baclofen: a series of 52 cases. Br J Neurosurg 18:240–245

11. Follett KA, Burchiel K, Deer T, Dupen S, Prager J, Turner MS. Et al (2003) Prevention of intrathecal drug delivery catheter-related complications. Neuromodulation 6:32–41

12. Gallichio JE (2004) Pharmacologic management of spasticity following stroke. Phys Ther 84:973–981

13. Goldstein EM (2001) Spasticity management: an overview. J Child Neurol 16: 16–23

14. Gooch JL, Oberg WA, Grams B, Ward LA, Walker ML (2003) Complications of intrathecal Baclofen pumps in children. Pediatr Neurosurg 39:1–6

15. Ibrahim M, Wurpei J, Gladson B (2003) Intrathecal Baclofen: a new treatment approach for severe spasticity in patients with stroke. J Neurol Phys Ther 27:142–148

16. Institute For Neurology Neurosurgery (2004) Rhizotomy. Retrieved August 16, 2005, from http://nyneruosurgery.org/cp/thizhist.html

17. Krach LE (2001) Pharmacotherapy of spasticity: oral medications and intrathecal Baclofen. J Child Neurol 16:31–36

18. Moss SD, Manwaring KH (1992) Relief of spasticity for children with cerebral palsy using selective posterior rhizotomy. Phoenix Child Hosp Pediatr Rev 4:5–11

19. O'Donnell M, Armstrong R (1997) Pharmacologic interventions for management of spasticity in cerebral palsy. Ment Retard Dev Disabil Res Rev 3:204–211

20. Plassat R, Verbe BP, Menei P, Menegalli D, Mathe JF, Richard I (2004) Treatment of spasticity with intrathecal Baclofen administration: long-term follow-up, review of 40 patients. Spinal Cord 42:686–693

21. Rizzo MA, Hadjimichael OC, Preinigherova J, Vollmer TL (2004) Prevalence and treatment of spasticity reported by multiple sclerosis patients. Mult Scler 10:589–595

22. Roscigno CI (2002) Addressing spasticity-related pain in children with spastic cerebral palsy. J Neurosci Nurs 34:123–133

23. Sheean G (2002) The pathophysiology of spasticity. Eur J Neurol 9:3–9

24. Stallings VA, Cronk CE, Zemel BS, Charney EB (1995) Body composition in children with spastic quadriplegic cerebral palsy. J Pediatr 126:833–839

25. Vanek ZF (2003) Spasticity. eMedicine Neurology. Retrieved May 21, 2004, from http://www.emedicine.com/neuro/topic706.htm

26. Vitztum C, Olney B (2000) Intrathecal Baclofen therapy and the child with cerebral palsy. Orthop Nurs 19:43–48

27. Von Koch CS, Park TS, Steinbok P, Smyth M, Peacock WJ (2001) Selective posterior rhizotomy and intrathecal Baclofen for the treatment of spasticity. Pediatr Neurosurg 35:57–65

28. Walton K (2003) Management of patients with spasticity: a practical approach. Pract Neurol 3:342–353

# Infections of the Central Nervous System

*George Marcus Galvan*

**12**

## Contents

## Brain Abscess, Epidural Abscess, Subdural Empyema

Intracranial suppurative (pus forming) processes can be divided into three categories based on the distinct anatomical areas in which the infection occurs. These areas, from superficial to deep, are the epidural space, subdural space, and parenchyma tissue. This section will focus on these processes and their relationships to one another.

## Etiology

Approximately 1500–2500 cases of brain abscess occur every year in the United States among all age groups, with 25–44% of these cases occurring in children less than 15 years of age [11]. The incidence for both subdural empyema and epidural abscess combined approximates 13–25% of all intracranial infections, with epidural abscesses being rare [16]. The incidence of all intracranial suppurative processes was thought to be declining due to improved antibiotic therapy, but it actually may be on the rise as a result of the increased occurrence of neurosurgical procedures, improved imaging techniques, and increased population of immunosuppressed patients [11]. The infective process depends on: (1) the quantity of microorganisms that are involved, (2) their virulence, (3) the immunological status of the patient, and (4) the timeliness of clinical diagnosis and treatment [16].

All three types of infections originate from many different sources, which include contiguous site infections (i.e., chronic otitis media, mastoiditis, dental procedures, sinusitis, or ruptured dermoid tumor), distant pathologic states (i.e., cyanotic congenital heart disease, chronic lung infections, pulmonary arteriovenous fistulae from Osler-Weber-Rendu Syndrome), head trauma (e.g., open depressed skull fractures, gunshot wound), neurosurgical procedures, or from cryptogenic sources [21]. The most common etiology for brain abscesses is hematogenous, while contiguous spread is seen more in subdural empyemas and epidural abscesses. It is not surprising that no source can be found in 25% of the cases. Those with congenital heart disease, especially tetralogy of Fallot, will have an increased risk of abscess, at approximately 4–7%, due to the lack of filtering provided by the lungs and hypoxic brain tissue, which is favorable for abscess formation [10]. Brain abscess rarely occurs in children less than 2 years of age, but if seen, it is usually secondary to Gram-negative, citrobacter, or group B streptococcus meningitis [2,11].

## Pathophysiology

Contiguous spread of an infection to the brain leads to an area of infection adjacent to the source. This is evidenced by the fact that a brain abscess, or subdural empyema, from otitis media will most likely occur in the temporal lobe, while those originating from the frontal or ethmoid sinus will occur in the frontal lobe. This type of spread results from direct extension through the bone, between bony sutures, or via extension through venous structures [11]. Epidural abscesses can occur in conjunction with osteomyelitis of the skull. Common organisms of contiguous spread include *Streptococcus, Staphylococcus, Bacteroides,* and *Pseudomonas* species [16].

Hematological spread usually originates from a cardiac or pulmonary source, and usually extends through the distribution of the middle cerebral artery. This type of spread tends to form at the gray–white matter junction, and abscesses due to this process are usually multiple, which makes this type unique. Common organisms include *Streptococcus, Staphylococcus,* and *Hemophilus* species [25].

Head trauma and neurosurgical procedures produce abscesses and empyemas, which contain organisms native to the skin. This includes *Staphylococcus, Streptococcus,* and Gram-negative species. Fungal infective processes are rare in the child and are usually associated with AIDS or immunological suppression after organ transplantation, chemotherapy, or from congenital disease [18].

There are four stages of abscess maturation. Days 1–3 consist of early inflammatory changes, with some necrosis and edema. Days 4–9 are characterized by increased inflammatory changes as fibroblasts and leukocytes are recruited to the area of central necrosis and edema. Early capsule formation begins on days 10–13, with maturation complete on day 14 [11].

## Presenting Symptoms

The nurse should look for objective signs and symptoms, such as fever, headache, and focal neurological deficit. Neurological deficit, including cranial nerve palsies, hemiparesis, or decreased mental status, can occur in up to 50% of cases. Most problems seen are due to increased intracranial pressure (ICP), and can result in vomiting, lethargy, and even seizures.

While interviewing the patient or the family, it is important to recognize any recent or chronic infections, especially of the head, ears, nose, or throat. Also inquire about fevers, headache, nasal or ear drainage, and earache. For infants, you will need to determine if there are any signs of failure to thrive (i.e., poor growth, lack of appetite, or delay in development).

Nurses should note any recent dental procedures, head trauma, or neurosurgical or otolaryngology procedures. Furthermore, the caregiver needs to inquire about history regarding congenital disease, immune deficiency history, as well as sick contacts.

On exam, note the general appearance of the child. Document whether the child is interactive, lethargic, or irritable. Inspect and palpate the skull for tenderness, trauma, or swelling. Check the ears for drainage, and look at the mouth and throat for exudate, erythema, dental caries, or swelling. Be sure to perform a full cranial nerves exam, look for asymmetry or dysfunction. In an infant, inspect for reactivity of the pupils, check for conjugate gaze, measure head circumference, and note whether the fontanels are bulging or if the sutures are splayed. Assess motor strength and sensation in all four extremities. If the child has concurrent meningitis, you may notice neck stiffness or photophobia. Auscultate the heart for murmurs, clicks, or dysarrhythmias. Observe for clues of right-to-left heart shunting such as cyanosis, clubbing, and tachypnea.

### Diagnostic Tests

Initial testing will involve obtaining a serum white blood count (WBC), blood cultures, erythrocyte sedimentation rate (ESR), and C-reactive protein (CRP). Unfortunately, the serum WBC may be normal or mildly elevated in 60–70% of cases, while blood cultures are usually negative. ESR will become elevated, but may be normal in some cases, such as congenital cyanotic heart disease, whereas polycythemia lowers the ESR. CRP becomes elevated with any type of infection and is more of an acute-phase protein than ESR, but is nonspecific like ESR [10]. The yield of a lumbar puncture depends on whether the infection is in contact with the intracranial cerebrospinal fluid (CSF) spaces. A lumbar puncture may reveal an elevated WBC, decreased glucose, elevated protein, or isolation of infective organism, all of which provide valuable information indicating an infective process. If a lumbar puncture is to be considered, it must be done with caution due to the concern of herniation, especially in the presence of increased ICP.

In infants, cranial ultrasonography may reveal fluid collections with echogenic boundaries. However, contrasted head computed tomography (CT) or magnetic resonance imaging (MRI) are better studies, with MRI being preferable due to superior visualization of brain matter and fluid collections (Figs. 12.1 and 12.2). Contrast enhancement will vary depending on maturation of abscess and whether steroids were administered, which may decrease contrast uptake, thus decreasing contrast enhancement. MRI spectroscopy and a leukocyte scan (radioactive labeling of a patient's WBC and reinjecting into the patient) are able to further confirm the diagnosis when CT or MRI leaves uncertainty in diagnosis. Finally, operative biopsy sampling or excision will bring forth a diagnosis and in most cases identify the pathogen.

### Treatment Options

For brain abscesses, surgical treatment is usually indicated. It becomes required for decreasing mental status, deteriorating neurologic exam, marked mass effect, location near the ventricles, failure of lesions to improve with 1–2 weeks of antibiotic therapy, or the need to obtain organism for culture and sensitivities. Surgical treatment consists of needle aspiration or excision. Medical management may be considered if

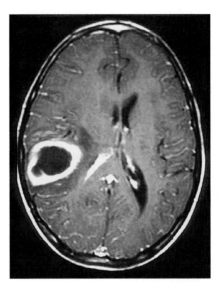

**Fig. 12.1.** T-1 weighted magnetic resonance imaging (MRI) scan with contrast demonstrating a ring-enhancing lesion suspicious for intracranial abscess

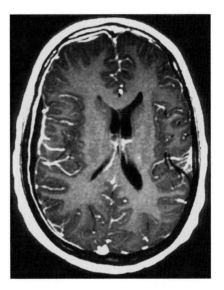

**Fig. 12.2.** T-1 weighted MRI scan with contrast-revealing, right-sided enhancement along the cortical surface of the brain with a hypointense (dark-appearing) fluid collection representing a subdural empyema

treatment is begun early in the infection, improvement is seen with initiation of treatment, the lesions are smaller than 3 cm, or if the abscess is located in an eloquent brain area.

For subdural empyemas and epidural abscesses, surgical treatment is indicated in most cases. The surgical therapy can range from simple burr holes to a

large craniotomy, with possible conversion to a craniectomy if the bone flap is infected. In infants with
subdural empyemas, medical management usually
suffices, but in certain cases transfontanel needle aspiration or burr holes are needed.

Antibiotic therapy should be started immediately
upon determination of intracranial infection. Initial
antibiotics for empiric therapy for all intracranial
suppurative processes should include the following:
vancomycin, a third-generation cephalosporin, and
metronidazole [15]. Once the bacteria is cultured and
identified, antibiotic therapy is tailored to suit. Intravenous antibiotic therapy is usually needed for 6–
8 weeks, with some recommending 2–3 months of
additional oral antibiotic therapy once intravenous
treatment has concluded.

A distinctive form of posttraumatic brain abscess
seen in children results from penetrating injuries to
the orbital region, as well as other areas of the skull.
These injuries are caused by such things as pencil tips,
wooden sticks, wooden toys, and lawn darts. Treatment involves prompt surgical debridement. To prevent meningitis or abscess following a penetrating
brain injury, prophylactic antibiotic therapy should
consist of either a broad-spectrum cephalosporin
with good blood–brain barrier penetration, or nafcillin. The general guideline for duration is 5 days, with
adjustments made based on the extent of injury. If an
abscess is suspected from a penetrating brain injury,
then the antibiotic regimen should be changed to
vancomycin, metronidazole, and ceftazidime for a
time course of approximately 6–8 weeks [22].

## Nursing Care

Nursing care is focused on observation of the patient, with special attention paid to the neurological
exam. Serial exams will allow the nurse to distinguish any signs of deterioration. Age-appropriate
neurological exams are key to the nursing care of
these patients. Alertness, mental status, cranial
nerve exam (especially pupil reactivity), motor and
sensory testing, reflexes, and fever curves will help
dictate care. Monitor incisions or wounds, inspect
for increasing tenderness, erythema, drainage, and
dehiscence. Ensure proper and timely delivery of antibiotics. Monitor fluid and electrolyte status closely,
since this can change drastically with deleterious effects. Attempt to keep the head of the bed raised to at
least 30° to help protect against elevated ICP, and
provide a quiet environment that does not overstim-
ulate the patient. Be sure that all caregivers and visi-
tors undergo thorough hand washing before and after visiting.

## Patient and Family Education

Upon discharge to home, educate the patient and
family to monitor for any type of change in neurological status. For infants, family should call the physician if they detect any change in alertness, difficulty
in arousing, irritability, decreased feeding, bulging
fontanels, seizures, or intractable vomiting. The family should also note fevers, and any temperature
greater than 100.5°F (approximately 38°C) warrants a
call to the physician. The patients should be kept away
from sick contacts during their convalescence. Discharge instructions should cover wound care, activity,
follow-up, and medications.

## Outcome

The prognosis for survival and neurological morbidity depends on the patient's level of consciousness at
the time of initiation of therapy [18]. If the patient is
unconscious at time of presentation, the mortality
rate reaches up to 50%, but if the patient is awake the
mortality drops to less than 10%. This statistic does
not apply to epidural abscesses, which tend to be associated with minimal risk of mortality [16]. With
today's diagnostic tools, neurosurgical intervention,
and antibiotics, the overall mortality rate has dropped
to 10%. Unfortunately, morbidity remains a problem,
with patients experiencing permanent deficit or seizures in up to 50% of cases [10]. The younger population, especially those under 2 years of age, has a high
risk of learning disability. Recurrence happens at a
rate of less than 10% [18].

In summary, treatment consists of antibiotic therapy, as well as surgical intervention when indicated,
and time is essential because rapid intervention leads
to improved outcome.

## Neurocysticercosis

Neurocysticercosis is a distinct infective process of the human brain by *Taenia solium*. It dates back to the time of ancient Greece, where it was known as the disease of the swine. Since the 17th century, it has been recognized as a disease that affects humans, and only since the second half of the 19th century has this pathogen been studied and understood. It is one of the few conditions included in a list of potentially eradicable infectious diseases of public health concern, but it still remains a problem in our world today [5].

## Etiology

For years the disease has been endemic to Eastern Europe, Asia, and Latin America [3]. The World Health Organization estimates that 50,000 people die each year, worldwide, from neurocysticercosis. Due to increased migration and people traveling to endemic areas, the incidence of this disease is on the rise in the United States [5]. Neurocysticercosis is currently one of the most common parasitic diseases of the central nervous system (CNS) in the United States, and is a leading cause of epilepsy among Hispanic children living in United States metropolitan areas along the Mexican border [9]. *T. solium* is the parasite responsible for Neurocysticercosis. The pig is the intermediate host, where ingested larvae cysts embed themselves in the pig's muscle. Ingestion of this pork by humans will result only in adult tapeworm manifestation in the gastrointestinal (GI) tract, known as taeniasis. Neurocysticercosis results from the next stage of the parasite, where the adult tapeworms lay eggs. These eggs are passed out of the human GI tract and are transmitted by the fecal-oral route. Vegetable matter may become contaminated when untreated sewage is used as a fertilizer. It is also known that flies play a significant role in the dispersion of eggs, since they can ingest the eggs and expel these same eggs 48 h later [16]. Once ingested, the eggs will enter and cross over the GI tract into the bloodstream, where they are free to penetrate different organ systems [3,5].

## Pathophysiology

Upon reaching the human GI tract, the egg's thin outer membrane will dissolve, releasing the inner oncosphere or larvae. The oncospheres readily cross the intestinal lining, but are usually destroyed by the immune system. They will escape the defenses of the host if they reach immunologically privileged sites, such as the CNS or eyes. In the CNS, the larvae tend to lodge in the small arterioles at the gray–white interface of the cerebral hemispheres and at the leptomeninges [2,3]. However, the larvae can invade any part of the CNS, and once they invade, they will each mature into a cysticercus with a lifespan of approximately 18 months. The cysticercus is characterized by a head, body, four suckers, and some 20 pairs of hooks arranged as a crown [3].

The immunological response to the cysticercus lays the foundation for what is known as neurocysticercosis, and manifests pathological changes like gliosis, necrosis, vasculitis, blockage of CSF drainage, meningitis, intracranial hypertension, and demyelination. The types of infestation can be categorized according to location. These are parenchymal, meningeal, intraventricular, spinal, or mixed. Even once the cysticercus has died, inflammatory reactions can continue to occur for years.

## Presenting Symptoms

The most common presenting symptoms are seizures and intracranial hypertension. Parenchymal forms manifest as convulsive disorders, motor or sensory deficit, or deterioration of consciousness. Meningeal involvement presents with photophobia, headache, nausea, vomiting, nuchal rigidity, cranial nerve palsies (particularly cranial nerves II, V, VI, and VII), and possibly hydrocephalus. Intraventricular infestation may manifest as intermittent acute hydrocephalus, which may result in loss of consciousness with position changes [3]. Spinal involvement has not been documented in children, but presents in adults as motor or sensory deficits, with a combination of upper motor and lower motor neuron pathology.

## Diagnostic Tests

The diagnosis is made on the combination of radiographic demonstration of a cyst and serological evidence. CT and MRI scans can accurately show the lesions of neurocysticercosis, with MRI having better sensitivity and CT being more readily available. In ac-

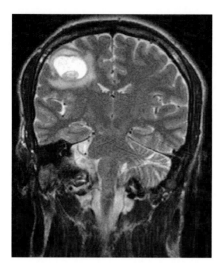

**Fig. 12.3.** T-2 weighted MRI scan showing a cystic lesion in the right parietal lobe with a nodule on the inferior aspect, which represents the larvae of *Taenia solium*

tive disease, a ring-enhancing cyst is noted on CT or MRI, which may have surrounding edema. On these images, the larvae can sometimes be seen within the walls of the cyst (Fig. 12.3).

An enzyme-linked immunoelectrotransfer blot for detection of antibodies to *T. solium* can be performed on either CSF or serum to achieve a diagnosis. This type of testing has a sensitivity of 98% and specificity of 100%, but in patients with only a single brain lesion, up to 30% test negative [6,19]. CSF enzyme-linked immunosorbent assay for detection of antibodies or antigens to *T. solium* is also available and has a sensitivity of 87% and a specificity of 95% [20].

## Treatment Options

The usual treatment for active disease is medical management with antiparasitic drugs. Brain lesions with no evidence of active disease, as evident by calcifications, typically require no antiparasitic treatment. The two main antiparasitic drugs used today are albendazole (15 mg/kg/day) and praziquantel (100 mg/kg/day). The efficacy for both is as high as 90%, but albendazole is preferred due to fewer side effects, lower cost, and higher CSF concentrations [3]. In cases of encephalitis and intracranial hypertension, antiparasitic therapy is contraindicated because treatment may cause exacerbation of cerebral swelling and edema, leading to herniation and death [9]. Other medi-

cal management focuses on antiepileptic drugs (AEDs), steroids, analgesics, and osmotic agents. Steroids play a significant role in the initiation of antiparasitic therapy, since the destruction of the cysticerci may lead to significant and devastating inflammatory responses, resulting in increased ICP and even death. Steroids also help alleviate symptoms such as nausea, vomiting, and headache during antiparasitic therapy.

Surgical therapy is indicated for the removal of space-occupying lesions causing significant mass effect and for the removal of seizure foci that are refractory to AEDs. Endoscopic removal is an option for ventricular lesions, and CSF diversion is often needed to treat communicating or obstructive hydrocephalus. In the case of obstructive hydrocephalus due to intraventricular neurocysticercosis, an attempt should be made to remove the lesion before shunting.

## Nursing Care

Nursing care is essential during the administration of antiparasitic agents. One must be on guard for signs of increased ICP, such as lethargy, vomiting, increasing headache, and unresponsiveness. Steroid administration should be initiated prior to antiparasitic therapy. Seizure precautions should be enforced to protect the child from injury. Analgesics will play a major role, since many will experience headaches during antiparasitic therapy.

## Patient and Family Education

Education will focus on medications, since the child may be discharged on an AED, as well as an antiparasitic agent or steroids. Neurocysticercosis can cause rapid deterioration, which can ultimately result in death. During discharge education, this needs to be emphasized, and the family should be instructed to seek immediate medical attention for any change in neurological status. Since a large proportion of pediatric patients inflicted with neurocysticercosis may be of Hispanic descent or from some other part of world beside the USA, an interpreter may be needed to help overcome the communication barrier. In addition, cultural issues may need to be addressed, and special help may be sought from the hospital or community to help bridge any gaps. The family members should be screened for disease, especially if the family comes from an endemic part of the world. Also, the patient and family should be taught how the disease is transmitted. Education should focus on frequent hand washing and sanitary handling of food. If the family and patient plan to travel to endemic areas, or areas with poor sanitation, caution should be undertaken in the consumption of foods from unsanitary restaurants or street vendors.

## Outcome

If neurocysticercosis is treated properly, a cure rate of 90% can be achieved in children. Even with cure, the child may have problems with epilepsy or hydrocephalus. With proper treatment, lesions will often disappear, seizures will resolve, and imaging studies will normalize. For these patients, AEDs may be tapered off in 2 years [9]. However, in one study there was a reported rate of 50% for seizure recurrence following cessation of AEDs after 2 years of treatment, indicating that the effects of neurocysticercosis on epilepsy may be life-long [17]. This may be the result of a permanent structural abnormality caused by neurocysticercosis that is responsible for the seizure foci. The long-term effects of this condition on mental and cognitive development are not known for certain, but it is suspected that it plays a negative role. The real cure will not come from the treatment of the disease, but only with the eradication of the parasite.

## Shunt Infections

Shunts continue to be the mainstay of treatment for hydrocephalus. These devices have reduced the morbidity and mortality of hydrocephalus, but can become the target of infection. When this occurs, the child may suffer serious negative consequences, and treatment is needed immediately. The care of patients experiencing a shunt infection is, unfortunately, a common event that nurses will encounter often in a neurosurgical setting.

## Etiology

The incidence of shunt malfunction is approximately 30% over 1 year, with shunt occlusion being the pri-

mary cause, followed secondarily by shunt infection. North American infection rates average between 5 and 15%, with 7% being the most cited number [24]. Shunt infections most often result from colonization of the device by normally nonpathogenic skin flora. They usually occur soon after placement, with 70% of shunt infections occurring within 2 months of placement and 80% within 6 months [7,8,14,23]. The main risk factors for shunt infection that have consistently been reported in the literature are length of procedure, skin condition, presence of open neural tube defect, and younger age. For example, in the case of an infant born with myelomeningocele, waiting until the infant is 2 weeks old may significantly reduce the infection risk [10]. Other implicated risk factors include etiology of hydrocephalus, number of shunt revisions, site of shunt revision, type of shunt, concomitant infection, condition of the skin, and number of people in the operating room [3].

## Pathophysiology

Shunt infections are unique from other types of CNS infections because they involve a foreign body. Often the shunt becomes colonized at time of placement. Infection can also occur from wound breakdown, retrograde colonization from the distal end, or hematogenous seeding. The bacteria are able to adhere to the foreign body and secrete glycolipids, which help protect the bacteria from host defenses [2]. More than two-thirds of shunt infections are caused by staphylococcal species. The most common is *Staphylococcus epidermidis*, followed by *Staphylococcus aureus*. Approximately 6-20% of infections are from Gram-negative bacilli, such as *Escherichia coli* and *Klebsiella* species. In neonates, the common pathogens are *Escherichia coli* and *Streptococcus hemoliticus* [10].

## Presenting Symptoms

Symptoms at presentation consist of headache, fever, chills, lethargy, nausea, vomiting, anorexia, irritability, mental status changes, and abdominal or pleural pain (depending on the location of the distal end of the shunt). In neonates, the presentation may manifest as apneic spells, anemia, hepatosplenomegaly, and neck stiffness [10]. A patient may present with tenderness, erythema, or cellulitis over the shunt tract. Shunt nephritis is unique to a ventriculovascular shunt in which immune complexes are deposited in the renal glomeruli causing proteinuria and hematuria.

## Diagnostic Tests

Initial evaluation begins with serum WBC, ESR, CRP, and blood cultures. In 25% of shunt infections, the WBC will be normal, while in another 33% it will be greater than 20,000 cells/mm [16]. ESR and CRP are nonspecific, but are rarely normal in shunt infections. Blood cultures will be positive in about 33% of shunt infections, unless the distal end is in a vascular structure, which brings the rate of positive cultures to 90% [10]. Collection of CSF via a shunt tap is desirable, since the fluid collected is in direct contact with the shunt. The fluid is sent for glucose, protein, cell count with differential, Gram stain, and culture. CSF studies suggestive for infection include low glucose, high protein, and elevated WBC (Table 12.1). A positive Gram stain or culture is diagnostic. Head CT is not useful to determine infection, but can show worsening hydrocephalus, indicating shunt malfunction secondary to possible infection. Ultrasound or CT of the abdomen may useful to determine if a peritoneal cyst, also known as pseudocyst, is present, which is suggestive of infection. If infection of a ventriculoatrial shunt is suspected, a 24-h urine collection for quantitative protein is obtained along with blood cultures, a complete blood count, and evaluation of CRP levels.

## Treatment Options

Medical management with antibiotics alone has a low success rate and requires weeks to months of treatment. Typical treatment requires initiation of antibiotics and removal or externalization of the shunt system. When the shunt is removed, CSF drainage can be provided by means of an external ventricular drain, intermittent ventricular taps, or lumbar punctures in the case of a communicating hydrocephalus. If the shunt is externalized, it is done distal to the site of ventricular insertion, usually at the level of the clavicle. Initial antibiotic therapy consists of vancomycin, rifampin, and a third-generation cephalosporin or aminoglycoside. Once cultures and sensitivities return, antibiotic therapy can be tailored to the organism. Intraventricular injection of preservative-free antibiotics via an externalized shunt or external ventricular drain is utilized in conjunction with systemic intravenous therapy to further enhance treatment. The patient is reimplanted with a new shunt based on the preference of the surgeon. The criteria usually considered on when to reimplant include serial negative CSF cultures, absence of fevers, and completion of antibiotics after negative CSF cultures.

## Nursing Care

Antibiotic therapy must remain on a tight schedule with no interruptions in treatment. Delay or missed antibiotics could lead to resurgence of the pathogen and delay the time for reimplantation. If the child's shunt is externalized, or an external ventricular drain is placed, care should be taken to keep the exit site clean and dry. It is acceptable to place antibiotic or Betadine ointment on the wound initially, but more than 3 days of this treatment may cause the skin to macerate and prevent good healing. It is best to keep it clean and dry, and to keep it covered with a sterile occlusive dressing, especially if the child is likely to pick at and touch the

**Table 12.1.** Cerebrospinal fluid (*CSF*) values according to age [8]. *WBC* White blood cell count

| Age group | WBC/mm³ | Protein (mg/dl) | Glucose (mg/dl) | Glucose ratio (CSF:plasma) |
|---|---|---|---|---|
| Premature infant | 10 | 150 | 20–65 | 0.5–1.6 |
| Term infant | 7–8 | 80 | 30–120 | 0.4–2.5 |
| Infant 1–12 months | 5–6 | 15–80 | | |
| Infant 1–2 years | 2–3 | 15 | | |
| Young child | 2–3 | 20 | | |
| Child 5–15 years | 2–3 | 25 | | |
| Adolescent and adult | 3 | 30 | 40–80 | 0.5 |

wound or catheter. Keeping the child occupied through playtime, schoolwork, or child-life activities will help distract the child during their hospitalization. Pain and irritability are issues with shunt infections, and the child may experience headaches and fevers. Treatment with acetaminophen and ibuprofen helps to alleviate these symptoms in most children, but occasionally you may need to employ stronger agents, such as hydrocodone, morphine, or nalbuphine.

## Patient and Family Education

It is vital to instruct parents and patients on the warning signs of shunt infections. Fever, headache, lethargy, anorexia, nausea, vomiting, irritability, and redness along the shunt track are all possible signs of oncoming shunt infection. After the shunt is revised, inform the family that infection recurrence is highest during the first 6 months, so constant surveillance is needed during this critical time. If the child is to be discharged on antibiotics, careful instruction needs to be given on proper delivery and schedule. Instructions on wound care and activity, as well as follow-up will ensure a smooth transition from the hospital to home.

## Outcome

With proper and timely treatment, most children do well. History of a shunt infection predisposes a child to future shunt infections and malfunction, as opposed to those without a history [13]. Chronic and repeated shunt infections are associated with intellectual, psychological, and neurological deficits, but little evidence supports this outcome for a single infection that is treated promptly and successfully [2,4,13]. Instruct parents to look for signs of developmental delay, and encourage them to seek assistance quickly if such issues arise.

Parents may ask about the need for oral prophylactic antibiotics for their child undergoing dental procedures, since this is associated with transient bacteremia. There is no simple answer, and the literature is varied with no prospective randomized controlled studies [1,12,15]. Generally, if the shunt is nonvascular in nature (i.e., ventriculoperitoneal or ventriculopleural) and the child is undergoing routine dental cleaning, then antibiotics are not needed. If the child has a vascular shunt, such as a ventricu-

loatrial shunt, then prophylactic antibiotics should always be used. Exceptions for use of prophylactic antibiotics in children with nonvascular shunts are those undergoing dental procedures beyond simple preventive measures and cleaning, those with poor dental hygiene, and those with history of previous shunt infections. Many physicians use subacute bacterial endocarditis prophylaxis as recommended by the American Heart Association.

## Postoperative Infections

Postoperative infections are always a concern, but can usually be prevented. Nursing plays a big role in this process.

## Etiology

The etiology for postoperative infections depends on anatomical location of the infection. Keep in the mind the "five Ws" of postoperative fevers: wind, water, wound, walking, and wonder drug. The timing after surgery when a fever occurs dictates which process is the most likely culprit. For wind, this usually refers to lung processes, which occur in the first 48 h postoperatively. Atelectasis is the source and, if not properly addressed, will evolve into pneumonia by postoperative days 3–5. For water, this involves urinary processes from indwelling Foley catheters, which become the source of fevers around postoperative days 3–5. Wound processes, such as wound infection and meningitis, can also present by postoperative days 3–5, while abscesses present later in the hospital course, usually starting after postoperative day 10. Walking refers to deep venous thrombosis and thrombophlebitis, which are a common finding in adults during postoperative days 6–10, but less common with the pediatric population. Wonder drug does not refer to an infective process, but simply refers to mediations that can cause fever in patients, such as phenytoin, or medications that induce an allergic reaction.

## Pathophysiology

The usual source for infection is bacterial, with viral and fungal being less likely. Pulmonary processes occur due to underinflation of the lungs postoperatively, but can result from aspiration. The pathogen will vary depending on the mechanism involved. Urinary process occurs due to the Foley catheter acting as conduit for bacteria to enter, or from urinary retention, which can result, for example, from opioid use. Sepsis can arise from initial introduction of bacteria into the circulatory system from a central venous catheter, but can also arise from a secondary source such as complex urinary tract infection. Postoperative wound infections occur from introduction of bacteria into the surgical bed during surgery. Skin flora are usually the culprit, but other pathogens not native to the skin are also implicated.

## Diagnostic Tests

The initial evaluation involves fever curves and a WBC with differential. Further testing involves blood culture, urinalysis, urine culture, sputum culture, and chest x-ray. If a postoperative CNS infection such as meningitis is suspected, a lumbar puncture can be diagnostic. Other studies for postoperative wound infections may include a wound culture, needle aspiration of fluid, CT with contrast, MRI with contrast, or a leukocyte scan.

## Treatment Options

The best treatment is prevention. Immediate mobilization after surgery, removal of indwelling catheters, and initiation of functional pulmonary toilet are key maneuvers in this preventive effort. Once infection is diagnosed, antibiotic therapy is indicated and should be tailored to the causative pathogen. If the infection involves the wound, surgical incision, drainage, and debridement may be indicated. In the unfortunate case of an infected prosthesis, such as a shunt or spinal hardware, removal is usually the treatment, as a foreign body can produce a breeding ground for bacteria.

## Nursing Care

Nursing care has the main responsibility of prevention. This involves ambulating or getting the patient up into a chair in the immediate postoperative period. Some children refuse to use incentive spirometry or are too young to do so. Encouraging the children to blow soap bubbles, a pinwheel, or a party horn also helps to expand the lungs and prevent atelectasis. Removal of indwelling devices, such as Foley catheters, arterial blood pressure lines, and central venous catheters in a timely manner is essential. Surgical dressing should be left intact until the surgeon does the initial dressing change. If the initial dressing becomes soiled or is saturated, the physician should be notified immediately. In some cases, it suffices to keep the wound open to the air after the initial surgical dressing is removed, but in other situations where the incision can become contaminated from bodily fluids, or if the patients continues to touch the incision, a dry dressing may be in order. If vigilance from the nursing staff or parents is not effective in preventing a child from touching his wound, elbow restraints or mitten gloves may be utilized. Avoid frequent use of wound ointments because they can delay healing or cause wound breakdown. Antibiotics need to be kept on a tight time schedule and antipyretics such as acetaminophen and ibuprofen are utilized to keep the patient comfortable. Routine use of antipyretics is not recommended because it may mask fevers and blunt the body's attempt to rid itself of infection.

## Patient and Family Education

Instructing the family and patient on signs of infection will assist in early detection. Postoperative wound care should be a primary focus on discharge teaching. Problems with wounds that require reporting to the physician include erythema, drainage, increased pain, fever, and dehiscence. If the patient is to be discharged on antibiotics, teaching regarding the administration, timeliness, and duration should be addressed.

## Outcome

Postoperative infections resolve with proper and timely treatment. The morbidity and mortality remain low, except in cases where detection and treatment were delayed.

## Pediatric Practice Pearls

■ In the presentation of fever, headache, and focal neurological deficit, nurses must be suspicious for an infective intracranial process.

■ Neurocysticercosis can occur anywhere in the CNS, and its presentation usually manifests as seizures or symptoms and signs related to increased ICP.

■ *T. solium* is the parasite responsible for neurocysticercosis, and its transmission occurs via the fecal-oral route seen with the improper handling of foods.

■ The number one cause of shunt malfunction is shunt occlusion, followed by shunt infection.

■ The average incidence of shunt infection is approximately 7%.

■ In neonates, infection may manifest as apneic spells, anemia, hepatosplenomegaly, and neck stiffness.

■ Once the infection is cleared, the shunt can be reimplanted, but the child will be at a higher risk for future infections.

■ Most postoperative infections are preventable.

■ Maintain good pulmonary toilet, encourage incentive spirometry as well as deep breathing and coughing, and mobilize the patient as soon as possible

■ When appropriate, remove all indwelling catheters and tubes promptly.

■ Report fevers immediately, avoid the routine use of antipyretics because this will mask fevers, therefore causing the clinician delay in detection.

## References

1. Acs G, Cozzi E (1992) Antibiotic prophylaxis for patients with hydrocephalus shunts: a survey of pediatric dentistry and neurosurgery program directors. Pediatr Dent 14:246–50
2. Albright AE, Pollack IF, Adelson PD (1999) Principles and Principles of Pediatric Neurosurgery. Thieme, New York, NY, pp 1177–1183 and 1203–1246
3. Choux M, Concezio DR, Hockley A, Walker M (1999) Pediatric Neurosurgery. Churchill Livingstone, New York, NY, pp623–631 and 640–647
4. Fobe JL (1999) IQ in hydrocephalus and myelomeningocele. Implications of surgical treatment. Arq Neuropsiquiatr 57:44–50
5. Garcia HH, Del Brutto OH (2005) Neurocysticercosis: updated concepts about an old disease. Lancet Neurol 4:653–661
6. Garcia HH, Martinez M, Gilman R, et al (1991) Diagnosis of cysticercosis in endemic regions. Lancet 338:549–551
7. Gardner P, Leipzig T, Phillips P (1985) Infections of central nervous system shunts. Med Clin North Am 69:297–314
8. George R, Leibrock L, Epstein M (1979) Long-term analysis of cerebrospinal fluid shunt infections: a 25 year experience. J Neurosurg 51:804–811
9. Gershon AA, Hotez PJ, Katz SL (2004) Krugman's Infectious Diseases of Children. Mosby, St Louis, MO, pp 235–236
10. Greenberg, MS (2006) Handbook of Neurosurgery. Thieme, New York, NY, pp 172, 214–216, 217–225, and 236–238
11. Heilpern KL, Lorber B (1996) Focal intracranial infections. Infect Dis Clin North Am 10:879–898
12. Helpin ML, Rosenberg HM, Sayany Z, Sanford RA (1998) Antibiotic prophylaxis in dental patients with ventriculo-peritoneal shunts: a pilot study. ASDC J Dent Child 65:244–247
13. Kanev PM, Sheehan JM (2003) Reflections on shunt infection. Pediatr Neurosurg 39:285–290
14. Keutcher TR, Mealey J (1979) Long term results after ventriculoatrial and ventriculoperitoneal shunting for infantile hydrocephalus. J Neurosurg 50:179–186
15. Long SS, Pickering LK, Prober CG (2003) Principles and Practice of Pediatric Infectious Diseases. Churchill Livingstone, New York, NY, pp 309–310
16. McLone DG (2001) Pediatric Neurosurgery: Surgery of the Developing Nervous System. WB Saunders, Philadelphia, pp 515–520, 973–989, and 1011–1012
17. Nash TE, Del Brutto OH, Butman JA (2004) Calcific neurocysticercosis and epileptogenesis. Neurology 62:1934–1938
18. Osenbach R, Loftus C (1992) Diagnosis and management of brain abscess. Neurosurg Clin North Am 3:403–420
19. Richards E, Schantz PM (1991) Laboratory diagnosis of cysticercosis. Clin Lab Med 11:1011–1028
20. Rosas N, Sotelo J, Nieto D (1986) ELISA in the diagnosis of neurocysticercosis. Arch Neurol 43:353–356
21. Saez-Llorens X (2003) Brain abscess in children. Semin Pediatr Infect Dis 14:108–114
22. Schmidek HH, Roberts DW (2006) Operative Neurosurgical Techniques: Indication, Methods, and Results. Saunders Elsevier, Philadelphia, PA, pp 91 and 1591–1596
23. Schoembaum SC, Gardner P, Shillito J. Infections of cerebrospinal fluid shunts: epidemiology, clinical manifestations and therapy. J Infect Dis 131:543–552
24. Sciubba DM, Stuart RM, McGirt MJ, Woodworth GF, Samdani A, Carson B, Jallo GI (2005) Effect on antibiotic-impregnated shunt catheters in decreasing the incidence of shunt infection in the treatment of hydrocephalus. J Neurosurg 103:131–136
25. Tekkok IH, Erbengi A (1992) Management of brain abscess in children: review of 130 cases over a period of 21 years. Childs Nerv Syst 8:411–416

# Subject Index